Mindful Birthing

Praise for *Mindful Birthing* and Nancy Bardacke

"Bringing mindfulness to the birthing process has everything to recommend it: it can reduce fear and stress and make the experience more rewarding for all involved. All that's required is to practice the techniques that Nancy Bardacke explains so clearly in this book. What's more, you will find they apply just as well to parenting and to all aspects of life."

—Andrew Weil, MD, *New York Times* bestselling author

"Beautifully written. This is a rare thing, a genuine breakthrough moment in the field of childbirth and parenting. Combining ancient wisdom and modern evidence-based science, the practices in this book will change your life. A must buy for expectant parents, for midwives and other professionals involved in birthing, and also for any of us who want a glimpse of what great mindfulness teaching can offer us."

—Mark Williams, bestselling author of *The Mindful Way through Depression*

"*Mindful Birthing* is a unique, positive, and welcome contribution to the world of birthing. I often recognize Nancy's students during their labor process when I am attending on the obstetrical unit by their enthusiastic embrace of their labor, by their focus, and by their amazing ability to cope with unexpected challenges. I highly recommend this book to all pregnant women."

—Patricia A. Robertson, MD, professor and attending obstetrician, University of California, San Francisco

"As a mother-to-be, I learned to mindfully embrace the uncertainties of birth and parenting through Nancy's teachings. As an obstetrician, I felt inspired to integrate these methods into my practice. Nancy's wisdom, humor, and compassion flow throughout her new book, imparting her depth of experience in an approachable manner. This is at the top of my recommended reading list for all of my patients."

—Sarah Wilson, MD, University of California, San Francisco

"Until *Mindful Birthing*, good techniques for helping you experience the unpredictable changes of pregnancy and birth with resilience had not been available. The process of pregnancy, birth, and parenting is transformed from a series of stressful changes to a joyful journey by using the mindfulness techniques in this book. This book supersedes every other book written for pregnant women."

—Tekoa L. King, CNM, MPH, deputy editor of
Journal of Midwifery & Women's Health

"*Mindful Birthing* develops a unique blend of meditation, yoga, and scientific information into a user-friendly approach to maternity care and life changes after childbirth. It is a practical way to approach the many potential technologic intrusions that are so much a part of modern-day obstetrics."

—Douglas W. Laube, MD, former president of the
American College of Obstetricians and Gynecologists

"Nancy has brought together her life dimensions as wife, mother, grandmother, midwife, and mindfulness practitioner into a book for birthing parents, but it is also about the life skills that will benefit each of us as we progress through our own personal journey. Science, story, and skill-building are woven together, seamlessly engaging the reader to pay attention to the breath and just 'be.' What a gift!"

—Sharon Schindler Rising, midwife and CEO of
Centering Healthcare Institute

MINDFUL BIRTHING

*Training the Mind, Body, and Heart
for Childbirth and Beyond*

NANCY BARDACKE, CNM

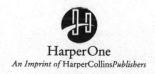

HarperOne
An Imprint of HarperCollins*Publishers*

MINDFUL BIRTHING: *Training the Mind, Body, and Heart for Childbirth and Beyond.* Copyright © 2012 by Nancy Bardacke. All rights reserved. Printed in the United States of America. No part of this book may be used or reproduced in any manner whatsoever without written permission except in the case of brief quotations embodied in critical articles and reviews. For information address HarperCollins Publishers, 10 East 53rd Street, New York, NY 10022.

HarperCollins books may be purchased for educational, business, or sales promotional use. For information please write: Special Markets Department, HarperCollins Publishers, 10 East 53rd Street, New York, NY 10022.

HarperCollins website: http://www.harpercollins.com

HarperCollins®, 📖®, and HarperOne™ are trademarks of HarperCollins Publishers.

FIRST EDITION

Illustrations, excluding those on pages 272 and 276, by Logan Granger
Designed by Adrianna Sutton

Library of Congress Cataloging-in-Publication Data

Bardacke, Nancy.
Mindful birthing : training the mind, body, and heart for childbirth and beyond / by Nancy Bardacke. — 1st ed.
p.   cm.
ISBN 978-0-06-196395-7
1. Pregnancy—Psychological aspects—Popular works. 2. Childbirth—Psychological aspects—Popular works. 3. Mind and body—Popular works. 4. Parent and child—Popular works. I. Title.
RG560.B36 2012
618.2—dc23   2012002470

13 14 15 16 RRD(H) 10 9 8 7 6 5 4 3 2

*To all parents everywhere
for birthing and nurturing the future
in this very moment*

Contents

Acknowledgments

COUNTLESS PEOPLE contributed to making this book a reality and I feel grateful to each one of them in a very particular way. First and foremost, enormous and heartfelt gratitude goes to Jon Kabat-Zinn, PhD. His genius created a form—the eight-week Mindfulness-Based Stress Reduction (MBSR) course—and with it a language and way of teaching that has made the practice of mindfulness accessible to innumerable people all over the world, transforming lives and easing suffering. Jon's unwavering support over the years for adapting the Mindfulness-Based Stress Reduction course to the needs of expectant parents has been invaluable, and without his directive to write this book, and his belief that I could in fact do so, I would never even have attempted it. Anyone who has ever heard Jon teach, read his books, or listened to his guided meditations, will easily hear his words echo throughout *Mindful Birthing*, for as a student, I have absorbed them into my being and then, to the best of my ability, transformed them into the Mindfulness-Based Childbirth and Parenting (MBCP) program.

I wish to thank Saki Santorelli, EdD, director of the Center for Mindfulness (CFM) at UMass Medical Center, for his beautiful teachings, friendship, and extraordinary work at the flagship Center for Mindfulness at UMass Medical Center, and for the invitation to speak at the CFM Conference in 2004, which proved to be such a catalytic event. Tremendous appreciation as well to the incredibly dedicated community of friends and colleagues who teach mindfulness programs in all their iterations worldwide—and to all the pioneering researchers for their profound commitment to understanding how mindfulness actually decreases suffering and increases our capacity for happiness, health, and wellbeing.

A deep bow of gratitude to my dear friend and teacher Ferris Urbanowski, MA, whose joyful energy, huge heart, wise counsel, and deep understanding of the importance of teaching mindfulness to expectant parents have been an inspiration and a precious gift to me over the years. Ferris also read the manuscript in its entirety and offered important and insightful suggestions.

I am deeply indebted to Bob Stahl, PhD, my first mentor, who invited me to teach the MBSR course in the program he founded at El Camino Hospital in Mountain View, California, so many years ago. Bob's initial guidance, and his later mentoring with regard to training others to teach MBCP, has been invaluable. Heartfelt thanks to the incredible community of mindfulness teachers, particularly Amy Saltzman, Joanne Martin Braun, Patrick Thornton, Tom Williams, Catherine Guta, Margaret Cullen, Mary Wade, Steve Flowers, Mark Neenan, Bonnie O'Brien Jonsson, Mark Abramson, Renee Burgard, Steve Alper, Bob Kalayjian, and Dennis Warren—who each in their own way gave support in the early years, and for their continuing support now.

Writing *Mindful Birthing* has in itself entailed a very long pregnancy, labor, and birth, and many book midwives have been involved along the way. Thank you to Dorothy Wall, Caroline Pincus, and Michael Ellsberg, for help during the book proposal phase, and to my dear friend Barbara Gates for her wise suggestions in the early drafts.

I am very grateful to Sharon Salzberg, who listened so carefully to what the MBCP program was about at a fortuitous breakfast meeting in Seattle and then guided me to my agent, Linda Loewenthal at David Black Literary Agency. Linda immediately saw the value of the MBCP program and worked tirelessly to shepherd *Mindful Birthing* through the tangled territory of the publishing world, ultimately helping it find a wonderfully supportive home at HarperCollins/HarperOne.

There is no doubt that the lead midwife for the writing of *Mindful Birthing* has been my editor and friend, Peter Guzzardi, who has been unfailingly present throughout the nearly three years it took to bring these words to the page. With his extraordinary editorial skills, his deep understanding of what I was trying to accomplish, and his own experiences of being a father of three, Peter guided and encouraged me with consummate skill and kindness through the many stages of the writing process, while still allowing me to find my own way. Our work resulted in a collaboration that was incredibly productive, instructive, and filled with many moments of laughter. I can't imagine having written *Mindful Birthing* any other way.

I also owe deep gratitude to Jeanette Perez, my editor at HarperOne, for her keen intelligence, enthusiasm, and infinite patience. A new mother herself, Jeanette has been consistent in her encouragement and her unqualified belief in this book's potential to benefit many. In addition to Jeanette, I have been fortunate to have a dedicated "birth team" at HarperOne that included Gideon Weil, Melinda Mullin, Mandy Chahal, Suzanne Quist, Jacqueline Berkman, and the artistry of Michele Wetherbee and Madeleine Budnick, who designed the lovely book cover. I appreciate the keen interest, guidance, enthusiasm, and the ease with which we have all worked together. I also want to thank my caring friend Barry Boyce, extraordinary editor and writer for his guidance, knowledge, and wisdom when it was very much needed.

Deep and heartfelt gratitude to my friend Tussi Kluge, a passionate force for goodness in this world, who so generously offered the gift of her home in Featheridge, Virginia, as a refuge for writing my first draft, and for her continuing support of mind and body in so many ways. To Myla Kabat-Zinn, a heartfelt thank-you for insights, encouragement, and caring support of *Mindful Birthing* and the development of the MBCP program. Much appreciation to Christiane Wolf, MD, for her obstetrician's eyes, her depth of mindfulness practice, the joy of teaching together, and for reading parts of the manuscript and giving important feedback. And to Catherine Polan Orzech, MA, LMFT, for her vibrant energy and passion for teaching and working with the MBCP program in all its many dimensions, a most sincere thank-you. Deep and continuing gratitude to my dear, kind friend Elizabeth Cohen for our friendship over the years and her steadfast support for the MBCP program in so many ways.

Toward the end of my writing efforts, two people appeared who made essential contributions to *Mindful Birthing*. I have deep gratitude for Logan Granger, with his incredible talent, commitment to mindfulness practice, and experience as a newly birthed MBCP father, who worked with ingenuity, intelligence, and tireless patience to create the book's wonderful illustrations and diagrams. Indispensible Kimberly Streeter, doula, passionate birth advocate, and technological aficionado, appeared just when she was needed most, giving support in ways I didn't even know I needed.

Of course the MBCP program and this book wouldn't exist without all the extraordinary expectant parents who signed up, showed up, and did the very real work of learning and practicing mindfulness as a way to prepare for the birth of their babies—and then encouraged other expectant parents to attend the course and do the same. As any teacher knows, it is really the student who teaches the teacher, and I have perhaps learned more from these parents both before and after they gave birth than from anyone else in this whole process. For me, their commitment to birthing and parenting their children with awareness and kindness is a wondrous bright spot in a world that sorely needs it. A particularly heartfelt thank-you to Brooke and Todd Kerpelman, for sharing with me the birth experiences of Dylan and Sydney, and then allowing me to write about them. Because of their openness of heart, the ripples from Dylan's all-too-short life may bring comfort to others.

A special thank-you goes to Ben Lovejoy and Mary Fairfield who attended the MBCP class to prepare for the birth of their daughter, Fiona, almost ten years ago. Ben insisted I needed a website long before I had any idea what an important tool it would be, and his creativity, design, and artistry have served MBCP beautifully for many, many years. If that weren't enough, Ben and Mary generously offered me space in their home for almost a year so I could continue to teach after a fire destroyed much of mine. My sincerest thank-you to my friend Judith Thomas, who for many years made it possible for MBCP all-day retreats to be held on the beautiful campus of the East Bay Waldorf School, and a special thank-you to meditation teacher Gregory Kramer, for his insightful teachings and for giving the MBCP program organizational shelter in the very early days.

I have had the enormous good fortune to benefit from many truly gifted meditation teachers over the past thirty years. A specific practice instruction, a teaching story that opened the mind and heart, a turn of phrase that continues to live within me—all contribute now to the teaching that emerges in the MBCP classroom. Thank you to extraordinary teachers Sharon Salzberg, Joseph Goldstein, Jack Kornfield, Sylvia Boorstein, James Baraz, Ajhan Amero, Yvonne Rand, Tsyokni Rinpoche, Christina Feldman, and Christopher Titmuss—and to Thich Nhat Hanh, who guided me through my first and still vivid eating and walking meditations at Green Gulch Farm Zen Center so long ago.

Thank you to Donald Moyer, my very first yoga teacher, whose classes I attended throughout the pregnancy with my second son in 1978; to Robin Sale for her early guidance regarding prenatal yoga; and to Marisa Torrigino, whose suggestions regarding the MBCP yoga sequence were so very helpful.

While MBCP has been my passion for the past eighteen years, it has been fueled by my first calling, midwifery. Appreciation goes out to the amazingly dedicated community of midwives I have been honored to learn from and work with over the decades—in homes, birth centers, hospitals, and educational programs—who serve women and families with dedication, presence, and caring during the process of bringing children into this world in all its multidimensional aspects of mind, body, and heart. Particular gratitude to Rosemary Mann, CNM; Susan Leibel, CNM; and Judith Flannegan, CNM; for their foresight in creating the nurse-midwifery education program at San Francisco General Hospital in the late 1970s and for welcoming me there as a passionate midwifery student. To them and to so many others too numerous to name—from obstetricians to labor and delivery nurses, therapists, and prenatal yoga instructors who have referred expectant families to the MBCP program over the years, very deep gratitude.

I especially want to acknowledge and thank my sister midwife and treasured friend, Tekoa King, CNM, who was my first midwifery partner in a hospital setting and who has given so generously of her time, wisdom, and knowledge whenever it was needed during the writing process. Tekoa read parts of this manuscript and provided invaluable feedback. Deep thanks to Sharon Rising, CNM, for a special friendship, inspiration, and our wonderful collaboration in the Centering with Mindfulness Skills project; and to Margy Hutchison, CNM; Laurie Jurkiewicz, CNM; and Deena Mallareddy, CNM, for the joy of working together on the research study. Many thanks to my friend and colleague Judy Cuneo, MD, one of a growing number of obstetricians who are using the lens of integrative medicine to re-examine the care currently being offered to the healthy pregnant woman and her baby, for her strong commitment to the MBCP program, and for reading sections of the manuscript and providing helpful feedback.

Over the years I have also had the good fortune to learn from some of the pioneers in the field of childbirth and early parenting, and for their teaching I am very grateful. Michel Odent, MD, deeply influenced my perspective on normal birth during the week I spent with him and the midwives in Pithiviers, France, in 1979. And a deep debt of gratitude goes to teachers and friends Marshall Klaus, MD, and Phyllis Klaus, MFT, LCSW, who first taught me about the importance of mother-infant attachment from the very first moments of birth.

My gratitude extends even further into the past, to my teachers of anthropology at UC Berkeley. Thank you especially to Professors May N. Diaz, Gerald D. Berreman, and Jack Potter for education in a field that allows for asking universal and fundamental questions regarding human beings as an evolving species within nature and culture, for reinforcing my understanding that there is a common humanity regardless of the many different ways the human mind can understand this world, and for allowing me to explore these areas in my early studies. This foundational education has been a backdrop for my practice of midwifery, and mindfulness teaching has served me well for all that was to come.

Deep gratitude extends to Susan Folkman, PhD, former director of the UCSF Osher Center for Integrative Medicine (OCIM), who first welcomed the MBCP program there, and to Margaret Chesney, PhD, the current director of the OCIM, for her ongoing kindness and support of the MBCP program. If something beyond gratitude is possible, it goes to Kevin Barrows, MD, director of clinical programs at the OCIM, whose enthusiasm was crucial to birthing the MBCP program at the Osher Center, and who continues to be an unfailing advocate for the program and for bringing mindfulness into the lives of parents and children. And my deepest admiration, respect, and affection to Larissa Duncan, PhD, who has guided the thriving MBCP research program, for being a true partner of heart and mind, and for her feedback after reading the manuscript. My appreciation extends to Amy Cowgill, group programs coordinator at the Osher Center, who so skillfully facilitates the day-to-day work that actually brings expectant parents into the MBCP classroom, and to all the clinicians and staff at the Osher Center for our shared understanding and commitment to the healing that is possible through integrative medicine.

As the MBCP program has begun to move outward into the world, I am deeply indebted to the amazing people who have come into my life with gifts of friendship and kindness, particularly Professor Mark Williams, the extraordinary director of the Oxford Mindfulness Centre (OMC) at Oxford University, whose unqualified support of MBCP has been absolutely key to me personally and to bringing MBCP work to the United Kingdom. To the talented, openhearted, and dedicated Maret Dymond, PhD, who leads the MBCP work at the OMC, what more can I say but thank you for the great pleasure of working together, as well as a heartfelt thank-you to Sian Warriner, consultant midwife at the John Radcliff Hospital in Oxford, whose investigations into integrative medicine and mindfulness in relationship to pregnancy, childbirth, and early parenting have resulted in a collaboration that is already bringing great benefit.

For the gift of friendship and support from my lifelong and very dear friends Terry Winograd and Carol Hutner-Winograd, MD, who early on saw the value of this work, the simple words "thank you" can't begin to express the appreciation I truly feel. And to my dear friends, Sue Trupin and Sue Sandson, a sincere thank-you for their patience with my absences during these writing years.

If our children are our mindfulness teachers, as I believe they are, this is just one more important reason I am thankful for my remarkable son Ted; my loving daughter-in-law, Naomi; and my two extraordinary grandsons, Niko and Ry, all of whom bring enormous joy into my life by their very being. The same is true of my son Mo: I am grateful for the sweetness of who he is, and most recently for his caring and kindness in reviewing several chapters of *Mindful Birthing* for medical accuracy. And to my stepsons, Daisuke and Kaitaro, thanksgiving for their delightfully surprising ways of being in this life, and to Kaitaro and his partner, Elena, a thank-you for the sensitive use of their video recording skills in support of MBCP. A loving thank-you to my dear mother, Frances Sturner, for the gift of life itself, and much appreciation to my kind sister, Judy, and her always supportive husband, Chuck Parnes, who have taken on the bulk of the work of caring for my mother during this writing. And to my very dear stepsister, Bonnie Sturner-Silton, who has been a steady loving presence throughout the writing process, and throughout so much of my life, a heartfelt thank-you.

None of this—the MBCP program or this book—would have been called into being without the boundless love and care I receive from my husband and partner in this life, Kenji Muro. A gifted writer himself, Kenji urged me to attend a talk by Jon Kabat-Zinn one rainy Friday evening nearly two decades ago, and later, when it proved so difficult to teach MBCP classes in a hospital setting, encouraged me to bring the classes right into the living room of our home. For these and countless other reasons—from the unquestioning support during the writing process to the meals he prepared to keep me going—my eternal love and gratitude.

Foreword

EVERY ONCE IN A WHILE a book comes along that is truly useful for a specific purpose, and yet, in using it for that purpose, repurposes you and transforms how you see and move in and understand your life and the world. *Mindful Birthing* is one of those books.

As the reader, you are no doubt coming to this book seeking information, expert advice, and perspective, and for an up-to-date and evidence-based orientation toward pregnancy and bringing your new baby into the world in a way that will be most in accord with your aspirations and wishes. You have come to the right place in that regard. However, because the Mindfulness-Based Childbirth and Parenting (MBCP) program is, as the name suggests, grounded in mindfulness, it also offers you—whoever you are, alone or together with your partner—something far more than mere information, no matter how useful. Mindful birthing offers a practical and systematic way to be in expanded relationship to yourself and your own experience, using pregnancy and birth and what follows from them as the raw material and the curriculum for this adventure, that is, the mystery of our lives unfolding and of new life developing and emerging out of us.

You couldn't place yourself in better hands. If we all have a particular and unique genius and calling—and I believe that we do—then mindful birthing is certainly Nancy Bardacke's. The MBCP program she developed and has conducted for more than one thousand expectant parents over the years is the distillation of that genius and calling. The world is very lucky to have MBCP available in this form now, and I hope that it will spread far and wide in our culture as a powerful support for pregnant couples and new parents.

With this book, the MBCP program and the mindfulness skills it encourages you to cultivate through ongoing practice are now available as if you were participants in Nancy's classes. You will come to see and feel how Nancy is truly a midwife. In fact, she will be midwifing *you* through a very special time in your lives—if you choose wholeheartedly to take on the curriculum, including the various carefully crafted practices she introduces and guides you in. Without taking on the full program in this way, the benefits you will read about here in the stories of other couples will likely remain an abstraction or simply something to be hoped for. If your intention is to realize the benefits of this approach, there is no other way than to "join her class" and throw yourself or yourselves into what is being offered, to take her advice, yes, for sure, but even more importantly, to practice mindfulness in all the specific ways that she recommends and assigns for homework—and then let life itself assume the role of the real teacher here, moment by moment by moment. For, like it or not, it is anyway. Nancy is very convincing on this score, and in a very winning way, as you will see.

The occasion of having a baby is a very special opportunity for learning mindfulness and for experiencing how deep, healing, transformative, and downright useful the systematic cultivation of mindfulness and heartfulness can be in the face of all the challenges that arise at this particular stage of your life. Nancy's voice is wise and compassionate, but also tough—not at all romantic. The book is a bit like a user-friendly and empowering how-to-survive-in-the-wilderness manual with an accompanying training regimen. Only in this case, it is how to *thrive* in the face of the unknown: the hospital culture if you are having a hospital birth, the risks and benefits of epidurals and other medical technologies, your own fears, issues between partners, strategies for dealing with outer as well as inner stresses, metaphorical and literal contractions (a big theme throughout the book), pain and other intense sensations, as well as strong emotions, all framed by the much larger perspective of your own innate wisdom and the innate wisdom of the body and of life itself. All these program elements, potentially a bit intimidating, are delightfully leavened by Nancy's wry sense of humor.

The bottom line, of course, is to be prepared. This book—and the curriculum it invites you to engage in—covers all that, and hits all the right notes, tonally, emotionally, and factually. At the same time, it also takes things much deeper, providing a container and a context within which everybody—you and the class participants—has an opportunity to befriend uncertainty and meet it with full awareness, clarity, and togetherness with their partner. In order to undertake such a momentous challenge wisely, the process has to be infused with and grounded in kindness and self-compassion. And indeed, the book is suffused with kindness and caring, and with ways to *cultivate* greater kindness and caring for yourself and for your baby and partner.

One more virtue of this book is that, through the vivid interchanges between Nancy and the participants in her groups, through their comments and questions and her responses, you have the benefit of a kind of ongoing consultation with her, as if she were a trusted friend. This aspect of the book can help a lot in terms of both information and attitudes. But part of Nancy's message is that, in actuality, the trusted friend is reality itself and your relationship to it, nurtured, deepened, and informed by your own systematic cultivation of mindfulness during the entire process of pregnancy, birth, and beyond. Here is what one father says about it:

> My initial thought when I began the class was that this would be a birth class that I might get something else out of. What it's ended up being for me is a life-perspective-altering class that's going to help with our birth. Leaving the class now, it's a complete reversal. It's not about the birth anymore. It's going to help us with the birth, but it's not about the birth. It's about our lives.

Nancy's love of the female body and of the miracle of pregnancy and birth and the exquisite biological orchestration that underlies the process may at turns bring both smiles of amazement and tears of poignancy as you read. It certainly did for me in many places. The wonder of it all never grows old and is never far away for us, given that we are embodied creatures, all having been born out of our mothers, and now likely parents-to-be or already parents, and even for some of us, grandparents. The most important thing is to allow ourselves to be fully present for it. Here is Nancy to tell you how. I wish you all the best in this ongoing adventure of life unfolding.

Jon Kabat-Zinn
Lexington, Massachusetts
January 16, 2012

Introduction

"I'M PREGNANT!" Where were you when those words first flashed through your mind? Sitting in a doctor's office or in a lab waiting room? Holding a phone in your hand or a little stick that had just changed colors? Or did you wake up one morning feeling queasy and you "just knew"? However it happened, there you were, a cascade of thoughts and a flood of emotions streaming through your pregnant mind and body. How many times throughout history have women all over the world experienced this moment? Billions. And now it's your turn. A transformative process of mind, body, and heart has begun.

And now you've picked up this book. However it came into your hands, chances are good that you're looking for some guidance or information or something yet unnamed that can help you navigate the territory of pregnancy, birth, and early parenting. As a midwife for more than four decades, I've had the privilege of accompanying thousands of women and their partners through pregnancy and childbirth—in hospitals, at birthing centers, and in their homes. And in more ways than I can name, these experiences have taught me extraordinary lessons about life itself. They have also led me to develop what you will be reading about in this book: the Mindfulness-Based Childbirth and Parenting program (MBCP), a childbirth preparation course for expectant parents based on the life skill of mindfulness.

WHAT IS MINDFULNESS?

Mindfulness can be defined as "the awareness that arises from paying attention, on purpose, in the present moment, and non-judgmentally."[1]

Mindfulness is cultivated through meditation practice, and, through the mindfulness practices outlined in this book, you will develop skills that can help you navigate the uncharted waters that lie ahead with more joy, kindness, awareness, calm, and wisdom than you might have otherwise.

Although mindfulness is a universal capacity of the human mind, unless we intentionally choose to cultivate it, we can spend much of our lives on automatic pilot, sleepwalking through life rather than being fully present for it. Taking the time to learn mindfulness through meditation practice now can help you more skillfully manage the inevitable stresses of pregnancy and the irreducible element of uncertainty of the birthing process. More than that, mindfulness meditation can help you manage the intense sensations of childbirth we usually call pain, increasing your confidence and decreasing the fears that so often accompany this profound journey into the unknown. And mindfulness can help you cultivate lifelong inner skills for healthy living, wise parenting, and loving partnership.

I clearly remember the moment I decided to teach mindfulness skills to expectant families. It was 1994, and I was attending a weeklong training retreat for health professionals with Jon Kabat-Zinn, PhD, and Saki Santorelli, EdD, at Mount Madonna Center in Watsonville, California. Jon had founded the pioneering Mindfulness-Based Stress Reduction (MBSR) program at the University of Massachusetts Medical Center in 1979, and since then he and his colleagues had taught the ancient Buddhist practice of mindfulness meditation to thousands of patients in a hospital setting. Through the program, ordinary people who were suffering from a wide variety of health challenges, such as chronic pain, anxiety, insomnia, high blood pressure, depression, asthma, migraines, diabetes, cancer, and the everyday stress of work and family life, were finding profound ways to come to terms with pain and illness in their lives.

I had discovered meditation practice twelve years earlier, in 1982, and it had become invaluable in my work as a midwife, wife, and mother-stepmother of four children. Having heard of Jon's work for many years through meditation networks, I was eager to learn how he and others were bringing the benefits of mindfulness practice out of the meditation halls and into the hospital setting. Jon's book *Full Catastrophe Living* had been published, along with several groundbreaking studies on the beneficial effects of mindfulness meditation for chronic pain and anxiety. Mindfulness-Based

Stress Reduction had been featured on the Bill Moyers TV series *Healing and the Mind,* setting off an explosion of interest in meditation practice and the then-nascent field of mind-body medicine.

More than one hundred healthcare professionals from all over the world attended the 1994 retreat, and as we sat on cushions in a spacious, light-filled meditation hall overlooking the town of Watsonville with the Pacific Ocean beyond it, we experienced this groundbreaking work firsthand. That week with Jon and Saki was truly transformative.

On the fourth day of the retreat we had just completed twenty-four hours of silent meditation practice. Jon was speaking about the mind-body connection when in one sudden, unexpected, electric moment, something shifted. In that instant I saw a way to integrate everything I was most passionate about—midwifery, meditation practice, and my intense curiosity about the mind-body connection—and offer it to those I served. I knew what I wanted to do—or, more accurately, felt utterly compelled to do. I set my intention to teach mindfulness skills to expectant parents as a way to work with the physical and emotional stresses of pregnancy, the pain and fear of childbirth, and the lifelong journey of parenting that lay ahead.

At the end of the retreat I approached Saki and told him what I wanted to do. "You can only teach what you know," came his sage reply, and I took it to heart. I went home and redoubled my commitment to daily meditation practice. I attended more silent meditation retreats and professional trainings and became part of an extraordinary community of mindfulness practitioners dedicated to bringing the benefits of mindfulness practice into health care and society at large. I found a mentor and now friend, Bob Stahl, PhD, who not only understood and supported my desire to offer mindfulness skills to expectant couples but also gave me the opportunity to actually teach the Mindfulness-Based Stress Reduction course for several years in the program he founded at El Camino Hospital in Mountain View, California.

Although I had no idea what a mindfulness course for expectant parents would look like, my intention never wavered. When I confessed to Jon that I didn't know what I was doing, his words of encouragement were "Just trust your own practice. You'll find your way." By 1998 I was ready to begin formally adapting the MBSR course into a Mindfulness-Based Childbirth and Parenting (MBCP) program.

At that time childbirth education focused primarily on providing expectant parents with a lot of information in a short period of time, in keeping with the faster pace of contemporary life. This emphasis on information fit well with obstetrical practices that were increasingly relying on technology in childbirth. In that context I wondered if I wasn't just a little bit nuts to offer a nine-week childbirth preparation course that focused on teaching life skills and that asked pregnant women and their partners to slow down, sit down, and look within.

Since teaching mindfulness meditation to expectant parents was completely new, I spoke at length with each woman or couple before they signed up, explaining that taking the course required their commitment to a daily meditation practice for a half hour a day, six days a week. I would often say, "The class is challenging, but giving birth and raising a child *without* a mindfulness practice is a lot more challenging!"

Now, fourteen years and sixty-eight courses later, more than a thousand expectant parents have participated in MBCP courses. What I have witnessed goes far beyond anything I ever could have imagined. Pregnant women and their partners often tell me that after taking the course they feel a lot more confident about childbirth and parenting; one woman laughed and said she was having "fewer panic attacks and more excitement attacks." Partners consistently report feeling more connected to each other and able to communicate more effectively. In emails and phone calls after babies are born, I hear expressions of enormous gratitude for the mindfulness skills that helped these new parents meet their birth experience however it unfolded.

At reunions, women who wanted a birth with minimal or no medication reported that mindfulness practice helped them cope with the pain of labor, allowing them to open to the birthing process moment by moment rather than fighting against it. When a labor or birth didn't unfold as they had hoped, women and their partners described how they used their mindfulness skills to manage the unwished-for and to help them make wise decisions in the moment. Though there were sometimes feelings of disappointment or sadness, the emotional tools developed in mindfulness practice helped them move through those feelings with compassion and grace. As one new mother commented after an unexpected cesarean birth, "Mindfulness doesn't give you the birth experience you want, but it gives you a way to fall in love with the birth experience you get."

At class reunions partners also express their appreciation for the way mindfulness helped them be fully present during the birth process. Perhaps most gratifying are the reports from new parents about how they continue to use mindfulness practice beyond the birth itself, as a way to fully experience the wonder of having a new baby and to weather the early postpartum period, when interrupted sleep, unexpected challenges with breastfeeding, and the stress of caring for a crying baby can take their toll. As one new mother succinctly put it, "Thank you, Nancy. We now know how to deal not only with the contractions of labor, but with the contractions of life!"

These days, expectant parents from MBCP courses create online communities where they announce the arrival of their baby, share their birth experiences, and provide a supportive place to turn to with questions and concerns. Much to my delight, many of these groups continue to meet, sometimes for years, meditating together and sharing the many ways they work at using mindfulness to raise their children with awareness, kindness, wisdom, and compassion, all right in the midst of "the full catastrophe" of everyday life.

HOW TO USE THIS BOOK

Pregnancy and childbirth have much to teach us when we know how to listen to their lessons with our minds, bodies, and hearts. This book is an invitation to use the life-changing process you are living right now as an opportunity for self-discovery, inner growth, and transformation. After all, you are living through the most transformative period in the adult life cycle, and your life—and the life of your partner—will never again be the same. So why not learn as much as you can from the process?

I have written this book to make it possible for you and your partner to gain some of the same benefits from mindfulness practice as those who participate in the nine-week Mindfulness-Based Childbirth and Parenting course and as an additional resource for those taking the course with an MBCP instructor. Whether you are new to meditation or are an experienced practitioner, you might want to read through the entire book first to get a sense of the territory we will be exploring. Then if you're not taking the course with a teacher, you and your partner can turn to Chapter 21 and follow the MBCP course outline week by week. Practical questions about meditation—such as when and where to practice—are answered there.

While some of us are very good at learning from a book (that's how my husband, Kenji, learned to swim when he was twenty-six years old), it can be quite helpful to have the guidance of a skilled meditation instructor. Although the number is growing, at present there are only a handful of trained MBCP instructors in the United States or abroad. (If you are interested in becoming an MBCP instructor, please see the information in Appendix B.) Finding an MBCP course in your area is ideal, but if one isn't available, you and your partner might consider attending a general Mindfulness-Based Stress Reduction (MBSR) course and then supplementing it with the information and practices in this book. Please see Appendix B for how to find an MBCP course.

Another option could be to seek out other expectant parents interested in learning mindfulness practice for pregnancy and childbirth and create your own childbirth preparation course. Having a supportive community as each of you does this inner work could make the journey that much more enjoyable. To help with the weekly meditation practices, you could order the audio guided meditations used in the MBCP course (see the resources listed in Appendix B). The audio guides may be particularly helpful for learning the yoga sequence.

A third option would be just to read the book, taking in what you find interesting or useful and letting the rest go. However, to become more mindful and less stressed in your life, there is no substitute for your own formal meditation practice. Without practice, the information given here will remain just that: information. In a way, meditation practice is a lot like giving birth and parenting: you can learn *about* it from a book, but it is the experience itself that is the real teacher.

However you decide to use *Mindful Birthing*, it is my deepest wish that you find something of value in these pages, something that will serve you well during the everyday joys and inevitable challenges of birthing and parenting that lie ahead.

CHAPTER 1

Everything's Changing!

Everything is impermanent: happiness, sorrow, a great meal,
a powerful empire, what we're feeling, the people around us,
ourselves. Meditation helps us comprehend this fact—perhaps
the basic truth of human existence. . . .
—Sharon Salzberg

THE SIGN ON my front door reads "Welcome. The door is open. Please come right in." It's the first session of the Mindfulness-Based Childbirth and Parenting course, and my living room has been transformed into a classroom: chairs form a circle, and my notebook, list of participants, and teaching supplies for the evening sit on a small table next to my chair. The hot water urn for tea is full; crackers, cheese, peanut butter, and apples for our break-time snack are ready in the kitchen; clean towels hang in the bathroom.

I always look forward to this night. By now I have spoken by phone, sometimes at length, with each pregnant woman and her partner. They have told me a bit about themselves—how they found the class and what prompted them to sign up. I know some of the circumstances surrounding their pregnancy—when they are due, where they intend to deliver (in a hospital, a birth center, or at home), and who their healthcare provider is. I also know how old they are, the kind of work they do, and any particular concerns they have about their pregnancy, birth, or the health of their baby.

For my part I've taken great care to explain that this is not your usual childbirth education course, that the heart of what we will be doing together over the next nine weeks is learning and practicing mindfulness. We'll learn how the mind directly affects the physiology of labor and how the capacity to be in the present moment can be a critical skill for giving birth. We'll learn ways to work with pain during labor, for most women in the process of giving birth, whether they intend to use pain medication or not, will experience some powerfully intense physical sensations we usually call pain. We'll also explore helpful positions for laboring and birthing, partner skills for supporting the pregnant woman through the birth process, breastfeeding basics, and how to manage the physical and emotional needs of the postpartum family. Partners may be coming to understand that they themselves need these mindfulness skills for they too will be having a birth experience and becoming a parent.

Occasionally during the phone call a pregnant woman will say something about wanting "a natural childbirth." If that comes up, I gently explain to her that from a mindfulness perspective, every birth is natural. It's natural for a baby to grow inside its mother's body, it's natural for a baby to be born, and it's natural for people to want to help with the process. That being said, if her intention is to birth with minimal to no medical interventions, she will definitely be learning skills for that—as well as skills for being in a hospital environment where people might want to help a little too much—and skills to work with however the birth might unfold, for there just isn't any way to predict the future.

Vicki and Matt are the first to arrive. Short, with curly, dark hair and a round belly barely contained by a blue stretch top, Vicki bubbles with life. Matt has a solid, quiet presence, as if in counterbalance to Vicki's vivacious energy. I know from our phone conversation that they are newly married and very happy to be pregnant.

I also know that this has been a stressful time for them. Right after they found out that Vicki was pregnant, Matt's company unexpectedly transferred him from the East Coast to the San Francisco Bay Area. Now they are subletting a tiny apartment in a new city without friends or family while Matt works long hours in a new job. Vicki, who gave up the job she loved as a second-grade schoolteacher, misses her close-knit family, particularly her mother. Matt's occasional migraine headaches are becoming more frequent. Knowing how much the two of them are dealing with, I'm very glad they decided to sign up.

I feel an immediate connection with Kristin, who arrives next with her husband, Peter. An obstetrician at the local county hospital, Kristin wears the familiar green hospital scrubs, which take me back to my own hospital workdays and nights. She looks tired. Over the phone Kristin confided that as someone who knows all the things that can go wrong, she is worried about giving birth and scared about handling the pain. "I know I just have to do something about my fears. I need to prepare emotionally—kind of get my mind around what's happening in a healthier way."

Kristin's husband, Peter, is looking for ways to manage *his* stress. Later this evening he will surprise the class with his openness by saying, "I have a lot of pressure at work right now, with a big deadline right before the baby is due. Kristin and I snap at each other more than we used to, which makes us both really unhappy. I know it's because of the stress, and I'm hoping this class can help calm us down."

While I'm giving Peter and Kristin name tags and directions to the bathroom, the front door opens again. Petite and blonde, Elizabeth seems shy, and her husband, Doug, towers above her. Married for nine years, they had planned on becoming pregnant long before now, but an unexpected period of infertility intervened. When I spoke with Elizabeth on the phone she told me that she and Doug call this their miracle baby. Though she prefers to give birth without medication, Elizabeth confessed that all the drugs and procedures she went through to become pregnant have shaken her confidence in her body's ability to give birth. "I'd like to go into labor believing that even though my body had difficulty getting pregnant, it still knows how to birth a baby. I think this class could help me do that."

In addition to the usual reasons, Doug is looking forward to class because an old back injury from his high school football days has flared up and settled into chronic pain. "I want to be able to crawl around on the floor and play with my kid," he told me on the phone, "and not have to take so many painkillers. I've heard that maybe this class can help with pain."

As seven o'clock approaches the front door swings open more frequently, so I'm kept busy greeting couples. Monica has been sent to the MBCP course by her obstetrician, who thinks mindfulness practice might help her cope with the emotional ups and downs of her pregnancy. "I'm a pretty anxious person," she confided during our phone call, "and pregnancy has really given me something to be anxious about. I'd like to learn ways to calm down." Kathy, Monica's partner, is definitely on board with this.

Emily and Hameed are having family challenges. After much deliberation they've decided to give birth at home with a midwife. This decision is causing quite a stir in Emily's family, particularly with Emily's father, a doctor. Knowing that she won't have the option of drugs or an epidural at home, Emily is especially interested in the skills we will be learning for managing pain during labor.

I'm delighted when Cara and Luis arrive. The daughter of my childhood friend Deborah, Cara was born into my hands thirty-two years ago, and I am thrilled to be helping one of "my babies" give birth herself, an occasion that will make my friend a grandmother for the first time.

Stephanie and Eric arrive next. Earlier in the year Stephanie went through a difficult miscarriage. Now well into the second half of her pregnancy, she confesses that the fear of another loss is still never far away. She also tells me she is worried because she didn't handle the pain of the miscarriage very well, and Eric had a really hard time seeing her in so much pain. "I'm hoping mindfulness practice will help us find some peace of mind. We'd really like to enjoy being pregnant, but I think we're both pretty worried."

Tomiko and Greg are last to arrive. Tomiko, pregnant with their second baby, reports that both she and Greg were very unhappy with their hospital experience three years earlier, when their son, Kai, was born. "It was a long, hard labor, and by the end, with all the drugs and tubes and machines, I felt like I wasn't even participating anymore. We want to do it differently this time. And if we can pick up a few pointers on how to use mindfulness to parent an energetic three-year-old, that would be great too."

Standing at the entrance to the living room, I watch as everyone settles, then take my place in the circle. The room falls quiet.

"Hello and welcome. I am delighted that you're here tonight. Thank you for coming."

After a short introduction telling them how I came to be sitting in the teacher's chair, I continue.

"When I chatted on the phone with each of you, we talked about the commitment you're making to practice meditation. I know how busy you are, and it can be a real challenge to take up a formal meditation practice, no doubt about it. So I want to honor the fact that you are choosing to make this commitment. The good news is that we'll all be taking on this challenge together, so we can support each other as we go along. Ultimately, though, each of us is responsible for our own practice. I can be your 'mindfulness midwife'—I can guide you, support you, believe in you, encourage you, even love you—but I can't meditate for you, and I can't have your baby for you. That part is up to you. What I can do is assure you that you'll get as much out of our time together as you put into it. And remember that you're learning skills you can use for the rest of your life."

SO WHAT IS MINDFULNESS?

We explored the question of mindfulness briefly in the introduction, but let's take a closer look. What exactly is mindfulness, and why would you want to take the time to learn it now, during pregnancy? Mindfulness, as we saw, is the awareness that arises from paying attention, on purpose,

in the present moment, and non-judgmentally. Mindfulness can be cultivated through ancient meditation practices that were developed and have
been practiced throughout Asia for some twenty-five hundred years. Although the practices you'll be learning are rooted in the Buddhist tradition,
mindfulness is a universal capacity of the human mind, a skill that can be
learned independent of any particular religious, spiritual, or cultural tradition. No one has to become a Buddhist to reap the benefits of mindfulness
meditation. All you have to do is practice, and you will become more mindful. It's that simple—even if it isn't always easy.

To understand this better, let's contrast mindfulness with mind*less*ness.
When we're not mindful, we're often on automatic pilot, sleepwalking
through life. Have you ever missed an exit on the freeway or walked from
one room to the next only to forget why you went there in the first place?
That's an experience of autopilot, of *not* being present with your experience.

If you begin to really pay attention, you'll soon discover that much of
the time your mind is caught up in thinking about the past or the future.
You may be remembering something your partner did last week or an
event that took place in your family years ago, or you may be planning for
or fantasizing about what lies ahead. When we're lost in these thoughts we
are not fully in our life in the present moment. Not that there's anything
wrong with this. Certainly with a baby on the way, you're thinking about
the future a lot. It's just that now, the present moment, is where your life
actually takes place; it's the only time you have to learn, to grow, and to be
fully alive. If you are constantly rehearsing for the future or rehashing the
past, you're missing this moment of your life, which is the only moment
you ever really have.

Learning to be fully present is a skill, and like any skill, it takes practice.
Sometimes the present moment isn't an easy place to be—like when you're
laboring to birth a baby. And so we practice meditation to learn how to be
present with things as they are, however they are, even when they are
challenging. And what we discover is that when we spend more time in the
present, life becomes richer, more interesting, and certainly less stressful.
Being pregnant and giving birth are moment-to-moment experiences; babies and children definitely live in the present, and the present moment is
absolutely where parenting takes place. So perhaps it makes sense to learn
and practice the skill of being present now.

Those of us who teach this way of training the mind sometimes say that
practicing mindfulness is like weaving a parachute. We don't wait until
we're ready to jump out of the airplane to begin weaving; we work day in

and day out making the parachute so that when the time comes to jump, the parachute may actually hold us. It's not so far-fetched to compare the experience of childbirth to jumping out of an airplane. By practicing mindfulness now, during pregnancy, we learn some skills to help us find moments of joy during the jump and perhaps help us come in for a soft landing.

THE BENEFITS OF MINDFULNESS MEDITATION

Learning meditation is not just a good idea. Research repeatedly shows that it offers tremendous benefits for our physical and mental wellbeing.

Numerous psychological studies have shown that regular meditators are happier and more contented than average. These are not just important results in themselves but have huge medical significance, as such positive emotions are linked to a longer and healthier life.

- Anxiety, depression, and irritability all decrease with regular sessions of meditation. Memory also improves, reaction times become faster, and mental and physical stamina increase.
- Regular meditators enjoy better and more fulfilling relationships.
- Studies worldwide have found that meditation reduces the key indicators of chronic stress, including hypertension.
- Meditation has also been found to be effective in reducing the impact of serious conditions, such as chronic pain and cancer, and it can even help to relieve drug and alcohol dependence.
- Studies have now shown that meditation bolsters the immune system and thus helps to fight off colds, flu, and other diseases.[1]

Back with the class that has gathered in my home, we begin a dialogue about all the changes becoming pregnant has brought into these couples' lives. Vicki is the first to speak, telling us how amazed she is by all the changes in her body. Always proud of being thin, for the first time in her life she has had to buy a bra. "I actually have breasts now!" she says, and the room fills with good-natured laughter. Others describe how their body is asking them to slow down, and they share the wonder of feeling their baby moving in their belly or note an increasing desire to spend more time at home instead of being constantly on the go.

With the moment of conception a profound biological process has been set in motion. Of course our body is always changing, but because it changes so quickly and dramatically when we're pregnant, we have a special opportunity to look deeply into the nature of change. Pregnancy is a very fluid state—literally—and as your blood volume increases and you create an ocean of amniotic fluid in your womb, emotions can wash over you. Tears may flow unexpectedly—and more frequently. An encounter with a sad story on the evening news or even a sappy TV commercial can leave you weeping as the radical hormonal shifts of pregnancy have their way.

Jessica leans forward in her chair and laughingly tells us, "I've totally changed what I eat. I've given up foods I used to love, and I'm finding myself craving foods I never dreamed of eating before." Hameed describes new feelings of protectiveness toward Emily and says he has been talking with his dad a lot about what it's like to be a father.

Pregnancy also brings new demands on your time. In addition to everything else, now you've got prenatal appointments and lab tests to schedule, research and shopping to do for essentials like a baby stroller and a car seat. Pregnancy and parenting books start piling up on the bedside table with little time to actually read them. Regular exercise, if not already a part of your lifestyle, is no longer something you can put off until later.

And then there's the matter of changes to your living space. Where are you going to put the changing table and the diapers and the baby clothes and all the toys that have started to arrive from generous friends and excited grandparents? Suddenly the space you have been using as your home office or a guest room has to morph into a baby's room, which of course needs to be painted, so there you are on the Internet researching the health impact of paint fumes during pregnancy. Or you may start wondering, "Do we have *enough* space?" Maybe it *is* time to move or to remodel.

Even though these enormous changes are due to a very happy upcoming event, the fact that they're all happening at the same time can be stressful. And this stress can be exacerbated by the clock ticking: the phrase "before the baby comes" serves as a constant reminder that time pressure is here in a big way.

All sorts of new questions compete for your attention. Where and how do you really want to live now? Nearer to parents and family? If so, whose family? What does your partner want? What kind of home do you want to create together? What kind of community do you want to raise your child or children in?

And how about finances? You and your partner may be accustomed to—or dependent on—two incomes, and now you have to consider the impact of one of you taking time off to care for your baby or the added expense of paying someone to provide childcare.

Stressful? You bet.

Work and career issues loom large as well. The pressure is on to finish projects or classes and exams or to train someone to take over your job while you're on maternity leave. The topic of work prompts Kristin to speak up. "I love my job at the hospital," she says, "and I'm going to take about four months off for maternity leave, but I just can't imagine how I'll manage breastfeeding when I go back to work. What if I'm in the middle of pumping and someone starts to deliver *their* baby?"

Pregnancy often prompts us to reflect more deeply on how we were parented and the kind of family we were raised in. When I mention that mindfulness practice has the power to change intergenerational family patterns, Emily, who has been quiet until then, sits up. Running her hand through her dark hair, she says in a clear voice, "That's why I'm here. I'm not at all scared about giving birth, but a part of me is pretty scared about becoming a mother. I *so* don't want to be the kind of mother my mother was for me! I think mindfulness practice might help me with that."

I sometimes hear both women and men say they're afraid of how their relationship will change once they have a baby. Doug voices this concern. "We're so used to being in charge of how we spend our time. It's not going to be like that anymore."

Your relationship may be based on notions of fairness and equality, sharing cooking and chores, and even earning similar amounts of money. But now there's a new reality: one of you can barely put on her shoes because there's a baby growing in her body. Most often primary responsibility for taking care of the baby falls, at least in the beginning, on the mother. Making money falls, at least temporarily, to the partner. Traditional roles make their appearance, much to the surprise—and sometimes dismay—of both partners. Mindfulness practice can help us adjust as we come to understand the new realities that are a part of family-making. It can also help us be present, listen attentively, and see each other's needs more clearly as we seek to find new common ground.

You may have noticed how pregnancy is changing your relationships with parents, siblings, and in-laws. Suddenly parents call more often, asking about your health and the health of your baby. You are giving birth not only to your child but also perhaps to a grandchild, niece, nephew, cousin, or sibling. Pregnancy can enhance the closeness of family if relationships are already positive, but it can also bring old unresolved issues to the surface. Fortunately, the birth of a child can be an opportunity to grow, change, and even move toward healing long-strained relationships. Everyone's world is changing with the arrival of this new being.

As your interests shift, you may notice a change in your relationship with friends. Stephanie describes this as a fork in the road. "We are the first in our crowd to have a baby. Our friends can't understand why Eric and I don't want to go out for a late-night drink or a movie anymore. It's like they are living another kind of life, a life we are becoming less and less interested in."

Your pregnancy itself can bring additional stress. While the vast majority of pregnancies are healthy, sometimes conditions arise that cause concerns about your health or the health of your baby. An unexpected test result can bring sleepless nights. A bout of uterine contractions or an incident of unexpected spotting can sometimes require you to change your life immediately and dramatically, forcing you to slow down or even stop working earlier than you expected. Even if you're blessed with a normal, healthy, and uneventful pregnancy, the common discomforts of a pregnant body—bouts of heartburn, leg cramps, swollen legs or feet—while not exactly debilitating, can certainly be stressful.

And then there is the growing awareness that the physical and emotional challenges of giving birth are not far away. I still remember a moment more than forty years ago when I was about thirty weeks pregnant and the obvious hit me. "Wait a minute," I thought. "In order for this baby to get here, it's going to have to come out of *there*!" Yes, the only way out is through. And certainly giving birth, as remarkable and joyous an event as it can be, can be pretty stressful too.

Mindfulness, paying attention in each moment as this transformational life process unfolds, is the best tool I know for meeting these completely normal yet tremendous changes during pregnancy with greater equanimity and for easing your worries about childbirth and parenting. As you expand your capacity to be mindful, you may find a way to become more resilient in the face of change, to increase your wonder at the miracle happening inside your body in this very moment, and to cultivate joy as you bring new life into this world.

Our classroom conversation about change, stress, pregnancy, childbirth, and the benefits of mindfulness practice has lasted over an hour. The faces

I see are more open now, bodies are more relaxed. Seeing themselves reflected in each other, this group of strangers has begun the transformation into an interconnected whole, linked by the common bond of pregnancy and the decision to learn and practice mindfulness to help them through the process of becoming parents.

And so we begin.

CHAPTER 2

Inner Preparation for Childbirth and Beyond

We have to study with our warm heart, not just with our brain.
—Shunyru Suzuki

IT'S THE second class of the MBCP course, and tonight we will learn a bit more about each other and go deeper into mindfulness practice. Once everyone has settled comfortably, I begin.

"I'd like to invite each of you to join me in a little guided reflection. Allow your eyes to close if you feel comfortable doing so, and come to the sensations of breathing. Taking a moment now, imagine yourself standing beside a well. Perhaps it's a well you've seen before, or one that you imagine right now. Notice the landscape around this well, the weather, the temperature of the air. Looking at the ground by your feet, pick up a stone. Feel its weight, its texture against the skin of the palm of your hand. Now, holding the stone over the opening of the well, let it become a question. And the question is: 'Why am I here?'" I pause for some moments, letting the words of the question sink in.

"And allowing the stone to drop into the well, notice if an answer comes with the first splash, as the stone hits the water. And just wait. Wait for the stone to drop deeper into the well. See if another answer arises, perhaps from a deeper place. Imagine the stone falling all the way to the bottom of the well and settling there. Just allow an answer to arise if one is ready to do so. There is no right answer, and even no answer at all is a kind of answer."

The classroom is silent. After a time I ring the bells and everyone opens their eyes. Through the sharing that follows, we come to a better understanding of who each of us is and what has brought us to this moment in this room. Benefiting from seeing each other in an expanded context, we can now do the same with our mindfulness practice.

FOUNDATIONAL ATTITUDES OF
MINDFULNESS PRACTICE

Cultivating certain attitudes of mind is part of the training in mindfulness and can help you get the most out of your meditation practice, giving you some touch-points to refer to when questions or obstacles arise. These attitudes are beginner's mind, non-judging, patience, non-striving, trust, acknowledgment, letting be, and kindness. Each of these attitudes relies on the others, so working on one enhances them all. You might think about the practice of mindfulness as cultivating a garden, a garden that flourishes when certain conditions are met: rich soil, plentiful sun, and adequate water. Holding these eight attitudes in mind, reflecting upon them, and cultivating them will nourish, support, and strengthen your practice and your capacity for becoming more awake and aware in each moment of your life.

Beginner's Mind

Most of the time we see life through the lens of preconceived ideas based on past experiences, abstract concepts, or future expectations. By contrast, beginner's mind helps us bring a fresh, unbiased, open perspective to our moments as we are living them. Cultivating beginner's mind helps us to experience each moment as it truly is: new, unique, and impermanent, a time that will never be lived again.

In beginner's mind, we bring simple curiosity to whatever we are experiencing now, thereby cultivating a mind that may be less filled with fearful thoughts about the future or unhappy thoughts about the past. By strengthening beginner's mind in pregnancy, you may find you are able to maintain that curiosity right through the experience of childbirth itself. As you come to experience that no two breaths are the same, and no two meditation experiences are the same, you can come to understand that no two contractions in labor are the same and that each labor and birthing experience is unique. Letting go of preconceived ideas about childbirth—your own ideas or those of others—*you become free to discover for yourself* what giving birth is all about.

While some aspects of childbirth are common to everyone, your birth experience will be yours alone—different from your mother's or your sister's or your friend's. It will be unlike your own previous labor or labors, if you've had them. It will be different from anything you've read about in a book, watched on TV, or seen in a video. Your labor will be as unique as you are in this moment, and practicing beginner's mind in meditation can help you truly understand this.

Beginner's mind has a close cousin, "don't-know" mind. During pregnancy, we often meet the unexpected—for example, a test result that indicates anemia or something potentially more serious, or perhaps a baby in a breech position (feet or butt first), which opens up wholly unexpected questions about how your baby might be born. In the process of giving birth, surprise is inevitable: surprise that *this* is the moment your water breaks, that *this* is the moment you feel the urge to push, that *this* is what it feels like to have your baby emerging from your body. When you experience the present moment with don't-know mind, understanding that this moment is the only moment that can truly be known, all your expectations, ideas, and fantasies about the future drop away, and you experience the present moment with a mind that is *open to what is*. Don't-know mind, a state in which we can be aware of hopes and expectations without rigidly clinging to them, helps us cultivate a mental resilience that can serve us well—in childbirth and in life.

Coming to terms with the truth of uncertainty, of not knowing what the next moment might bring, can sometimes feel scary, at least to begin with. Amy confessed to everyone early in her MBCP course that she really didn't like not knowing what would happen. She described herself as "a control freak" and told us that her way of coping with her anxieties about the uncertainty of the future was to make lots of lists and plans.

One evening Amy said, "I started to get really anxious during the meditation tonight." When I asked her what she had been thinking just before she started to feel anxious, she answered, "Well, I was wondering how long this was going to last. Then the phrase 'don't know' popped into my head, and I came back to the breath. Then my mind started worrying again about how long the meditation was going to last. And again I thought, 'don't know,' and came back to the breath. I just kept doing that the whole meditation. And it worked. The anxiety was still there, but I didn't feel so caught up in it. It was amazing to see how my mind was making me anxious and to know that I had a way to interrupt it. I can see how this could be totally useful during childbirth!"

The attitudes of beginner's mind and don't-know mind can be particularly helpful if you have given birth before, especially if the experience was challenging or not what you wished for. Though it may seem obvious, it is worth stating: *it is absolutely impossible to have the same birth experience twice.*

By training the mind to return to the present moment each time the mind drifts back into memories, we can use beginner's mind to find freedom from our fears of repeating a previous difficulty in childbirth. It isn't easy, and it definitely takes practice—and it is definitely possible.

For the birth of their first child, Kimberly and Tyrone had planned for a minimum of medical intervention. However, an unexpected drop in the baby's heart rate right after Kimberly's water broke created a very different scenario. Several measures were quickly tried to no avail, and Kimberly was rushed to the delivery room where baby Ryan was delivered by emergency cesarean surgery. Though she and Ryan were both physically fine after the birth, Kimberly never really recovered emotionally from the fear she experienced during the delivery.

When she became pregnant again, Kimberly sought out a physician and a hospital that would support her desire for a vaginal birth after a cesarean (VBAC). Even though she was told by her doctor that it was extremely unlikely that anything like the first birth would happen again, Kimberly often found herself revisiting the frightening memories of Ryan's birth. When she signed up for the MBCP course she told me that she was looking for some emotional tools to help her. "I wasn't afraid before or during Ryan's birth; the fear started when they rushed me into surgery. Now I just worry that something like that will happen again. I know I have some emotional work to do to get ready for this birth, and I think mindfulness practice can help me." Tyrone, who had been pretty frightened during Ryan's birth too, concurred.

As Kimberly and Tyrone learned to spend more time in the present moment, they both reported being much less fearful. "I'm not sure I can explain it," Kimberly told us one night in class, "but I just feel more at ease about this labor now—and about everything." At the reunion class Kimberly said, "Remember how scared I was? Well, the water broke at almost the exact same time in labor as it did in my labor with Ryan, and I could feel myself beginning to get afraid. So I said to the nurse, who was an absolute angel, 'I'm starting to feel scared because this is where everything bad started to happen last time, but I can see what my mind is doing, and I'm just not going there.' The nurse smiled and said, 'Good idea. Just stay here in the moment with me.'"

"I couldn't believe she said that!" Kimberly went on. "I thought, that's exactly what I learned in class! It was pretty incredible. The fearful thought just came, I saw it, felt it, and chose to let it go. I just stayed in the moment with my breath and the sensations in my body and did what I needed to do. The pushing sensations were pretty amazing—you know I missed that part last time. I felt Ava's head coming through my pelvic bones from the inside. I couldn't think of anything besides the sensations I was feeling. It was very intense, but I could definitely handle it. I wouldn't have missed it for the world!"

Non-judging

Whether we are aware of it or not, the mind is constantly generating thoughts. The thinking mind, the part of our brain that in evolutionary terms developed most recently, has evolved to, well, think! It's a perpetual analyst, a problem-solving, drop-of-the-hat fix-it specialist, and though it can be very creative in the tales it projects and the fantasies it becomes attached to, it can be amazingly inaccurate when it comes to perceiving reality.

Our thoughts are often reactions to our experience of the moment. We can be so very quick to judge things as good or bad according to whether we find them pleasurable or painful. For most of us this is a very strong habit, and it establishes us firmly in our stories about our likes and dislikes.

With mindfulness practice you become more familiar with the various patterns of your mind, including one of the most common patterns for many of us: self-judgment. Because mindfulness allows us to take a step away from our stories (psychologists call it decentering), we are less likely to get caught up in an endless loop of painful judgments about either ourselves or others. Mindful awareness helps us to recognize thoughts, even self-judging ones, as mental events arising and passing, like clouds in the sky. This makes it possible to see that *we are not our thoughts,* which is a tremendously liberating insight!

With mindfulness practice you can learn that you don't have to *believe* all the painful, judging thoughts that arise in your mind. And when you become aware of judging thoughts, you certainly don't have to add another layer of unkind thoughts, like, "Oh, here I go, I'm judging again." You also don't have to make up a story about yourself, like, "I'm such a judgmental person," which is just more judgmental thinking. Instead, you can learn how to non-judgmentally observe your thoughts without becoming caught up in them. Coming back to the breath with gentleness and kindness, over and over again, we learn how to dwell in a space of non-judging.

Lisa had struggled with weight gain all her life, and although she was at her normal weight when she became pregnant, the pounds she put on during pregnancy reawakened her old judging thought patterns about being overweight. Through mindfulness practice Lisa became aware that her judging thoughts were especially harsh when she went to her prenatal yoga class. Looking around the room at the other women, she found her mind unfavorably comparing her body to theirs.

"I kept telling myself that I was fat and ugly, that all the work I had done to lose weight before I was pregnant was wasted, that I was as big as a house and always would be. The judging thoughts got so bad that I started thinking about giving up yoga class, even though I really liked how it made me feel."

But one day something happened to Lisa in yoga class. "We were practicing hip openers, and my judging thoughts were so loud I could barely hear the instructor. Then all of a sudden I realized I could draw on my mindfulness practice. So each time I became aware of a judging thought, I let it go and came back to the sensations in my body. It wasn't easy, but I kept doing it, over and over. And after a while the thoughts weren't so loud. And they weren't coming as often. By the end of the class they were still annoying, but they had lost a lot of their charge. I realized that as long as I stayed in the moment and in my body, I could handle this judging mind of mine! And now I know how to go to yoga class and not feel so bad about myself. It's just another opportunity to practice!"

If we have a strong attachment to how we want our birth experience to be, and it turns out to be far from those hopes and dreams, the judging mind can really have a field day. We can judge our labor as if it was a test we failed, or we can get caught up in a loop of anger and blame, passing judgment on ourselves, our support team, or our healthcare providers. While anger or disappointment may be understandable—we are, after all, human—they only create suffering for ourselves. Mindfulness offers us another option.

The judging mind can also be a significant factor in postpartum depression, particularly for women with a history of depression. One of the antidotes to the judging mind is kindness for ourselves and others, and we can cultivate that particular attitude with a meditation practice called Lovingkindness. Cultivating kindness for ourselves and others is so important that all of Chapter 14 is devoted to it.

Patience

Patience is the understanding that events unfold at their own pace and not necessarily on a timetable of our own choosing. And pregnancy and childbirth are excellent teachers of this lesson. For all sorts of reasons we may want, or at least think we want, things to happen on a certain schedule. Modern life conditions us to expect immediate results, and when a click of a switch (or a mouse) doesn't bring immediate satisfaction, we get frustrated or upset. When it comes to meditation practice, we may also want immediate results. This sense of urgency to get somewhere other than where we are is just another way the mind creates unhappiness.

Mindfulness practice helps us learn patience. If you diligently keep at your practice, over time you may gradually notice not only that everything around you is constantly changing, but that you are changing too. For reasons you can't seem to explain, old triggers just don't seem to affect you as much as they used to. And with that often comes a new inner sense that things are okay, just as they are.

Allowing things to unfold in their own time is particularly helpful in relation to your due date, which is of course only a guess based on averages. If your due date comes and goes, you may be very glad you've cultivated the wisdom of patience.

Your patience may also help your healthcare providers be more patient. Although a shift is taking place within the field of obstetrics, the majority of healthcare providers for pregnant women, at least in the United States, are living and practicing in the fast lane, on Industrial Time. Measuring time in this way is often at odds with the pace of biological processes, which take place in Horticultural Time.[1] (We'll learn more about Industrial Time and Horticultural Time in Chapter 6.)

Recognizing when impatience is driving action, either in ourselves or in a healthcare provider, can help us make wise choices during pregnancy and labor. Of course patience needs to be tempered by intelligence. Midwives sometimes describe patience as "watchful waiting" or "the art of doing nothing well." Both phrases imply intelligent patience, an appropriate balance between being and doing.

Whoever first said that patience is the highest form of love may have been thinking about parenting. When you feel like you're about to lose it with your two-year-old, who insists on having his food cut in triangles not squares, or with your partner, who in your opinion doesn't see what needs to be done in the present moment, you can use the breath to practice the wisdom of patience. And of course becoming familiar with the unpleasant feelings that accompany impatience can help you bring compassion to your parenting when a fidgety child is caught up in the throes of her own impatience.

Non-striving

Striving is a component of trying, of "efforting" to get somewhere, of achieving a goal. In mindfulness practice there is nothing to achieve, nothing to get, and nowhere to go. Instead, you are cultivating another way of being, learning how to be fully aware of exactly where and how you are in this very moment, even if the moment is painful or you don't like it, because in this moment, this is your reality. A non-striving attitude can be especially valuable during childbirth. As you will see, allowing things to be exactly as they are during labor actually creates the optimal mind-body condition for your body to open, change, and give birth.

And as we will discuss in more detail later, the inverse is also true: the mind that resists the labor process, wanting things to be other than they are, sets up conditions that can lead to a less-than-optimal mind-body state during childbirth. Paradoxically, in labor non-striving will bring us closer to exactly where we want to go.

Labor has two phases. The first is the *allowing phase*, when the cervix is opening to full dilation. The second is the *bringing forth* phase, when the urge to bear down and push your baby out takes over. In the allowing phase, the more we can just be in the moment and let the energy of birth move through our being, the easier the process will be. In the bringing forth phase, though it may seem as if we're striving, we're actually cooperating with the body to do the work it already knows how to do.

If your mind is striving to get somewhere other than where you are in any stage of labor, resisting the truth of the present moment, energy is being dissipated or lost. It is a non-striving, focused mind cooperating with the body's efforts in the moment that can best help you birth your baby.

Trust (as Self-Reliance)

Learning to listen to ourselves is also a key element of mindfulness practice. You are the ultimate authority on your experience, and learning how to trust your inner wisdom is the path to what is best for you in birthing, parenting, or the general conduct of your life. As you practice mindfulness, the capacity to trust yourself grows, and inner strength, confidence, and self-reliance emerge, helping you take full responsibility for your choices and your actions.

This kind of trust is not about anything external. It's not about "trusting the birth process" or "trusting your body," for if you adopt this way of thinking and your birth doesn't go as you wish or expect, you may find yourself rushing headlong into the pain of the judging mind. Mindfulness practice offers a different kind of trust—*a trust in yourself, a trust that you can handle whatever unfolds during pregnancy, in your birth experience, or with your baby, no matter how challenging, difficult, painful, scary, or far from what you imagined it might be.* As Simone said after her birth experience, "The birth didn't happen at all as we expected, and we are perfectly content with how it actually was." Mindfulness can hold anything and everything. Nothing is left out.

Acknowledgment (Moving Toward Acceptance)

In meditation practice, when we bring awareness to our moment-to-moment experience without trying to change anything, run away, or deny what is happening, we are practicing *acknowledgment of things as they are.* This doesn't mean we have to *like* things as they are. Instead, acknowledgment becomes a starting point for us to clearly see a situation as it is. Once we can see clearly, without the mind being so clouded by reactive emotions or judgments, a greater range of options opens up. In time, as we work with what is real, we may come to accept even very painful emotions or situations. And with acceptance comes a kind of inner peace.

A few years before becoming pregnant, Grace was in a serious car accident. Her shoulder had required several surgeries, and her left hip had been replaced. Grace felt she had been through more than her share of medical procedures and really wanted to give birth without medical intervention. Although Grace's obstetrician, whom she liked and trusted, was a bit concerned about the limited range of motion in Grace's hip, she was hopeful that Grace could deliver vaginally. Then, at thirty-two weeks, her doctor discovered that Grace's baby was in a breech presentation, and because of Grace's hip condition her doctor wasn't comfortable attempting a vaginal breech delivery. She told Grace that unless the baby turned on its own, or she was able to turn the baby manually at about thirty-six weeks, she was afraid that Grace would have to have a cesarean birth.

Understandably upset, Grace sprang into action. She searched the Internet. She talked to her husband and her friends. She practiced a yoga posture her yoga teacher suggested might help the baby turn around. She saw an acupuncturist and a chiropractor. She visualized the baby turning, talked to it, and asked the baby to turn head down. Grace became consumed with finding a way to fix the situation.

During this time Grace also continued her meditation practice. Each time she sat she observed the contractions in her mind and body and noticed how much she was resisting things as they were. She watched as thoughts, mostly worries about having another surgery or memories of past surgeries, raced through her mind. She didn't deny or repress the very real feelings she was experiencing—fear in her belly and disappointment in her chest.

At thirty-six weeks, Grace's doctor tried to turn the baby without success. Still caught in resistance to things as they were, Grace began to despair. She *really* did not want a cesarean birth. Still she continued her meditation practice. One morning as she sat, the phrase "it is what it is" came to her. She let the phrase go, and it came again. And then again.

"I don't know how it happened, but suddenly I got it. I really *felt* what those words meant. I mean, I felt it in my body. I also realized that this birth was not just about me—it was about what was best for the baby too. My doctor was thinking about what was best for both of us. Then I experienced an incredible sense of peace. It wasn't like I was happy with the situation or that I suddenly *wanted* the cesarean. But something shifted. I saw the bigger picture and let go of my fierce attachment to a vaginal delivery. It didn't happen all at once. It was a process. But by acknowledging the reality of the situation and my feelings, I found some acceptance of things as they were. It was such a relief!"

Grace's story shows us that acknowledging things as they are doesn't mean we don't work to change things. Far from it. Acknowledgment, seeing the situation as it is, is an intelligent *starting point* for change. If we can't see a situation clearly as it is—if instead we are caught up in our attachment to how we *want* things to be or resistance to things as they are—we have less creative energy and clear seeing for finding skillful strategies for change, and then for doing the nitty-gritty, moment-to-moment work that change requires.

Letting Be

An important element in acknowledging and eventually coming to terms with things as they are is letting be. When we want something very badly, when we are very attached—be it to a person, an object, an idea, or a fantasy of the way we want things to be—we hold on, often quite tightly. It is this *attachment* to the way we wish things to be that can pose some of life's greatest challenges.

Usually we try to avoid unpleasant situations by denying them, running away from them, or fighting them. In fact, our entire life can revolve around trying to avoid what we don't like and clinging to what we do like. Now there's nothing wrong with this. It's totally human. But unfortunately it's also a recipe for suffering. We cannot control everything, and there is no way we can prevent external circumstances from bringing us some things we don't like. Cultivating mindful awareness, however, offers us another way. With mindfulness, we can turn *toward* the difficult or unwanted and find a way to let it be, as Grace did.

It's interesting to discover that the more we resist the way things are, the more suffering we create for ourselves. It's a paradox summed up in the saying "that which you resist, persists." Coming to terms with things as they are, even if unwanted or painful, gives us a completely different way to approach the challenges of life. In fact, this is the heart of our mindfulness practice for working with pain and fear in childbirth.

Approaching birth from this perspective does not mean that you will not have preferences or that you will passively accept care that is offered if you have doubts about its wisdom. Quite the contrary. It means you will have skills for giving yourself the best chance to get what you want, to work with that which you may not want, and to come to terms with the way things actually unfold. A tall order, but I've seen it happen time and again. (We will cover this aspect of birthing extensively in Chapter 16.)

Kindness

In class I often say that mindfulness practice is ultimately about kindness—kindness toward ourselves and kindness toward others in this life as it is. In fact, we begin to cultivate kindness in the very first meditation instructions on the breath. First you are asked to bring awareness to the sensations of breathing wherever you feel them most vividly in the body—at the belly, at the nostrils, or at the chest. Then you let your attention rest there, feeling the breath as it comes and goes. And when the mind wanders away from the breath, as it will inevitably do, you notice where the mind has gone, and letting go of those thoughts, you *gently and kindly* escort the attention back to the breath.

This quality of kindness inherent in mindfulness practice is cultivated as an antidote to the difficult mind-states we human beings are so prone to—fear, anger, envy, greed, judgment, and all the variations on those themes. Over and over we cultivate kindness, moving in the direction of greater compassion and acceptance. We observe the thinking mind and all the unkind thoughts it can generate toward ourselves and others, and we interrupt that cycle. We acknowledge an unkind thought, and with *kindness* we bring our attention back to the breath. Over and over again. If the mind wanders fifty times in five minutes, we have fifty opportunities to cultivate kindness within ourselves. What a beautiful way to spend five minutes!

Being a parent is one of the most demanding jobs on the planet. In fact, giving birth is sometimes the easiest part of parenting. Though we may not think of preparing for childbirth as an opportunity to learn skills for parenting, that is in fact exactly what we are doing when we learn mindfulness during pregnancy. Cultivating kindness toward ourselves and others builds a strong foundation for wise, healthy birthing *and* parenting.

More than once, I've heard new parents say that they couldn't believe the hospital was sending them home with a baby to take care of when they knew they didn't have a clue about what they were doing. Babies don't come with a how-to manual; parenting is moment-to-moment on-the-job training. Knowing how to bring kindness to yourself, especially while you're coping with the very steep learning curve of being a new parent, can help a lot.

We human beings are sensitive creatures, and we all need lots and lots of kindness. When we get frightened or confused about which direction to take, sometimes we can find our way by asking, "What, in this moment, is most kind—for my baby—and for me?"

Chris's story provides an excellent example of the kindness that can emerge through mindfulness practice. Given the class assignment of bringing attention to a simple, routine activity of daily life, such as brushing teeth or washing dishes, Chris chose the activity of changing sixteen-month-old Kyle's diapers first thing in the morning. "Every morning when Kyle wakes up, he screams to get out of his crib. My morning routine is to get up and go get him. His diapers are always soaking wet, so the first thing I do is change him—and he just hates it. He screams and yells; every morning is a battle, and I have to fight to hold him down. I just couldn't understand why he kept doing this, why he didn't get used to the routine.

"But this week something different happened," Chris reported to the class. "When I heard Kyle crying, I went into his room and picked him up as usual, and all of a sudden I could see that what he wanted was a hug. I don't know how I knew it—maybe because I was more mindful—but I just did. So I said to myself, so what if he has wet diapers on for a little longer? I'll just hug him. Then Kyle started calling for Teresa. He wanted to hug her too. Again I let go of my agenda, and I carried him into our room. While he was cuddling with Teresa I went and got him his bottle, and as he was drinking it, I changed his diapers. He was totally relaxed and happy, and so was I. It was so simple! There was no terrible battle. And all because I was paying attention!"

Then Chris had a further insight. "I realized that I had been so intent on getting Kyle's diapers changed because when I was growing up that was my job. I'm the oldest of eight kids, and my responsibility was to manage the total chaos of getting everyone up, dressed, and ready for school in the morning. So when I was changing Kyle in the morning, I did what I had always done: impose order. I was on autopilot, totally unaware of my mind-set. But I see now that there is another, kinder way."

Now that we've explored the eight foundational attitudes of mind for mindfulness practice, let's go ahead and have a direct experience of the practice itself. The Raisin Meditation is one of my favorite teaching moments in the MBCP course, and you will have the opportunity to practice it in the next chapter.

CHAPTER 3

The World in a Raisin

When I look at amniotic fluid, I am looking at rain falling on
orange groves. I am looking at melon fields, potatoes in wet earth,
frost on pasture grasses. The blood of cows and chickens is in this tube.
The nectar gathered by bees and hummingbirds is in this tube.
Whatever is inside hummingbird eggs is also inside my womb.
Whatever is in the world's water is here in my hands.
—Sandra Steingraber

"WE COME TO know the world through our senses—seeing, touching, hearing, smelling, tasting—and through the knowing faculty of the mind. So tonight we will begin our mindfulness practice by bringing our full attention to these senses, one by one, as we experience eating one raisin mindfully."

As I look around at the expectant couples attending tonight's class, I see that I have their full attention. "You might find this meditation a little odd," I continue. "However, from a mindfulness perspective a little novelty can serve us well, waking us from habitual ways of seeing that can come between us and our direct experience of living. So tonight we are going to experiment with bringing beginner's mind to this experience, as if you were a newborn baby and had never seen a raisin before because, in truth, you have never seen *this* raisin before." I pick up the small bowl of raisins I have prepared for tonight's class and slowly walk around the circle, carefully spooning a raisin into each outstretched hand.

This simple meditation is often one of the most memorable practice experiences in our nine-week journey together as a class, demystifying meditation and clarifying our understanding of mindfulness. It may very well have the same effect on you. I encourage you to do the actual meditation practice now, but if you prefer to keep reading, please do make a commitment to come back to the Raisin Meditation at a later time. Of course, it's your choice, but remember, the only way to truly benefit from mindfulness is through the direct experience of practice.

⟶ THE RAISIN MEDITATION: PART ONE ⟵

*(Reader's Note: In the classroom I guide participants through this practice.
If you are practicing with your partner, you could take turns reading
the meditation aloud to each other.)*

When you are ready, pick up the raisin and look closely at this object in your hand. Taking your time, notice its shape, its color, its texture, and how the light reflects off its wrinkled surface and where it is absorbed. Observing the raisin from different angles, as if you were a scientist studying it with intense curiosity, look at every tiny detail of this particular raisin.

Now picking up the raisin, move it gently between your fingers. Is it soft and spongy? Is it hard? Does it feel rough or smooth or sticky to the touch? Notice every aspect of your experience of touching this raisin.

And now, bringing the raisin very close to your ear, roll the raisin between your fingers. Listen carefully. What do you hear? Crackling? Popping? If you notice that your mind is having thoughts, like, "This is really weird" or "What does listening to a raisin have to do with having a baby?," just notice those thoughts and let them go, gently shifting your attention back to noticing the sound of a raisin.

Now bringing the raisin to your nose, smell it. Taking your time, breathing in deeply. In this very moment, what is your experience of smelling a raisin? Notice if you can smell the odor from the raisin more clearly through one nostril than the other. If you become aware of thoughts, once again just notice them and let them go, bringing your attention back to smelling the raisin, right here, right now, in this very moment.

And now looking at the raisin once again, very slowly bringing the raisin to your lips. Feel your arm move as your hand approaches. As you see the raisin coming closer, pay close attention to what is happening inside your mouth. And when the raisin reaches your lips, closing your eyes, devoting your complete attention to the sensations at your lips. And when you are ready, allowing your tongue to take the raisin from your lips into your mouth. Noticing how the tongue knows exactly what to do with the raisin, how it positions the raisin between your teeth.

Being aware in this moment of any emotions that might be arising for you: perhaps impatience, desire, anticipation, resistance, or worry. Observing these emotions, acknowledge their presence, and then gently shift your attention back to the sensations in your mouth.

And when you are ready, I invite you to bite down on the raisin. Taste the flavor of the raisin bursting onto your tongue. Now, very, very slowly, chew the raisin. Chewing. Tasting. Chewing. Tasting.

And when you are ready, begin to swallow. Can you feel the raisin moving down your throat? Can you be aware of how many times you have to swallow to eat one raisin? And now noticing how the tongue moves into the crevices of the teeth, seeking out all the tiny pieces of the raisin. And noticing how the taste in your mouth is different now than before you bit into the raisin—being fully aware of this process of eating a raisin.

Now, when you are ready, if your eyes have been closed, please slowly open them.

If you followed the instructions above, you have just eaten one raisin *mindfully*, bringing focused attention to each moment, observing the three pillars of experience: body sensations, thoughts, and emotions. There is much to learn from this meditation, and after we practice it together in class we spend a good bit of time processing our experience. We will turn to that in a moment, but first there's another important aspect of this meditation: becoming aware of interconnectedness.

It can be helpful to think of mindful awareness as a lens. Sometimes we use it in a very focused way, as we just did with the raisin, using all our senses to observe every detail of our experience. And sometimes we widen the lens of mindfulness so that our awareness expands to take in the bigger picture. We nurture both of these aspects of awareness as we practice.

In this wider, more spacious view, we become aware of the larger context of being, in which we can see how everything is interconnected. Sometimes called "looking deeply," this aspect of practice helps us become aware of the multitude of causes and conditions that are a very real part of our experience in this very moment. If you would like to experience this more expansive view, I invite you to follow along with a second set of Raisin Meditation instructions. When you are finished, we'll reflect on what you might have observed in both practices.

⟶ THE RAISIN MEDITATION: PART TWO ⟵

Now, picking up another raisin, bring beginner's mind to this experience—for after all, this is a completely new raisin. Looking carefully, see if you can find the stem end of this raisin, its belly button. In this moment, taking time to reflect on this part of the raisin, for it can tell you a lot. It can tell you that at one time this raisin was attached to something larger than itself—to a vine. And that vine was nourished by the soil it grew in and by the sun and the rain. The vine and the grapes that grew on it experienced wind, cold, and warmth; at night the moon and stars gazed down on it, as did the sun by day.

When this grape reached a certain size it was picked by people, workers who had parents and perhaps children of their own, who had hopes and dreams and challenges in their lives, who were perhaps born in another country, whose first language may not have been English. They picked this grape and helped it through the drying process that transformed it into a raisin, after which it may have been packaged in a box or stored in a bulk container. Either way, human energy was used to move this raisin onto a truck, a truck that was the result of the labor of hundreds, perhaps thousands, of people. And a person drove this truck, using energy from the earth, from oil and gasoline that may have come from the far side of the planet, to transport this raisin to market.

When the truck arrived at its destination, more human beings expended energy to unload the raisin and carry it in its box or container to a shelf or a bin. And then you or someone in your household came along and picked up a box of raisins from the shelf or scooped up and bagged some raisins and carried them to the checkout register. There the cashier used more energy from the earth, this time in the form of electricity, to calculate the price for this raisin and all the other raisins that came along with it. You brought those raisins home, and now here you are with *this* raisin, this unique raisin that has had quite a remarkable journey to arrive here in your hand in this moment.

When we slow down and look deeply at this raisin, we can see that perhaps what a few minutes ago was just an ordinary raisin is not so ordinary after all. By expanding our awareness, we can actually see the earth and sun and stars and clouds and rain and oil and gas and electricity and all the people who played a part in bringing this raisin into our hand. Paying attention, looking deeply, we can see the entire web of life itself—a vast interconnectedness that includes the raisin, ourselves, our partner, and our baby. In this very moment we are holding the entire universe right here in our hand.

Now returning from this wide-angle view to the more concentrated focus we used before, eat this raisin as you did the first one—slowly, bringing concentrated attention to seeing, feeling, hearing, smelling, and tasting the raisin. If thoughts or emotions arise, just notice them, let them go, and return to the sensations of eating the raisin. Perhaps you are experiencing a deeper understanding of and appreciation for the existence of the raisin, including all the many causes and conditions that led to its being right here, right now.

Once you have finished chewing and swallowing the raisin, take a moment to look deeply once again. Reflect on the fact that your body, right in this moment, is one raisin heavier. And consider that the raisin you have just eaten is, in this moment, undergoing another transformation, this time inside your body. It's actually becoming a part of your body and ultimately a part of your baby's body.

Consider that raisins have a lot of iron in them, a mineral that comes from the earth. Iron is critical to our body's production of red blood cells, which we are in constant need of replenishing. Red blood cells carry oxygen to every cell and organ in our body. Taking iron into our body is particularly important when we are pregnant because we need lots of new red blood cells to take oxygen and nutrients to our baby's body through the placenta and the umbilical cord.

By slowing down and looking deeply at the raisin, we can see how this small, dark, wrinkled, sweet object that we have just eaten, with all its countless interconnections to the larger universe, has directly contributed to our own health and wellbeing and to the health and wellbeing of the next generation.

REFLECTIONS ON THE RAISIN MEDITATION

The simple elegance of the Raisin Meditation elicits wonderful observations and insights from expectant parents attending class. Someone says, "I don't think I ever really tasted a raisin before. I mean, this was the best raisin I ever ate!" Of course this triggers a rhetorical question: Was this really a special raisin, or was it the quality of attention we brought to the experience, the fact that we were really *there* for the eating of it, that made the taste so vivid?

Eating can be one of life's great joys. How many such moments of sheer delight are you missing every day because you're not really there for a bite of an apple or the taste of a peach? And how many other moments are you not fully experiencing, like the smell of the morning air as you step outside on your way to work or the delicate shape of the flower in your neighbor's garden that bloomed overnight? And how many joyful moments of your pregnancy are you missing because you are so busy rushing from one thing to the next?

Regardless of the physical discomforts—the nausea, the backaches, the shortness of breath—and all the uncertainties and worries you may be carrying about the future, if you take a moment to really see, you will find that in this very moment you are a living, breathing miracle, with a new human being growing inside of you! And if you are missing this miracle, how many more such moments will you miss during the process of childbirth and parenting?

Perhaps taking a moment to stop and ask, "Where does the joy of living exist anyway?," you may find that it exists in the sweet taste of an orange, the sudden smile that lights up your baby's face, the warmth of a hug from your partner or a friend, or the sweet smell of your baby's skin. When we practice mindfulness we become more awake and alive in the present moment, for ourselves and for our children.

I remember Claire, the mother of three-month-old Julian, telling me about the changes she observed in her own father after the baby was born. She said it was amazing how endlessly happy her father was to hold and play with his new granddaughter. It was so uncharacteristic of him, and she was both surprised and delighted by the change. One day he confided in her how thrilled he was to have a second chance with his granddaughter. When Claire asked what he meant, he said that he deeply regretted not having been there during so much of her childhood and that he had promised himself he was not going to have that regret with his granddaughter.

Perhaps one or the other or even both your parents were a bit like Claire's. Whole families can be raised without anyone being fully present for the experience and for each other. Past chances for shared moments of intimacy, joy, connection, and understanding are lost. Gone forever. But by cultivating mindfulness during pregnancy, you're giving yourself a far better chance of not having this particular regret about your own parenting.

In many ways the heart of parenting is about being fully present with our children. One way we can learn how to do this is by learning how to be fully present for and connected to ourselves in our own lives right now.

A DIRECT EXPERIENCE OF
THE MIND-BODY CONNECTION

Another experience that participants in the class report after the Raisin Meditation is "My mouth was salivating before the raisin even reached my lips!" If you actually practiced the Raisin Meditation instead of just reading about it, you may have had this experience too. This is an especially interesting observation because it is a direct experience of the mind-body connection. What do I mean by this? Well, you were looking at or smelling the raisin, right? And then you started bringing it to your lips. As you did so, you could feel more saliva flowing in your mouth. How did that happen? It happened because the mind perceived food coming, and in response to that *perception*, the body changed. In an instant, your body began making more saliva. You could quite accurately say, then, that the digestive process actually begins in the mind.

The critical point here is that *it was the mind that created the change in the body*. When we slow down enough to actually observe the workings of the mind-body phenomenon that we are, it is really quite extraordinary. The mind perceived the raisin coming toward the mouth and set in motion this amazingly complex process in the body—the release of fluids and all sorts of enzymes in anticipation of nourishment.

Perception matters. And it matters a lot. How we see things (or don't see them) has a tremendous impact on the workings of the body. The mind-body connection is very, very real. If you're afraid of dogs and you see one, your perception triggers a sudden rush of adrenaline into your bloodstream, putting your body on high alert. By contrast, if you like dogs and you see one, your perception of the very same stimulus—the sight of a dog—will trigger the release of oxytocin into your blood so that you feel friendly and happy. This mind-body dynamic is at work all the time, every moment of every day. And as we will learn, this has tremendous implications for the process of giving birth.

ENCOUNTERING RESISTANCE

As we share our experiences of the Raisin Meditation in class, Monica speaks up. "I had a really hard time with this meditation. Ever since I was a kid, I've hated raisins. I've always picked them out of muffins or cereal, stuff like that. So when you were coming around passing out the raisins I thought, 'Oh, no. What am I going to do?' I could see Kathy watching me, knowing how much I don't like raisins. But I decided to go along with the exercise.

"When the time came to put the raisin into my mouth, I really didn't want to. But I figured, 'What the heck, it's only a raisin, for heaven's sake.' So I put the raisin to my lips, and then let my tongue take it into my mouth, just like everybody else. And I was really surprised. When I bit into the raisin and really tasted it, it wasn't at all what I expected. In fact, it was almost good!"

I asked Monica, "How was the rest of the experience—the seeing, hearing, smelling, and becoming aware of interconnection?"

She replied, "I didn't have any trouble with those parts. I liked looking at the raisin, seeing all the wrinkles and the color. Feeling the squishiness of the raisin was kind of interesting. And listening to it, even though that was pretty weird, was fun. When I realized how much the raisin had been through, I was pretty amazed—and even grateful for it."

We can learn a lot from Monica's account. First of all, she strongly identified as being someone who "doesn't like raisins." From the very moment she found out a raisin was coming her way, her mind located her in a story about herself as a person who doesn't like raisins. And she began to conjure up worries about the future. She expected a very unpleasant experience, which she didn't want, but she was also curious and open enough to go along with the meditation and see what would happen. She was bringing beginner's mind to the experience.

What Monica discovered from eating the raisin mindfully was that it actually consisted of many moments. Some were interesting; some were odd; and in some moments she actually felt gratitude for a raisin! And when the time came for her to eat the raisin, her experience was not at all what she had expected.

Of course there is an obvious parallel here to childbirth. Like Monica with the raisin, most of us carry around a lot of preconceptions, expectations, ideas, beliefs, hopes, and fears—even long-standing ones—about childbirth. We worry about how much it will hurt and what might happen to us or to our baby, and we fantasize about how we would like our partner, our healthcare providers, and ourselves to behave during the experience itself.

As you can see from Monica's experience, with mindfulness practice, there is another way. What if you approach the experience of childbirth mindfully, like Monica did with the raisin, taking it one moment at a time? Might a whole different way of relating to childbirth be possible? What if you could shed your expectations and ideas about childbirth—everything you have read and heard about it—and just go through the experience with beginner's mind, moment by moment? In doing so, *you might discover that childbirth isn't what you think*. Perhaps it is possible, through the lens of mindfulness, to discover for yourself, through your moment-to-moment experience of living it, exactly what birthing a baby is for you.

Even if you've had a baby before, beginner's mind or don't-know mind can be a helpful way to approach your next birth experience. After all, you don't know what *this* childbirth will be like. So why not put your energy into learning to be in the *now*, becoming aware of and perhaps letting go of ideas and fears about the future, and then do the same thing as you go through labor? It could be a much more interesting and less stressful way to approach the whole experience.

INTERCONNECTION

Cultivating the capacity to be present brings all sorts of surprises, like Monica's feeling of gratitude for the raisin. Learning to be mindful can lead us to a kind of openheartedness, a sense of connection and caring—even for a raisin! If we can learn how to slow down and become more connected to the deeper aspects of ourselves, if we can be more present in our lives and access greater calm and ease within, caring and connection naturally arise. Mindfulness and the awareness of interconnectedness are already inside each of us, just waiting to come into fullness of being. All it takes is practice.

OF BABIES AND RAISINS:
A STORY OF MINDFULNESS IN ACTION

Not long after I began teaching mindfulness to expectant couples I was invited by a local hospital to give a two-hour presentation titled "Mindfulness and Stress Reduction for New Mothers." I was delighted by this invitation, and when I asked what size group to expect, I was told that it would be small—perhaps eight women and their babies. Being new at sharing mindfulness practice, I put considerable energy into thinking about and planning for the event. The morning I arrived, a cheery volunteer at the front desk escorted me to the classroom. What I saw stopped me in my tracks. The presentation room was *huge*, populated by *forty* women and their babies, ranging from three weeks to eight months of age.

To say things were chaotic would be an understatement. Mothers stood in small groups or sat on the floor, nursing, changing diapers, and trying to converse above the din. Babies squealed and fussed and cried as their mothers patted, rocked, walked, or bounced them. My first thought was, "So much for planning for the future!" Then I thought, "It is what it is. I'll just do the best I can."

I settled myself in the front of the room. A distraught woman sitting directly in front of me was offering her breast to a very unhappy baby in an attempt to soothe him while he arched his body away from her, screeching louder than before. Taking a deep breath, I started speaking quietly about cultivating mindfulness and the skill of being in the present moment. Those close to me stopped talking, and gradually, like a ripple moving outward, the silence spread as mothers turned their attention to the front of the room. The babies mostly continued their crying and fussing. One woman, whose baby was wailing inconsolably, got up and practically fled the room.

"So why don't we experiment with some mindfulness practice right now?" I continued, knowing that some women had no idea what in the world I was talking about. "It might help settle us and our babies." And so I began what would become the Raisin-Baby Meditation.

"Let's begin with ourselves. See if you can become aware of any body sensations right now—perhaps a place of tension or tightness or a holding of discomfort in your body. Notice any thoughts running through your mind, perhaps a worried thought about the baby, or a thought about what others might be thinking of you or your baby. Notice any emotions you might be feeling, perhaps anxiety, or distress, or protectiveness, or empathy, or self-consciousness, or ease."

Pausing, I allowed some time for the mothers to drop into practice, into the present moment.

"And now see if you can come to the breath, feeling the breath as a physical sensation, wherever you feel it most vividly, perhaps at the belly, or the nostrils, or the chest. Let the breath be an anchor to the present moment."

As my voice continued, the sounds in the room began to subside.

"Now I invite you to look at your baby. See your baby's face, her eyes, the miracle of her eyelashes, the turn of her nose, the shape of her mouth. Notice the color of her cheeks, the color and texture of her hair. Notice her expressions, perhaps of contentment, or of alert interest, or of distress. If your baby is fussing or crying, really look at your baby. As difficult as it might be, see your baby just as she is now. Notice any thoughts or emotions you might be experiencing in this present moment, and how powerfully you feel them. If your baby seems to need comforting and there is something you can do, do that now, slowly and gently, paying full attention to the action.

"Now let's explore the sense of touch. If your baby is in your arms, feel his weight, his warmth where he is in contact with your body, or the softness of his skin against your cheek. If your baby is asleep, perhaps you would like to close your eyes for some of this meditation practice too. If your baby is fussing or crying, feel the tension in his body under your hands, or against your body, as he wriggles or twists."

No doubt about it. The room was definitely quieter now.

"Now I invite you to smell your baby. If you are holding your baby, perhaps you can position her so that you can smell the hair on the top of her head. Really breathe in the smell of your baby, the smell at the crook of her neck, her cheek, or her hands.

"And if you become aware of any thoughts, thoughts like, 'Oh, I have to wash his hair tonight' or 'Do I smell a poopy diaper?' or 'I wonder if anyone here knows something I haven't tried yet for his cradle cap,' just notice those thoughts, let them go, and come back to the smell of your baby."

At this moment, the room was almost completely quiet, and I found myself wondering, "What are these mothers thinking? Do they think this is totally crazy? Do they think *I* am totally crazy?" But I too gently let the thoughts go and came back to this moment of leading these forty women with their babies in mindfulness practice.

"And if you are nursing your baby in this moment, feel the weight of the baby in your arms and the sensations of your baby's mouth and tongue moving against your nipple. Perhaps you can hear the rhythmic sounds of your baby swallowing. If your baby's hand reaches for your mouth, and if you are comfortable with it, allow your baby to put his hand in your mouth. Taste your baby's fingers, knowing that right now your baby is tasting the sweet milk flowing from your breasts, appreciating the fact that not only did your body nourish this being while he was inside you, your body is continuing to nourish him in this very moment. If you are feeding your baby with a bottle, appreciate the nourishment you provided your baby while he was growing inside your body, and acknowledge the care and nourishment you are continuing to give your baby in this very moment."

Except for the occasional squeal or snuffle, the room was now utterly silent: forty mothers, in silence, practicing mindfulness meditation, being totally present with their babies, in that very moment.

Finally I said, "And if you are ready, begin to move and stretch your body a bit. Raise your shoulders toward your ears, and let them drop down once or twice, or wriggle your fingers and toes, and if your eyes have been closed, slowly open them."

The eyes of the woman sitting directly in front of me, the one whose baby had been so unhappy when we began (and was now peacefully sleeping in her arms), flew open. "Oh, my god!" she exclaimed for all to hear. "They feel whatever we're feeling! If we're stressed out, they're stressed out! If we calm down, they calm down!"

I smiled. Mindfulness practice had worked its magic. It was a morning well spent.

CHAPTER 4

The Breath
A Friend for Life

*If the heart wanders or is distracted, bring it back to the point quite
gently. And even if you did nothing during the whole of your hour but
bring it back, though it went away every time you brought it back,
your hour would be well employed.*
—Saint Francis de Sales

WE ARE BORN on an in-breath, and we die on an out-breath. Meditation practice offers us an opportunity to look deeply at breathing, this often unnoticed and utterly remarkable process that keeps us alive. Breathing is a series of expansions and contractions. When you inhale, oxygen comes into your lungs, where tiny blood-filled capillaries allow for the exchange of the oxygen essential to life with the carbon dioxide your body no longer needs. In a process of give-and-take that begins at birth and continues until you die, the breath brings nourishment to your every cell, helping you produce the energy you need to run up the stairs, to think about what to make for dinner, to laugh with a friend, and to birth your baby into this world.

Newly oxygenated blood flows from the pulmonary vein in the lungs to another miracle of expansion and contraction: the heart. This amazing muscle pumps blood through the miles of arteries, veins, and capillaries of your circulatory system to every cell in your body. When we are pregnant the total amount of blood we carry in our arteries and veins increases by almost a liter. In addition to growing your baby, your pregnant body grows an entirely new organ, the placenta, which gives your baby access to the life-giving exchange of oxygen and carbon dioxide. When you are pregnant your lungs are literally your baby's lungs, and your heart pumps oxygen and nourishment to your baby living in the inner sea of amniotic fluid.

When we take time to reflect on breathing, we can see our interconnection to the great web of life, just as we did with the raisin. The oxygen
we breathe into our bodies comes from the trees and plants that surround
us, and the carbon dioxide we breathe out gives them life in a miraculous
symbiotic process.

Though all this is going on, moment by moment, whether we are aware
of it or not, whether we are pregnant or not, we usually give little thought
to the process of breathing. Unless we have a respiratory illness like a cold
or bronchitis or a chronic breathing condition like asthma, we usually take
the breath pretty much for granted.

Except when we begin to meditate.

MEDITATION AND BREATHING

While human beings have discovered many methods for increasing awareness and focusing the mind—including sounds (such as a prayer, or a mantra), visual images (like a mandala), or movement (as practiced in yoga or
tai chi)—one of the most universal meditation practices is bringing attention to the breath. There are many reasons for this. For one thing, there's
nothing special about breathing; after all, everyone does it. Yet without the
breath, we wouldn't be alive. In each moment the breath is both totally
ordinary and completely extraordinary. Just like giving birth.

The breath is also wonderfully portable, which makes it very convenient.
It goes where you go. Unlike your lunch or your cell phone, you can't leave
home without it. By focusing on the breath, we always have everything we
need to come fully into the present moment.

And because it is such a neutral event, the breath as a focus for meditation is also quite practical. You don't have to believe anything or adhere
to any dogma in order to pay attention to the breath. You just pay attention as best you can to the sensations of breathing as your breath flows in
and out of your body, moment by moment. This also allows meditation to
be a very private affair. Nobody needs to know if you are paying attention
to the breath—you can do it while you're in a meeting at the office or waiting in line at the supermarket or having a conversation with your partner
or child.

The breath can shift us out of our habitual Doing Mode and into a completely other way, which we can call Being Mode. In Doing Mode the mind
is endlessly thinking, analyzing, telling us stories about the past or the
future, setting goals, and trying to solve problems. Now there's nothing
wrong with this—it's helpful to make a shopping list before going to the

supermarket and to have some idea of how long it will take to drive to a dentist appointment; it's just that if we live only in Doing Mode, we are missing an important dimension of living.

Being Mode is another way of relating to the world: experiencing your thoughts, your emotions, and your body sensations directly, just as they are. In Being Mode you are not dependent on external conditions for happiness, ease, and wellbeing. Being Mode helps us see the world and ourselves through the lens of interconnection, wholeness, and compassion. It is this Being Mode that we cultivate in our mindfulness practice, and the breath can be the doorway through which we come to it—just being right here, right now.

The breath can be a touchstone for dropping into awareness at any moment; it means the mind always has a home, a refuge, a familiar place to return to again and again. By anchoring us in the present, the breath provides a way to step out of the thinking mind and into a place of calm, ease, and connection with ourselves, others, and the world around us. All of these aspects of the breath make it a perfect match for pregnancy and childbirth. If you showed up at the hospital in labor with nothing more than your breath, you would be just fine. And if you showed up with some training in paying attention to your breath, you would be even finer.

⌐ AWARENESS OF BREATHING MEDITATION ¬

If you would like to experiment with using the breath as a focus of attention, which I wholeheartedly recommend, here are some simple instructions. If you aren't able to practice at this time, make a commitment to yourself to return to this page later. See if you can practice this meditation for one minute; even a brief experience with paying attention to the breath will provide you with a reference point for understanding the rest of this chapter (and for that matter the rest of this book).

Settle your body into a comfortable position, in a chair or on a cushion on the floor. If you are sitting in a chair, place both feet flat on the floor, if that's comfortable for you. Feel the points of contact between the backs of your thighs and your buttocks and whatever you are sitting on. Gently allow your spine to lift upward from your lower back, letting it be straight but not rigid. If you are sitting in a chair, you can also experiment with sitting away from the back of the chair so that your spine is more upright. Let the crown of your head rise upward toward the ceiling and the sky above. It can be helpful to tilt the chin ever so slightly down and toward the chest, opening space in the back of the neck and allowing the head to balance easily.

Let your shoulders drop away from the ears, and gently slide your shoulder blades down your back, opening the chest. Let your arms hang loosely, finding a resting place for your hands—on your lap, thighs, or knees—palms facing upward or downward, whichever you prefer. If you are well along in your pregnancy, feel free to modify these instructions as needed to find a posture of ease, including lying on your side. Your comfort is more important than any posture you might take. You can practice with your eyes either open or closed. If you practice with your eyes open, let your gaze be soft, focusing on a spot on the floor a few feet in front of you.

Once settled in a comfortable position, bring your attention to the sensations of breathing, wherever you feel them most vividly in your body: perhaps at the belly, as it rises on the inhalation and falls on the exhalation; or at the nostrils, as the air passes in and then out; or perhaps at the chest, feeling the lungs and rib cage expanding and releasing. Wherever you choose to pay attention to the sensations of breathing, allow your attention to rest there as best you can, moment by moment. There is no need to change the breath in any way, no need to do anything or fix anything. However you are breathing right now—slow or fast, shallow or deep—is just fine. You are just sitting where you are, paying attention to the sensations of breathing, however they are, allowing the breath to come and go all on its own, moment by moment.

If at any time during this practice you feel the baby moving inside your belly, just allow your attention to shift to those sensations, feeling both the movements of the baby within and the movements of the breath at your belly, expanding on an inhalation and releasing on an exhalation. If you want to bring your hand to your belly as you practice, that's fine; if you do, feel the weight of your hand and perhaps some warmth from it against your belly as you breathe—breathing for yourself, breathing for your baby.

And each time you become aware that the mind has wandered away from the breath, as it inevitably will, that it has gotten caught up in thinking—commenting or judging, planning or speculating or remembering the past—gently take note of the thought of the moment and let it go, kindly and gently escorting the attention back to the breath, back to the sensations of breathing, at the belly or the nostrils or the chest, wherever you are experiencing the sensations of breathing most vividly. Just being here—breath by breath.

And when you become aware that the mind has wandered once again, gently and kindly return the attention to the breath again . . . and then again.

After a minute or so, wriggle your fingers and toes, stretch a bit, and, if your eyes have been closed, gently allow them to open.

This is one way to practice meditation: training the mind to be in the present moment.

TAKING REFUGE IN THE BREATH

After their birth experience, I ask mothers who took the MBCP course what was the most helpful thing they learned for giving birth. Far and away the most frequent answers are "the breath" and "being in the present moment." Interestingly, partners also say that "the breath" helped *them* most in dealing with their own experience of childbirth.

Gina's comments are typical. "I really used everything we practiced in class and at home. The breath helped me to stay focused and to take the experience one contraction at a time. It absolutely helped me work with the pain and to rest between contractions. And when I left the present moment, I had Tom to remind me of the breath and all the other tools we learned. That was especially helpful for the really intense part, when I wasn't sure I could keep going. Then I just kept thinking, 'One breath at a time.'"

Having learned how to use the breath as an anchor to the present moment, this couple applied that skill to their childbirth experience so that *there was no separation between their meditation practice and their labor experience.* They were in a dynamic relationship to the birthing process as it unfolded, moment by moment. Like the dancer who is one with the dance, their birthing *became* their meditation practice. And the breath was their refuge, just when they needed it most.

THE WANDERING MIND

These directions for practicing meditation are simple enough. You choose a place in your body where you can vividly feel the sensations of breathing then pay attention to those sensations. And you keep paying attention to them as best you can, moment by moment. When you notice that the mind has wandered away from the breath, as it will do, simply bring the attention gently back to the breath. That's pretty much it.

However, if you accepted the invitation to actually experience the Awareness of Breathing meditation, you probably discovered that following those simple instructions was not so easy. You may have had the experience of your mind wandering and then bringing it back to the breath. Maybe that happened to you a couple of times. Or a dozen times. Or a couple of dozen times, depending on how long you practiced. Not to worry. One of the most fundamental realizations people have when they begin to meditate is how much the mind seems to have a mind of its own. As Tenisha said in class one evening, "I never realized before how much chatter is going on in my head all the time. It just doesn't quit. I thought meditation was supposed to make my mind go blank—that I would be able to stop the thoughts and find some rest. But at this point I'm more aware of my thoughts than ever."

Tenisha is giving voice to one of the most common misconceptions about meditation: that meditation is about stopping your thoughts or making your mind go blank. If you believe this and you start meditating, then when the thoughts keep coming, you'll think you are "one of those people who can't meditate," or you'll think "meditation doesn't work for me" and that somehow you've failed. So let's be clear from the beginning. *Meditation practice is not about stopping thoughts; it's about finding that we can increase awareness and observe our thoughts—or for that matter, anything else in our inner experience, including our body sensations and our emotions—and establish a kind and gentle relationship with them.*

Remember, part of the instruction for Awareness of Breathing is to notice where the mind has gone when you become aware that your attention is no longer on the breath. This is where you can learn about particular habits or patterns of your mind—perhaps a habit of constant worry or a strong need to plan for the future or a habit of endlessly replaying an unhappy memory or a mind that harshly judges you or others. Our friend the breath is helping us get to know ourselves better and perhaps giving us a chance to make peace with this chattering mind, learning not to take these thoughts quite so seriously and thereby developing a friendlier, easier relationship with our mind.

As we become more familiar with our own mind, we can also come to know that it is not so different from everyone else's. If your mind is chattering away, jumping like a monkey from tree to tree (in fact, the wandering mind is sometimes called "monkey mind"), you can bet that most everyone else's mind is doing that too. This doesn't make us bad. It's just something that the human mind, especially the untrained one, does. And it does it a lot.

The point is, when we're *not aware* of this chatter it drives much of our behavior, whether we want it to or not. Monkey mind is particularly prevalent in twenty-first-century life; in the extreme we call it ADD or ADHD.

Through overscheduling and multitasking, we may be unwittingly encouraging this tendency of the mind and creating a tremendous source of stress for ourselves.

If you come to discover, for example, that you have a very strong habit of mind that plans for the future in a vain attempt to control it, you may be creating a lot of suffering for yourself. Not knowing what the future will bring, you can get caught up in all sorts of possibilities (usually negative), for the possibilities are as endless as the river of thoughts that pours from the thinking mind. This is what Mark Twain was alluding to when he said, "My life has been filled with many misfortunes, most of which never happened."

By paying attention to the breath, you can interrupt that habit of trying to use your thinking mind to do something that is in fact impossible to do—control the future. Instead, you can begin to come to terms with uncertainty and not knowing, which means learning how to live with more ease in the now.

THE POWER OF A MINDFUL PAUSE

When we begin to train the mind through meditation, new possibilities open up. Not only do we begin to become more familiar with the patterns of our mind, we discover that it's possible to free ourselves from them. Every time we realize we have become lost in thought, this is a moment of mindfulness, a moment of waking up. And in this moment we find we have a choice, *a choice about where we put our attention.* Rather than following a thought into an old, established groove, we discover—right in the present moment—that we can actually change a habit of mind.

Over time, and with practice, lots and lots of practice, we can break out of less-than-optimal patterns of mind and begin to find more and more choice-making moments in our daily life. This awareness then becomes a new way of being, a new way of relating to both our inner and outer experiences. As we practice, our lives become more interesting, vivid, and real. And we often become happier.

But that's not all. Researchers have found that as we become more mindful, we are actually laying down new neural pathways in the brain. Of course this takes time, commitment, and effort, but researchers have found that by deliberately choosing to bring your attention back to the breath in your meditation practice, in that very moment *you are literally using your mind to change your brain.*[1]

Through a phenomenon known as neuroplasticity, when you use awareness to interrupt unhelpful mental patterns you are actually creating new neural pathways in your brain. As the saying goes, "Neurons that fire to-gether wire together." If your neurons are frequently firing together in un-helpful repetitive patterns, such as being angry or frustrated, you get really good at anger and frustration. However, you can actually create new and more positive neural pathways by *choosing* to pay attention to something else. As you practice you come to feel different—steadier, more resilient, and less reactive to life's inevitable ups and downs—because you *are* differ-ent. You have used your mind to change your brain.

BEING WITH THE JUDGING MIND

One useful thing to notice in your meditation practice is the thought that arises immediately *after* the moment you wake up from the dream of the thinking mind. As perhaps you've seen already, in the moment after be-coming aware of thinking, the mind often has a judging thought—or a cas-cade of them. "Oh, there I go again; I'm thinking. Why can't I keep my attention on the breath? I can't do it, even though everyone else seems to be able to. I guess I'm hopeless at this." And on and on. Of course these are just more thoughts, the thinking mind falling into its pattern of con-structing a judging story about you. This self-judging habit may be a very old one, and there's no doubt that it can be very painful. Sometimes the judgments we pass on ourselves are remarkably cruel—far harsher than we would pass on anyone else.

So if judgmental thoughts arise about meditation practice—or anything else for that matter—the instruction is the same: notice the thought and return your attention to the breath. In the noticing, the awareness itself interrupts the cause of your suffering, the painful thought. And the con-sequence of this interruption is the dissolving and passing away of the thought. Like a bubble in a stream.

Remember, the meditation instructions are to kindly and gently bring your attention back to the breath—and rest there. In those moments we are actually learning how to befriend ourselves. We are discovering that we can find peace, kindness, and caring even in the presence of inner tur-bulence. We will explore this territory more deeply later on, but for now, just knowing that there is a way to uncouple from this painful self-judging can be truly liberating. Those judging thoughts, as familiar as they are, are just habits of mind. And habits of mind, even long-standing ones, can be changed. You are not your thoughts.

THERE'S NO SUCH THING AS A "GOOD" MEDITATION—AND THERE'S NO SUCH THING AS A "BAD" MEDITATION EITHER

When you have a pleasurable meditation experience, take care not to fall into the trap of becoming attached to the experience, thinking that it was a "good" meditation or that you are finally "doing it right" and will therefore strive to have the same experience again. In reality, there is no such thing as a good meditation. A meditation in which you were quite focused, when you experienced a degree of stillness and inner peace, is no better than a meditation in which the mind is quite agitated or the body is very uncomfortable. While you may certainly *prefer* a peaceful meditation (and an uncomplicated birth), that is just a preference for ease over discomfort, which is certainly understandable. But if you try to make the pleasurable happen each time you practice, thinking that you are not doing it right if it doesn't turn out that way, then you are setting yourself up to suffer—and to miss the opportunity to grow in inner strength, wisdom, and compassion, which is the point of our meditation practice.

Each time we practice, our meditation experience will be different because we are different. What we are learning is the letting go of the dualistic mind, the mind that separates the world into like and not like, into good and bad, and to step instead into conditional reality, the reality of how things are in any particular moment, whether in relation to a particular meditation or to giving birth or to any other aspect of life.

ALLOWING THE BREATH

For some of us, at least at the beginning, it may be a challenge to just allow the breath to come and go as it does. We are so conditioned to striving that when we sit down to meditate, the mind thinks there must be something to do. Unfamiliar with this mode of just "being with," we metaphorically lean forward, thinking we must change or fix something. But by learning to just feel the sensations of the breath, observing them and letting the breath be as it is, coming and going, we are actually cultivating equanimity, a quality that can play a welcome role in the rest of our life.

Having some experience of this mindful relationship to the breath, you can choose to drop into this way of being during labor. Allowing the sensations of the contractions to rise and ebb, you meet them with the same open, allowing awareness. Just as you allowed the breath to take care of itself during meditation practice, you allow the contractions of labor to take care of themselves. You can choose to observe the process of labor moving through your body because, like the breath, the sensations of labor are simply arising and passing. This is perhaps the greatest gift we can take from our meditation practice into our birthing experience.

THE RELATIONSHIP BETWEEN
BREATHING AND RELAXATION

A common experience reported by participants when they first practice Awareness of Breathing is a feeling of relaxation, either during the meditation or afterward. In fact, when we practice in class, at least in the beginning, it's not uncommon for participants to fall asleep. It's wonderful that people are discovering a precious inner resource for bringing ease to the mind-body, but it's also important to remember that paying attention to the breath in order to *do* anything, even to relax, is not the point. Relaxation is not the object of our practice, although it can be a welcome outcome. Relaxation is a natural by-product of our practice, the *result* of a calm, focused, and concentrated mind.

Discovering the breath as a resource for cultivating ease is particularly useful for those of us who have a history of distress about breathing. Stephanie had a history of asthma, for example, and after the Awareness of Breathing meditation on the first night of class she reported that paying attention to the breath brought up a lot of anxiety and upsetting memories of times in her childhood when she struggled to breathe. One of Stephanie's big worries about childbirth was that she would have an asthma attack during labor.

Because of her conditioned anxiety regarding the breath, Stephanie needed to approach the Awareness of Breathing meditation with special gentleness, care, and kindness toward herself. Together Stephanie and I decided that she would start by practicing Awareness of Breathing for only three minutes once a day rather than the longer periods assigned to the other expectant parents. Over time her anxiety diminished and she gradually increased the amount of time she spent practicing. Eventually she came to enjoy these moments of stillness and quiet with her breath. On the last night of class, as each person spoke about what they had learned, Stephanie shared how much her feelings about the breath had changed. "Now I am totally grateful that I have the breath to go through labor with me," she said.

THE BREATH, OUR BODIES, AND OUR EMOTIONS

Breathing is unique among our bodily functions in that it has both a voluntary and an involuntary aspect. For example, we can voluntarily take a deep breath and hold it, but if we go beyond a certain point, the involuntary aspect will take over: we pass out or momentarily lose consciousness, during which time we start breathing again; in its wisdom our body will override a decision by the mind.

The breath also changes with our emotional states. When we are relaxed and at ease, the breath is deep and regular, as it is when we sleep. When we are anxious or fearful, in distress or in pain, our breathing becomes shallow and rapid. We'll learn much more about the breath and its relationship to our nervous system in Chapter 6.

During pregnancy, the body's shape changes so dramatically that it should come as no surprise that this affects how we breathe. As your uterus gets larger, it causes the organs inside your abdominal cavity to rearrange themselves. Gradually the stomach and intestines are nudged upward under the diaphragm and back toward the spine. As a consequence, the diaphragm, the sheet of fibrous muscle under the ribs that moves down when we inhale and returns to its resting position when we exhale, has significantly less space available for movement. Most women find that their breathing becomes shallower, more constricted, or even labored during pregnancy. It can be a great relief to be able to breathe fully and deeply when, in the last month or so, the baby drops deeper into the pelvis, opening up more space under the ribs for the diaphragm to move freely once again.

It's interesting too to see how the body adapts to this decrease in space below the rib cage for diaphragmatic movement. The body still needs just as much oxygen as it did before pregnancy, in fact, more of it since there is now more blood to be oxygenated. To compensate for the loss of space, the circumference of the chest expands laterally. You may have noticed that you now need a bra that is larger around the rib cage. Yes, your body is expanding in many places, not just your belly!

As you become more mindful of the breath during pregnancy, you can take a more active role in your self-care. If you notice that you're feeling slightly anxious or out of sorts, perhaps it's simply due to the shallowness of your breathing as a result of the changes in your anatomy; stopping and taking a few deep breaths or doing some stretches to open the chest, as you will learn in the yoga sequence in Chapter 8, may help you regain your emotional equilibrium.

MINDFULNESS PRACTICE

In the MBCP program we start practicing Awareness of Breathing in our very first meeting, right after the Raisin Meditation. Now that you understand the importance of the breath in cultivating awareness, I invite you too to begin paying attention to it. Here are several suggestions for getting your meditation practice under way.

AWARENESS OF BREATHING: PRACTICE 1

Reread the instructions for Awareness of Breathing earlier in this chapter, and make the commitment to practice between five and fifteen minutes every day for one week. Do this whether you feel like doing it or not, whether you like it or not, and even if your mind is all over the place or you fall asleep every time you practice. The point here is not to have any particular experience but to see what it's like when your life includes a regular, daily meditation practice.

AWARENESS OF BREATHING: PRACTICE 2

Bring awareness to your breath throughout the day, whenever you can remember to do so; place your attention where you feel the breath most vividly in your body—perhaps at the belly or the nostrils or the chest. Do this for one or two breaths, more if possible. Observe, without judgment, what you are thinking and feeling in those moments of mindfulness. As best as you can, let your attention stay with your breath.

BEING WITH BABY PRACTICE

Let the baby's movements serve as a reminder to come to the breath throughout your day. As you bring attention to the baby's movements in your belly, see if you can also be aware of your breath at the belly as well—of the rising of the belly on the inhalation and the release of the belly on the exhalation. You may want to bring your hand to your belly as a way of becoming more aware of both the baby's movements and the movements of your breath. When your mind wanders, bring it back to the sensations of your breath, the feeling of your hand on your belly and of the movements of the baby. Though many women bring their hand or hands to their belly almost instinctively when the baby moves, see if you can bring awareness to this practice. Notice any thoughts or feelings that arise as you practice.

━ THE THREE-MINUTE BREATHING SPACE ━

STEP 1: BECOMING AWARE

At any time during your day, deliberately bring yourself into the present moment.[2] Adopt an erect and dignified posture, whether sitting or standing. If possible, close your eyes. Then, bringing your awareness to your inner experience, acknowledge it, asking, What is my experience *right now?*

- What thoughts are going through the mind? As best you can, acknowledge thoughts as mental events.
- What feelings or emotions are present? If they are pleasant, allow yourself to fully experience and enjoy them. If they are unpleasant, acknowledge and turn toward them, even if they are uncomfortable, painful, or unwanted.
- What body sensations are here right now? Perhaps do a quick Body Scan (you will learn this practice in the next chapter), noticing any sensations of contraction or tightness, acknowledging them without trying to change them in any way.

Do this for approximately one minute.

STEP 2: GATHERING AND FOCUSING ATTENTION

When you are ready, gathering in your attention, bringing it to the physical sensations of breathing, particularly the sensations of the breath at the belly. Noticing the sensations of stretching and expansion at the belly on the in-breath and the softening and releasing of the belly on the out-breath. Use each breath as an opportunity to anchor yourself in the present moment. If you experience the sensations of your baby moving within your belly, allow your attention to rest with those sensations as well as with the feeling of the breath, acknowledging that there is a person growing within your body, right here, right now. And if the mind wanders, gently and kindly escort your attention back to the breath at the belly. Be with your breath for as long as is appropriate given the context you are practicing in, sustaining awareness of the breath for one minute, or longer if you are able.

STEP 3: EXPANDING ATTENTION

Now widening the field of awareness around the breath so that it includes a sense of the body as a whole: your posture, your facial expressions, your whole body breathing alive, cradling another being within. If you become aware of any sensations of discomfort or tension, experiment with bringing your awareness right into that intensity, imagining that the breath can move into and around the sensations. In this way you are exploring the sensations, being with them, befriending them rather than trying to avoid or change them in any way. If there are no particular sensations calling for your attention, just be where you are, aware of the whole body, moment by moment. After one minute or so you can open your eyes, letting your attention expand outward, bringing this open awareness into the next moments of your life, just as it is.

For this meditation it can be helpful to see your awareness in the shape of an hourglass. Step 1 is the wide flare at the top of the hourglass, opening and acknowledging your present-moment experience, whatever it is. Step 2 is the narrowing neck of the hourglass, where you focus your attention on the physical sensations of breathing at the belly, grounding you in the present moment. Step 3 broadens your awareness into the base of the hourglass. You are opening to your whole being and coming back into life just as it is, gently but firmly stepping into this next moment of your life with awareness—grounded, dignified, and whole, just as you are.

The breath is both ordinary and miraculous. It is with us wherever we are, and just by becoming aware of it we can find moments of calm in any situation. Convenient, simple, and effective, becoming aware of the breath is one of the foundational practices for bringing more awareness into our lives.

CHAPTER 5

Practicing Embodiment
The Body Scan

We can bring an open and respectful attention to the
sensations that make up our bodily experience.
—Jack Kornfield

ALTHOUGH THE MIND often leaves the here and now, the body never does. In daily life, whenever you want to bring your attention back to the present, you can use various sensations in the body as an anchor, just the way you use the breath. The pressure of the soles of your feet on the ground as you stand in line at the post office; your bicep contracting as you lift the teakettle to pour a cup of tea; the rolling sensations in your belly created by the movements of the baby; the intense sensations of labor: becoming aware of any of these sensations can bring you right into the present moment. The body serves as a focus of practice that is personal, practical, and profound.

And so we come to the Body Scan, the formal meditation we practice during the first two weeks in the MBCP course. With the Body Scan, you cultivate mindfulness by slowly and systematically moving attention through the entire body, from the head to the feet, paying exquisite attention to the body sensations you are experiencing in the present moment. In practicing the Body Scan, you may find a way to appreciate your body and all that it does for you and your baby as well as inhabit it more fully.

"Folks, if you would, please push the chairs back against the wall, take a yoga mat, and find a place for yourself on the floor for our Body Scan practice." The room fills with the sounds of bustling and chairs scraping.

"If you're pregnant, lying on your side might be most comfortable. Do help yourself to some pillows—perhaps put one between your knees, one under your belly, and one under your head. If you aren't pregnant or very far along in your pregnancy, please lie on your back. Place your legs hip distance apart, feet gently falling away from each other. Loosen any constricting clothing around your waist, and put a pillow under your knees or thighs if you care to. Remember, let your body guide you to what's most comfortable. We're going to be on the floor for a bit, so if you think you might get chilly, feel free to use one of the blankets to cover yourself."

I too take a yoga mat as well as a pillow to put under my knees; I strained my back working in the garden this past weekend and need to take a bit of care with it tonight. Surveying the room, I watch as everyone settles on the floor next to their partner; then I dim the lights, lie down on my mat, and begin giving instructions for the Body Scan.

⤙ THE BODY SCAN ⤚

My suggestion to you is to read over the following instructions for the Body Scan once or twice, then settle yourself on your bed or the floor and practice the Body Scan too. If you and your partner are learning these practices together, you can take turns reading the instructions aloud to each other a time or two until you have learned the practice well enough to do it on your own.

For readers who are pregnant, if at any time during the Body Scan sensations of your baby moving within your belly become predominant, allow your awareness to shift to them; be with the sensations coming from your baby and the movements of the breath at the belly, just as you did when practicing Awareness of Breathing in the previous chapter. When your baby settles, resume the Body Scan practice, picking up wherever you left off when your baby's movements drew your attention. If you are using an audio guide for your practice, resume the Body Scan practice by returning your attention to the instructions you hear at the particular moment your baby quiets. If your baby is very active, your entire Body Scan practice could very well become a Being with Baby practice!

Once you have found a comfortable position on the floor, allow your eyes to close, if you are comfortable with this. If you prefer to keep them open, let your gaze soften as you turn your attention inward. Now, bringing your attention to the belly, notice the sensations of breathing as your belly rises on the inhalation and falls on the exhalation. Acknowledge the presence of your baby in your belly. If you have difficulty feeling the breath at the belly, you might bring your hand there for a few breaths to help you become more aware of those sensations.

Now, allowing your awareness to include the body as a whole, noticing points of contact as your weight presses against whatever surface you are lying on. See if you can allow yourself to sink fully into the surface beneath you, allowing it to do the work of holding your body. If you are lying on your side, becoming aware of the points of contact of the leg, the hip, the side of the torso, and the belly, noticing the pressure on the side of your arm, shoulder, and the side of your head. If you are lying on your back, bringing awareness to points of pressure at the heels, the backs of the legs, the buttocks, the upper back, and the back of your head.

And now, if you're ready, moving your awareness upward from the belly, perhaps feeling the breath rising and falling at the chest, noticing the sensations of air moving through your nostrils. As you shift your attention upward, allowing awareness to come to rest at the top of your head, about four fingerbreadths back from the hairline at your forehead. This was the soft spot on your skull when you were born, and it's the place where you will be able to feel a soft spot on your baby's head after she or he is born. Allow yourself to become aware of any sensations that might be present at this spot on your head, such as tingling or pressure or coolness. You may not be feeling anything at all, which is fine too. If that's the case, just allowing yourself the experience of "lack of sensation" or of "not feeling anything," which in fact is a kind of sensation.

And when you are ready, expanding your awareness over the entire top of the head. Once again, noticing whatever sensations are present, perhaps feeling pressure or throbbing or tightness or tingling. Now allowing the awareness to move, perhaps on an out-breath, to the right side of the head, directing your awareness from the top of the head downward, to where the skull meets the neck. Include the awareness of your right ear and any sensations you might be experiencing in or around your right ear. If you are lying on your right side, you will undoubtedly feel pressure on your right ear from the weight of your head against a surface.

Now shifting your awareness to the back of your head. If you're lying on your back, feel the pressure of your head against the surface beneath you. Notice the place where the pressure is greatest as well as the edges where the sensations of pressure gradually lessen and disappear. And when you are ready, moving your awareness to the left side of the head, including the left ear, proceeding just as you did for the right.

While you are practicing, whenever you notice that the mind has wandered away from the sensations of the body and has become caught up in thinking or planning or wondering or worrying about the past or the future, noticing this, and gently and kindly return your awareness to whatever part of the body you were paying attention to when the mind wandered off. Repeat this process over and over again, every time you become aware that the mind has wandered.

Now, shifting your awareness to the left temple, slowly sweep the awareness across your forehead and over to the right temple, and as you do so, become aware of any sensation, perhaps tension or tightness in the forehead, perhaps between the eyebrows. Moving the awareness downward, pay careful attention to sensations around the eyes, and then the cheeks, perhaps becoming aware of the cheekbones underneath the skin, the muscles of the jaw in front of the ears, and the nose, including the feeling inside the nostrils as air comes in on the inhalation and goes out on the exhalation. Now becoming aware of the mouth, focusing on the sensations in your lips, and the points of contact between the upper lip and lower lip. Letting your attention move to the sensations inside your mouth—the tongue, the teeth, moisture, the softness of the inner cheeks—lingering for a moment. Now letting go of your attention to the inside of the mouth, shifting awareness to the jawbone, and to the chin.

Now, slowly moving your attention under the chin and then to the front of the neck, feeling any sensations in your throat. Moving awareness to the right side of the neck, around to the back of the neck, and to the left side of the neck, taking time to experience whatever sensations are present.

Continue to move the focus of your awareness, shifting it to the upper shoulders, and the upper back, and into the shoulder joints, and all the way around the shoulder joints, including the armpits. Now moving your awareness simultaneously down both arms, all the while paying exquisite attention to whatever sensations are present in the upper arms, the elbows, the lower arms, the wrists, and the hands, noticing any tingling, warmth, coolness, itching, aching, ease, tightness, sensations of clothing against skin—or perhaps the absence of feeling.

Letting your awareness shift from your hands up to the collarbones and down into the rib cage—to the breastbone, the breasts, and the muscles between the ribs—feeling the front of the chest, the sides of the rib cage, the upper back, the midback, and the shoulder blades, all expanding as the lungs take in air on the inhalation and release it on the exhalation. Becoming aware of the heart beating inside your chest, and the rhythmic movement of the diaphragm as it invites the breath to enter and leave the body moment by moment.

All the while experiencing whatever sensations are present in the part of the body that is the object of awareness in this moment, remembering that there is no one right way to feel during this Body Scan; there is just what you are feeling right now. There is no need to change anything, even no need to relax. Just being aware is enough.

Now shifting attention down to the lower back. If tightness or tension is present, see if it softens as you direct the breath into the lower back on an inhalation and out on an exhalation. Does the tension ease a bit as you breathe out from your lower back? It may, or it may not; just observe with the curiosity of beginner's mind, being with any sensations that may be present in this very moment. And when you are ready, moving your awareness around to the abdomen, taking some time to fully acknowledge the presence of your baby growing within, exploring any sensations you may be experiencing in your belly. Notice any thoughts or emotions that may arise. If you are practicing the Body Scan and are not pregnant, explore any sensations you may be experiencing in your own belly as well as any thoughts or feelings that may arise in relation to the baby growing within your partner's body.

Now directing your awareness to the pelvic region—to the lower abdomen, the pubic bone, outward to the hips, and to the hip joints where the thighbones meet the pelvis. Letting your awareness shift around to the sacrum, becoming aware of the muscles of the buttocks, the anal region, the genitals, and the creases of the groin, pausing to devote some moments of attention to the pelvis—this remarkably flexible, expandable structure through which a baby can pass down and through and out in the process of being born.

Continuing to shift your awareness downward into the thighs—the fronts of the thighs, the sides and backs of the thighs, the soft inner thighs—then down to and around the knees, the calf muscles, the shins, and all the little bones that make up the ankles, and the tops of the feet, the heels, the soles of the feet, and the toes. Taking some time to explore all the sensations in your feet.

Now moving your awareness up from the feet through the body to your head, expanding your awareness to include a sense of the body as a whole, just as it is in this moment. And if you are pregnant, taking a few moments to appreciate that your body is cradling and nourishing a small new being within it. Allowing your attention to dwell for a few moments in a place of wholeness, of silence, of stillness, and perhaps of peace.

Now, returning your attention once again to the breath, following the arc of feeling the breath move upward to the head on the inhalation and downward through the whole body to the feet on the exhalation, in a gentle, rocking, full-body experience of breathing.

And when you are ready, return your awareness to the belly, to the rising of the belly on the inhalation and the falling of the belly on the exhalation, once again becoming aware of the baby within if you are pregnant. After a few breaths, and perhaps after offering some appreciation to yourself for taking this time to practice, begin to wiggle your fingers and toes, gently moving, stretching, and opening your eyes if they have been closed. Taking your time, rolling onto your side if you are on your back, and, using your arms, push yourself up to a sitting position.

THE BODY SCAN: CHALLENGES AND OPPORTUNITIES

The Body Scan can be both a challenging and extremely rewarding meditation. The main instruction for the Body Scan is to *feel into* or *fully experience the sensations in the body,* wherever you are focusing your attention, just as you did with the breath during your first Awareness of Breathing meditation. The instruction is not asking you to *think* about your breath or your mouth, your lungs or your heart, your hands or your feet. Nor is the instruction to visualize them in your mind's eye. The instruction is to *feel* them.

Falling Asleep

Falling asleep while practicing the Body Scan is common, especially in the beginning. While you may enjoy taking a lovely nap during the Body Scan, the practice of mindfulness is about *"falling awake,"* not falling asleep. If you experience sleepiness during the Body Scan, there are several ways to work with it. You might experiment with keeping your eyes open during the practice or sitting upright in a chair or lying on the floor rather than on a bed. You might even try practicing the Body Scan standing up! We tend to get sleepy if we are warm, so dressing lightly and making sure the temperature of the room is neutral or slightly cool are other things to consider if you consistently fall asleep while practicing. Also consider the time of day you have chosen to practice. If you are practicing in the evening, perhaps morning would be a better choice, when the mind is usually fresh and alert.

One question to ask yourself if you are continually falling asleep during the Body Scan is this: Are you getting enough sleep? The Body Scan may be helping you become aware of just how tired you actually are. If you suspect you are sleep deprived, as so many of us are these days, the wisest and kindest strategy may be to just accept your fatigue and go to sleep. Really enjoy your nap. Then, when you wake up, practice the Body Scan.

It is a significant act of self-care to assess the choices you are making in your life with regard to sleep. Research tells us that pregnant women who sleep six hours or less each night or who have severely disrupted sleep in late pregnancy have significantly longer labors and are more likely to have cesarean deliveries than women who sleep more and have less disrupted sleep before labor.[1] Not getting enough sleep definitely increases feelings of stress in daily life and is less than optimal for our general health and wellbeing.

The good news here is that in addition to being a body-awareness practice, the Body Scan can also be used as a tool for falling asleep. Pregnant women often report using it to fall back to sleep at night after getting up to pee. Some use it in labor, as you'll read about in the pain practices chapter, and new parents frequently report how grateful they are for the Body Scan during the sleep-challenged months after the baby is born—using it to rest during the day if they can't nap or to fall back asleep at night after nursing or comforting a crying baby.

Although it's fine to use the Body Scan to help you fall asleep, when you are first learning the Body Scan remember that the intention behind the practice is to learn a skill for being more awake and present in your life. Being clear about your *intention* when you practice is what it's all about; it sets the stage for the skillful use of the Body Scan.

A Moment of Mindfulness, Again and Again

The mind has a tendency to wander during the Body Scan, just as it does when we practice Awareness of Breathing or any other form of meditation. Remember, each time we become aware that the mind has wandered during the Body Scan, we are experiencing *a moment of mindfulness*, of waking up in the present moment to where our attention is. This is the moment we talked about in the last chapter, the moment when we can exercise *choice* about where we want to put our attention and how we want to use our mind. As pioneering psychologist William James put it, "My experience is what I agree to attend to. Only those items I notice shape my mind."

So when you're practicing the Body Scan and you notice the mind wandering, kindly and gently choose to bring your attention back to the sensations in the body you were attending to. This moment of choosing is as much a part of the practice as sustaining the attention on the primary object, be it the breath or other body sensations. In fact, this *is* the practice.

The Body Scan and Relaxation

What we are practicing in the Body Scan is a way to cultivate awareness through the mind's ability to concentrate, stabilize, and focus attention, using the sensations in the body in the present moment, *being with* our experience, whatever it might be. Though relaxation often occurs during the Body Scan, this relaxation is the result of a calm and focused mind. The Body Scan is not to be confused with the progressive relaxation exercises that are sometimes taught in childbirth classes. While we are practicing the Body Scan, it is important to remember that we are not trying to *do anything:* we're not even trying to relax. In the spirit of non-striving, we are not trying be anywhere other than where we are right now, experiencing what is.

The Breath and the Body Scan

Of course while you're practicing the Body Scan, you are still breathing. However, unless the instruction is to specifically focus on the sensations of the breath, let the breath recede into the background of your awareness, allowing the sensations you are attending to in other parts of the body move into the foreground. That said, some people find it useful to use the breath in various ways when practicing the Body Scan. Two of these ways are "breathing into" and "letting go."

Breathing Into: Experiment with breathing directly into whatever part of the body you are paying attention to on the inhalation and breathing out from it on the exhalation. It may help to imagine the breath traveling from the nose into the lungs and then all the way into whatever part of the body you choose and then back from that area into the lungs and out through the nose. This can be a particularly helpful way to work with pain or tension in the body during the Body Scan. Some women use the breath this way to work with pain during labor and find it quite effective.

Letting Go: Some people find it helpful to breathe in with awareness to a particular part of the body and then, on the out-breath, to shift the attention to the next area of the body. Coordinating attention and the breath in this way can help bring increased awareness to the process of letting go in the moment. For example, if you're paying attention to the lower back, see if you can intentionally breathe in with awareness to the lower back, and then intentionally let go of the lower back on the out-breath as you shift your attention to the abdominal area. Experiment with this approach. It may come in handy when you are in labor.

Painful or Unpleasant Sensations During the Body Scan

While we can and often do touch moments of deep relaxation and peace while practicing the Body Scan, sometimes pain or discomfort arises. Though it is completely natural not to want pain, experiencing it during the Body Scan offers us an opportunity to *increase our capacity to be with discomfort in the body* when it arises. This is obviously good preparation for the intense sensations of childbirth.

If discomfort arises during your Body Scan practice, there are many ways to work with it. If the discomfort is manageable, as it often is, you might practice bringing awareness directly into the sensation. With an attitude of open curiosity, shine the light of awareness on the unpleasant sensations, discovering and exploring the sensations that are actually present for you. Most often when we bring focused awareness directly into sensations, we find that they are not fixed or single entities but are in fact a composite of many different sensations, sensations that are continually changing, moment by moment. This is certainly true of labor contractions.

When practicing with discomfort during the Body Scan, see if you can experiment with using the breath as described earlier: breathing into, or letting go. Perhaps you will find one of these practices helpful enough to allow you to just stay and work with them. However, if your discomfort or pain becomes too intense, the wisest course may be to move your body a bit so that the pain lessens or stops. Only you will know what is most skillful for you in any particular moment. You might ask yourself, "Can I breathe with this sensation for just this breath? And then just this breath? And then this one?" Because in labor that's all you will be called upon to do (or, more accurately, not do): breathe and be with the intense sensations of the birthing process as they move through your mind-body, one breath at a time, one moment at a time.

If you do decide to move during the Body Scan in an attempt to lessen your discomfort, see if you can be aware of your *intention* to move before you move. Then move slowly and mindfully, carefully noticing if or how the unpleasant sensations change. In this way you are *responding* to discomfort or pain with mindful awareness rather than *reacting* automatically to it out of fear and distress, even when those emotions are present. In practicing the Body Scan, we are not repressing pain or discomfort or pretending it isn't there if it is. Rather, we are finding a way to have a different relationship to it. Holding our pain, our discomfort, our distress with kindness, in mindful awareness, we are learning to be with what is. And that makes all the difference.

The Beauty of an Itch

Pain is certainly not the only unpleasant sensation we may encounter during the Body Scan. Itching is another. Sometimes just *thinking* about itching sensations can cause them to arise. In this moment, as you read these words, is there any place on your body—your face or your hand or your arm or your neck—that itches? If so, can you experiment with bringing your attention to the sensation right now, breathing with it, and just letting it be?

Because it's difficult to find sensations that are like labor contractions—distinctly unpleasant feelings in the body that arise spontaneously, reach a peak, and pass like a wave—a normal itching sensation is a fabulous teacher in preparing for labor and delivery. If you pay very careful attention to an itch, you will notice that it arises unbidden, seemingly out of nowhere, gradually increases in intensity, and reaches a peak or crescendo. This last stage is when most of us scratch. There is nothing wrong with this; we've been reacting to itching sensations automatically for most of our lives.

However, when we're practicing mindfulness as training for labor, for being with things as they are even if they are unpleasant or painful, we have another option. In the stillness and quiet of practice we can just notice the presence of an itch and breathe with the sensation, as best we can, without reacting, without scratching or rubbing the itch. If we can do this, we might discover something extremely interesting—something that most people don't know. If we can hang in there and just breathe with itching sensations when they arise and just keep breathing with them as they increase in intensity, without scratching, the *itching sensations will go away, all on their own.* Just like a labor contraction, an itch arises spontaneously, reaches a peak, and then subsides. Not scratching an itch during meditation is great practice for the contractions of childbirth.

As you will learn in Chapter 7, "Mindfulness Practices for Being with Pain," there are many options for using mindfulness for working with the intense sensations of childbirth. Depending on your intentions and the circumstances surrounding your labor, mindfulness practice and a supportive birthing environment may be all you need. Or perhaps at some point you may want to respond to the sensations of labor by making a choice to use pain medication or an epidural. Only you will know in the moment what is a wise decision for you and your baby. Living with awareness is often called "the middle path," and being able to be present in the midst of an intense and challenging experience that includes physical pain is a quality to be valued and cultivated.

And so we practice.

The Dynamic Duo
Pain and Fear

PART ONE: PAIN

To diminish the suffering of pain, we need to make a crucial distinction between the pain of pain and the pain we create by our thoughts about the pain. Fear, anger, guilt, loneliness, and helplessness are all mental and emotional responses that can intensify pain.
—the Dalai Lama

IT'S 5:30 P.M., and I'm driving west over the Bay Bridge to the Osher Center for Integrative Medicine at the University of California, San Francisco, on my way to teach the third class, a pivotal one in the MBCP course. I'm particularly happy because this is perhaps my favorite class. The expectant parents have been practicing the Body Scan at home this past week, and I suspect that at least some of them have begun to wonder exactly how mindfulness practice is going to help them during childbirth. I know from past experience that by the time they leave class tonight there will be a significant shift in their perception of childbirth pain and that they will clearly understand how critical mindfulness skills are for maintaining the normal physiology of labor.

Tonight we will connect the dots.

CHILDBIRTH EDUCATION 101

When we strip away all the anticipation and fear of childbirth, we can see that the *mechanics* of labor and delivery are actually quite straightforward. In the third class I like to give a brief overview of how the process of childbirth typically unfolds before we take a look at it from a mind-body perspective.

I caution participants tonight to be careful about how they take in this information, humbly requesting that they not accept anything I say about childbirth (or anything else for that matter) as gospel, for the truth about mindfulness practice and birthing will come from their own experience as they live it. I also caution them to not let what I say become an expectation of what will happen for them, to which they may become attached. The truth is that I have no idea what their birth experience will be like—and neither do they. As the saying goes, "Expectations are suffering under construction."

Every woman's labor and birth is unique, and there is tremendous variation in the normal process. However, there are some universal features of the process that are undoubtedly helpful to know about. Since 85 to 90 percent of births fall in the normal range, for now we'll turn our attention to them—and explore how the *inner skills* you learn in mindfulness practice can help facilitate the normal physiologic process. Later, in Chapter 16, "Causes and Conditions: Navigating What Is," we'll take a look at some of the external factors—such as the person you have chosen as your healthcare provider, the place you intend to give birth, the other people who may be present (or absent), and the use of technology—that can also deeply affect the normal physiology of childbirth.

Normal Childbirth and Horticultural Time,
or It Takes as Long as It Takes

For all the scientific research on pregnancy and childbirth, it is still not known exactly what triggers the normal labor process to begin for a particular woman, and you can't know when your labor will begin either. (Even the timing of a scheduled induction or cesarean birth can get changed if your healthcare provider or the Labor and Delivery unit suddenly becomes too busy.) We do know the timing of labor has something to do with your baby, something to do with your placenta, something to do with the readiness of your body, and maybe even something to do with the barometric pressure on a particular day, but more than that is yet to be known. Put most simply, when conditions align for you and your baby's particular bodies, labor will begin.

Typically, pregnant women are given a due date based on their last menstrual period (if they know it) and perhaps some information from an ultrasound report. If you are reading this and you're pregnant, you almost certainly have a due date already. While this can be helpful, it's also important to know that a due date is a guesstimate; in reality, there is a five-week window of time, between thirty-seven and forty-two weeks, when it is totally normal for your baby to be born.

It can be a bit unsettling to realize that the certainty of your due date is an illusion, so during the very first meeting of the MBCP class I encourage couples to begin their mindfulness practice by becoming a bit more tentative about their due date, perhaps substituting for it by saying, "We're due sometime at the end of March" or "maybe around mid-April." This is a practice in itself, a way of beginning to live in don't-know mind, of discovering something about the nature of attachment, of getting a bit more comfortable living in the truth of uncertainty about the future.

Looking deeply at due dates is actually an opportunity to discover that pregnancy and childbirth take place in a kind of time that most of us, unless we tend a garden, are unfamiliar with: the realm of Horticultural Time. Horticultural Time is measured in a slower arc than we are accustomed to, a time span that is in harmony with the biology of living things: plants and their seasons, and humans in their life cycles of birth, growth, aging, and death. Horticultural Time is conditional time; whether or not we harvest a bountiful crop of tomatoes from our garden or apples from our apple tree depends on a multitude of causes and conditions—with many of them, as any farmer can tell you, well beyond our control.

Unfamiliar, and perhaps somewhat uncomfortable, with Horticultural Time, we try to put pregnancy, childbirth, and the growth and development of our children into the time frame we are most familiar with: Industrial Time. Industrial Time is based on the clock, with its exact calculations of seconds, minutes, and hours. Living on clock time these days often means living in the fast lane, which, while it may seem invigorating for a short period, usually feels pretty stressful.

The very existence of your due date can interfere with seeing the processes of pregnancy and birthing as being in harmony with Horticultural Time because you may come to see your due date in the same way you view a meeting at work, a scheduled airline flight, or an appointment for a haircut. Because Industrial Time fosters the illusion of certainty—after all, people do arrive at an appointed time for a meeting, airplanes do arrive on schedule more often than not, and you do usually show up for your haircut on time—we may create stress for ourselves by imposing the standards of Industrial Time on this biological process occurring in our body. Due dates, while undoubtedly helpful, can also encourage you and others around you to worry about the future—when the birth will actually happen, how many hours your labor will take, and so on.

While due dates are not bad, and we certainly don't want to throw away all that we have learned by looking at childbirth through the lens of Industrial Time, it can be helpful to remember that your body and your baby's body are living and growing in Horticultural Time. (In fact, as biological beings, we are *always* living in Horticultural Time, whether our mind knows it or not.) When our body begs us to slow down during pregnancy, when we realize we cannot predict the exact date of our birthing, when after birth our baby needs us to be in harmony with his or her rhythms of hunger and sleep and growth and change, we are being asked to become more intimate and in tune with Horticultural Time.

The Labor Process

EARLY LABOR

Due dates aside, we know that the labor process typically begins with mild, irregular, menstrual-like cramping that comes and goes about every ten to twenty minutes. We call this stage, which could take anywhere from several hours to a day or more, early labor. During early labor the cervix—the opening to the uterus—is softening, thinning, shortening, and beginning to open. Over time the cramping sensations in this stage become more frequent, regular, stronger, and of longer duration. Once this happens, they become what we call labor contractions.

Sometimes—perhaps 10 percent of the time—these irregular, menstrual-like cramping sensations are preceded by your bag of water, or amniotic sac, breaking. Healthcare providers and institutions take a variety of approaches to labor beginning this way, depending on their philosophy, which is expressed in protocols—everything from inducing labor within six to eight hours after the water breaks to waiting for as long as two days for labor to begin on its own. If your preference is to have a labor with minimal interventions, it's a good idea to have a conversation with your healthcare provider about how this situation is usually handled and what your options might be, if any. (In Chapter 16, "Causes and Conditions: Navigating What Is," you will learn a way to bring mindfulness into this conversation.)

FIRST STAGE OF LABOR

When your contractions are about four to five minutes apart, you are considered to be in the first stage of labor. With each contraction, the powerful muscle fibers of the uterus contract, pulling the cervix open just a bit more each time. From inside the uterus, your baby's head presses down on the cervix, which also helps it to open. Each contraction urges your baby downward through the bones of your pelvis. As time passes the contractions continue, getting stronger, more intense, and closer together.

TRANSITION

At a certain point your contractions are as intense and as close together as they are going to get. This phase of labor is called transition because you are transitioning from the first stage of labor, when the cervix is opening, to the second stage of labor, when you feel the urge to bear down and push your baby out. Typically, if your bag of water hasn't broken before now, it breaks during this time. During this transition, labor is often experienced as being at its most intense. This phase usually doesn't last very long—perhaps an hour or so.

Most often, by the time your cervix is completely open (it's usually called "complete dilation" or "ten centimeters"), your baby has moved down through the bones of your pelvis and is low enough so that his or her head begins to put pressure on stretch receptor nerves deep inside your vagina and around your rectal area. This pressure, which can build gradually or appear all at once, becomes quite powerful, creating in you an involuntary urge to bear down, usually several times with each contraction. Pressure and the urge to bear down are welcome signs that your baby is closer to being born.

SECOND STAGE OF LABOR

You know you're in the second stage of labor because the primary sensations are very different from what you've felt up to now. Many women describe these sensations as "wanting to poop." In fact, mindful pooping practice is a great way to prepare for this stage of labor, as you will learn in the next chapter.

The second stage, or the pushing phase, can last anywhere from a few pushes to several hours, depending on lots of variables, such as the size and position of your baby's head, the internal diameters of your pelvis, the force generated by your uterine muscle, the position or positions you are using during this stage, whether you have given birth before, and the level of energy you are able to bring to the process. Pushing with each contraction and resting when it is over, you engage in a rhythm of work and rest, work and rest. With each push, the muscles and tissues of your vagina and genital area stretch, expand, and then expand even more. With each contraction and each push, your baby's head descends just a bit; when you rest between pushes, your baby's head slides back into your vagina just a bit. And so it goes in the second stage, a lot of forward movement and a little bit back until much—but not all—of your baby's head is visible with your bearing down efforts.

In the last ten minutes or so before birth, there are usually some fairly intense sensations of burning as you push and your baby's head stretches the muscles and tissues around your vagina until the moment arrives when your baby's head does not slide back anymore. Your stretched and expanded vaginal tissues now encircle your baby's head like a crown, which is why this time is called "crowning." You and your baby are balanced on the threshold of birth.

Usually with the very next push your baby's head eases out. The crown of your baby's head appears first. Then the forehead. Then come the eyebrows, the closed eyes, the tiny ears, nose, mouth, and chin, leading to the magical, awe-inspiring moment when your baby's head and face become visible for the first time.

For you, the birthing woman, the arrival of your baby's head is usually accompanied by a profound bodily sense of relief and release. Though some women find it helpful to watch the birth of their baby's head in a mirror, many prefer to concentrate their full attention inward on the intense sensations they are experiencing and on the words of the midwife or doctor guiding them. Some women give voice to the intense sensations at the moment of birth with a powerful birth cry. Others are quiet and intensely focused, perhaps breathing deeply or gently blowing as their baby's head emerges. There is no one right way. There is only each woman's way of helping her baby through her body and out into the world.

Once your baby's head has emerged, there is still more birthing to be done. Usually after some moments of rest and one more contraction, the shoulders are born, after which the rest of your baby's body eases out into waiting hands—your partner's, the midwife's, the doctor's, or even your own. And within moments (or sometimes more) after the baby's torso is out of your body, another remarkable event occurs: your baby takes his or her first breath. If all is well, as it usually is, your baby can be placed skin-to-skin on your belly or into your arms—one of life's truly unforgettable moments.

THIRD STAGE OF LABOR

The third stage of labor usually comes within five to fifteen minutes after your baby's birth. With a gush of blood, one last strong contraction, or possibly two, and a sustained bearing down, the warm, soft placenta is born.

A THREE-MINUTE BREATHING SPACE

You've just finished reading one of a vast number of descriptions of the normal physiologic process of giving birth. Reading about it and imagining it happening to you and your baby may have stimulated all sorts of thoughts and feelings. Giving birth is not an academic exercise; it is an embodied experience that you too will pass through, in one way or another. Why not take a moment, right now, to practice the Three-Minute Breathing Space, which you learned in Chapter 4? Observe your thoughts. Notice your emotions. Feel the sensations in your body. Come to the breath. Perhaps you will discover something about yourself and how you are relating to the process of giving birth right now.

CHILDBIRTH CAN BE SIMPLE—
AND ALMOST ALWAYS PAINFUL

In the MBCP class it takes me about seven and a half minutes to explain the process of childbirth much as I did above. When I finish, there is often surprised laughter. It's not unusual for someone to say, "You make it sound so simple!"

Well, on one level, childbirth *is* simple—or at least it can be. So why then do we need childbirth education classes? What exactly do we need to get educated about before giving birth? Usually, when I ask a class these questions, there is silence. After a few moments of reflection, someone says something like, "Well, yes, it sounds pretty simple. But it also sounds like it hurts."

Exactly! Much like meditation practice, childbirth can be simple but not easy. In the case of childbirth, the process almost always involves some fairly intense physical sensations, which the vast majority of women call pain. This pain is one of the major factors that make childbirth not so easy. Now this is truly a wonderful place for us to begin, for by acknowledging that most women experience childbirth as painful, we can begin to work with things as they are.

There are a number of attitudes we can take toward the intense bodily sensations of childbirth. In my experience women approaching labor fall somewhere along a continuum. At one end are those whose approach to childbirth pain is "I don't want to feel any pain at all. Just give me whatever drugs you've got, and I'll be happy. I just want my baby, and the sooner the better." At the opposite end of the continuum are women whose attitude goes something like, "This is not a medical event but a natural process, and I want to fully experience it, even if it hurts. I don't want any pain medications whatsoever. In fact, I'm more afraid of the problems the drugs might cause me and my baby than I am of the pain."

Many women fall somewhere between. Wary of technology and medication, they would prefer to have a "natural childbirth," feeling that it is best for themselves and their baby, but they have very real doubts about whether they can handle the process. This is particularly true for women who have never given birth before.

Some women are clear at the outset that they intend to use an epidural, the most common form of pain management for childbirth in industrialized countries today. With an epidural, the body is numbed from below the breasts all the way down to the toes. (For more about epidurals, including their benefits and risks, see Chapter 16.) However, even if you intend to use an epidural, you will still have some amount of physical sensation during childbirth. During early labor you will experience pain before you get to the hospital. And when you do get to the hospital, you can't be sure what the situation will be. The anesthesiologist may be so busy that you'll have to wait for your epidural. Or perhaps the epidural won't be completely effective. Or your labor may go so quickly that you'll arrive at the hospital ready to give birth and there won't be time for an epidural. Even if you elect to have a scheduled cesarean birth, you will still have pain following the surgery. The causes and conditions specific to your body and to your baby's body in the moments of your labor—and all the other factors that can influence your particular birth experience—are ultimately uncertain, unknown, and unknowable, so it just makes good sense to learn some skills for handling physical pain before you give birth.

Of course, if your preference is to have minimal pain medication for childbirth, or none at all, then it certainly is wise to learn some skills for engaging the mind to work with pain. A preference *not* to have an epidural or pain medication means that, in fact, your preference *is* to experience the intense sensations of childbirth, or pain. Learning how to work with these intense sensations, to actually embrace childbirth pain, is no small matter, and mindfulness practice helps us acquire the skill to do exactly that.

Regardless of your current plans for how you will manage the pain of childbirth—with an epidural or other medications or with your partner's support, the help of a doula, a birthing tub or warm shower, or something else—you have a body that will have sensations, you have a mind that will have thoughts, and you will feel many emotions during the experience of giving birth. With mindfulness practice you can prepare for all the dimensions of giving birth, however your particular childbirth experience unfolds.

WHAT *IS* PAIN?

Having finished Childbirth Education 101, the general description of the labor process, we can now begin to explore one of the most fundamental questions about childbirth.

"Since one of the main challenges of childbirth is what we usually call pain, let's ask the question, 'What exactly *is* pain?' We know pain when we experience it. We know we don't *like* pain. And we know we don't *want* pain. But most of us, unless we are healthcare providers or have had a serious injury or illness, might have never stopped to ask ourselves, 'What *exactly is* pain?' "

When I ask this question, the class falls silent. After some dialogue we collectively arrive at a definition: pain is a strong sensation from somewhere in the body that occurs when specific nerve endings have been stimulated.

"And why do we have these painful sensations in the body?" I ask.

Usually someone replies, "So we know that something's wrong."

"Okay. So we could say that pain is trying to tell us something. The body can't talk to us in words, so it communicates through sensations, right?" Heads nod in agreement. "We could really say that pain is information. It's information being sent from the body to . . . where?" I ask.

"To the brain" is a typical response.

"Exactly. So we could say that *pain is information from the body to the brain.*

"And why do we need this information?" Silence . . . until someone finally says, "Because pain is telling us that something bad is happening."

"Yes. This is often true. So let's see how this sounds: *"Pain is information from the body to the mind that tells us to pay attention.* Will that work?"

More agreement. "Pain alerts us that something important is happening in our body. Again, we know we don't like pain. And when we have pain we wish we didn't, but in fact our ability to feel pain is a very *good* thing. People who are born without the ability to feel pain are in big trouble. They can seriously injure themselves and not even know it. The bottom line is we *need* pain. Pain can be lifesaving."

I encourage the class to take a closer look at exactly what pain in the body is communicating. "Throughout our lives, at least for most of us," I say, "pain in our body has basically meant one of two things. It has either been a signal that we are injured or a signal that we are ill. If we sprain an ankle, pain lets us know that we need to stop walking on it so we don't create more injury. If we have a headache and aching joints from a fever, these painful sensations are the body's way of telling us we need to rest so we can heal or that we need to take some medicine or seek medical advice. Pain in the body helps us take care of ourselves."

Okay, so far so good. The class agrees that pain is information from the body to the mind telling us to pay attention because an injury or an illness is present. "So now the question becomes, what about the pain of childbirth? Does the pain of childbirth signal an injury?" Several people shake their heads. "And does the pain of childbirth signal an illness?" Again, the consensus is no.

"So if the pain of childbirth is not a signal of injury or illness, what is it? How might we think about childbirth pain?"

TRANSFORMATIONAL PAIN, OR
EVERYTHING THAT HURTS IS NOT HARMFUL

To my way of thinking, we need a completely different category for the pain of childbirth, so I offer the concept of *transformational pain*. Transformational pain is *normal pain*. It is the pain of living in a mortal body, a body that exists in Horticultural Time, a body that is birthed, grows, at times experiences illness, the eventual pains of aging, and ultimately death. Physical pain is just part of the business of being alive. (Emotional pain is too, and we'll get to that in Part 2 of this chapter.) When we give birth, change is taking place very rapidly—anywhere from a few hours to a day or more—and when a body changes so quickly, we experience *intense transformational pain*.

You may be experiencing some milder forms of transformational pain right now, during your pregnancy. Swollen feet, heartburn, and an aching back all fit into that category. Sometimes it's not easy living inside a pregnant body, but you can use these pains and discomforts as opportunities to practice mindfulness and learn how to work with transformational pain.

Your baby will also experience transformational pain. When? When she or he is teething. Do we like that our baby experiences pain? No. Do we wish we could take the pain away? Of course. Do we try to alleviate the pain as best we can, by comforting our baby or perhaps giving something cold to chew or suck on? Absolutely. But does that pain signal that anything is *wrong*? Absolutely not. Just as we don't have to worry about teething pain, we needn't be concerned about childbirth pain, even though it certainly hurts. Nothing is wrong. Something in our body is profoundly changing, and as a result we experience normal transformational pain.

We don't ordinarily see our body as a continually changing entity, but in fact our body is changing all the time. We cycle through periods of hunger and satiety, hours of peak performance, and times of low energy—all day, every day. Our body's circadian rhythms are the work of an internalized twenty-four-hour biological clock that is keenly synchronized with the cycles of day and night, regulating a wide range of our biological processes, including hormones, body temperature, and sleep and wake cycles. We are also aging every day. The more mindful we become, the more aware we can be of this ever-present biological change. By observing the breath and watching the ebb and flow of sensations in our body as well as shifts in our thoughts and emotions, we become more and more aware that change is the only constant. Everything, from the body we are living in to the universe itself, is in constant, moment-to-moment transformation.

One of the gifts of pregnancy, childbirth, and becoming a parent is an opportunity to bring this particular universal truth front and center. Your body is transforming during pregnancy. It's transforming very rapidly during childbirth. Your baby will practically transform before your very eyes in the early days after birth and will continue to change day by day, month by month, and year by year. Your family is transforming. The world is transforming because a new human being is coming into it. Mindfulness practice helps us connect with the truth of transformational change and perhaps helps us to see childbirth in a new light: it certainly can be comforting to know that however long your labor lasts, it is not a permanent condition. Nothing is.

REACTING OR RESPONDING TO PAIN

Physical pain in human beings is actually a complex phenomenon, and in the MBCP classes we spend considerable time deconstructing it. Understanding the phenomenon we call pain and learning mindfulness skills to be with it are well worth your time and effort, for these are life skills that can help you not only work with childbirth pain but *any* pain you may experience in the future. This is true for partners as well.

When we look closely at pain, we see that it has three basic components: the sensory or *physical* component, which is how the pain actually feels in our body; the *affective* component, or the *emotions* we feel in relation to those sensations; and the *cognitive* component, or the *thoughts* that go through our mind about the pain. I can see all these components at work, for example, when I stub my toe. First I feel the sensory component of pain—a sharp sensation that gradually becomes a throbbing or dull ache. I am hardwired for this to happen: nerve cells in my toe send messages up to my brain. However, how I *relate* to those pain signals from my body, the thoughts and emotions I have in relation to the sensations, is *not* a matter of hardwiring; it's subject to how my mind *perceives* the sensations. And for this, mindfulness training is key.

Usually we relate to intense sensations in our body by simply reacting to them. When I stub my toe and feel the physical pain, my mind quickly floods with all sorts of reactive thoughts and emotions, the dominant one usually being fear. In reaction to the pain, my mind races into the future, filling itself with worry. ("Oh my God, is my toe broken?" "Oh, no, I have to get to that meeting at work today!") *Fear is always about the future, even if it's only about the next moment.* While there's nothing I can do about the pain signals being sent from the nerves in my toe to my brain, with mindfulness practice there is a lot I can do about how I perceive it—how I handle the thoughts and emotions that spring up in relation to that pain.

If I use mindfulness practice when I stub my toe, I feel the sensations and immediately come to the breath. Anchored in the breath and the present moment, I can *observe with awareness* the physical sensations in my toe as they move and change. I can also observe the thoughts and feelings that arise in relation to the sensations. In bringing mindful awareness to the pain, I have in that very moment stepped out of *reacting,* and instead found a way of *responding* to the unpleasant sensations in my toe.

Mindfulness practice gives us options for relating to the physical sensations we call pain. In the very observation of the pain, a tiny window of freedom has opened up in which you have the ability to *choose* how you will relate to the painful sensations in that moment—and in the next, and the next after that. With mindfulness you have brought an entirely new element into the pain-of-the-stubbed-toe equation, and because of that, you have *changed your relationship* to the sensation in your toe. And in doing so, you *actually experience the pain differently.* You still feel pain, but you are liberated from the reactivity of the mind.

This is how mindfulness practice can provide you with a different option in relationship to the pain of childbirth—or for that matter, any other pain in your life, physical or emotional. Breathing with the pain, bringing awareness to the pain, being with the pain, you are able to just be with things as they are.

It's important to realize that words are powerful and that when we call something "painful" we are bringing all our thoughts and ideas about pain, all our memories of it, and all our fearful associations, emotions, and projections about pain right into the present moment. In relation to childbirth, most all of us carry a story or idea about its pain, whether from tales told by family, friends, or the media or from our own previous experience. (Extraordinary midwife-activist Ina May Gaskin understood this years ago when she renamed labor contractions "rushes" in an attempt to separate childbirth pain from the pain of injury or illness.) As powerful as words are, they are still abstractions; they are not the thing itself. When we approach the pain of labor mindfully, we use mindful awareness to let go of all conceptions and stories created by the thinking mind (our own stories and those of others) and just experience the sensations as they are. In this way we experience what is real or true for us in the present moment.

This shift in perception is just one of the many important things we learn when we practice mindfulness: *that it is possible to uncouple the sensory component of pain from the emotional and cognitive components.* Our reaction to pain may be one of resistance—fighting it, contracting around or against it—basically bringing a fearful mind-set of "no" to the experience in the moment. Caught in our reactions to pain, we suffer.

Mindfulness practice offers us another way of approaching our childbirth experience and, for that matter, any challenging experience in life. Through mindfulness practice we can learn to hold *whatever* we are experiencing in the present moment in a space of open acceptance to things as they are, even if those things are unpleasant—and, yes, even painful. In that space of open acceptance, we find freedom, the freedom from endlessly struggling to escape from the unpleasant or endlessly grasping for what is pleasant. Right in the moment we find we have a choice, a choice not about whether to experience pain, but about *our relationship* to that pain or how we interpret it. *This is the difference between pain and suffering.* It is sometimes said about life that pain is inevitable, but suffering is optional. This can certainly be true about childbirth.

It's important to be clear here. Practicing mindfulness does not make the pain of labor go away. That's neither the intention nor the goal. Rather, *mindfulness helps us find an accepting, non-reactive relationship* to the intense physical sensations we are having in the present moment, a relationship we might not have known was possible.

THE PHYSICAL SENSATIONS OF CHILDBIRTH

In continuing to untangle thoughts and emotions from the physical sensations of childbirth, I ask expectant parents to recall a time when they were in pain and to offer some words to describe it. At first, they usually say something like "agony," or "terrible." I gently point out that these words describe the emotional reactions to pain. What we are looking to do now is to identify or name the *physical sensations,* the sensory component of pain—what pain actually *feels* like.

As they call out the words, I write them on a big whiteboard.

"Sharp," someone calls out.

"Throbbing," another says.

"Dull."

"Numbing."

"Cramping."

"Burning."

"Prickly."

"Stretching."

"Aching."

"Pulsing."

"Tearing."

"Stabbing."

"Tightness."

"Piercing."

"Stinging."

"Grinding."

Before long the whiteboard is covered with words that describe physical pain.

"Now," I ask, "how many of these sensations will you experience during childbirth? Remember, I'm talking about normal labor, the sensations of your uterus contracting and the baby actually coming through and out of your body, not the pain of a momentary leg cramp or the sharp sensation of a needle if someone draws blood from your arm or starts an IV."

"All of them!" many call out.

"Well, that's what most people think. But, no, that's not true," I reply. "You will most likely *not* feel all these sensations in childbirth. Though no one can say for sure what the sensations will feel like for you, you will most likely not feel sensations that are sharp, throbbing, dull, numb, prickly, stabbing, or pulsing. Or sensations that are piercing, stinging, or grinding." As I say each of these words, I erase them from the board.

When I come to "tearing" and "burning," I pause. "Now let's look at burning and tearing. During childbirth, some tissue inside or around your vagina could tear as the baby comes through. To prevent this, your midwife or doctor will work with you so that the baby's head is delivered slowly, giving time for the vaginal tissues to stretch. But sometimes, despite their best efforts and yours, tearing happens. Tearing *feels* like burning, which you will experience whether you tear or not. So we can get rid of 'tearing' and just leave 'burning,'" I say, as I wipe "tearing" from the list.

"And how about cramping and aching? Which is more intense?"

"Cramping" is the unanimous reply.

"Good." I quickly erase aching from the board.

"Now what does that leave us?" I ask.

Cramping. Stretching. Tightness. Pressure. Burning.

Five simple words are all that's left of the long list the class first came up with. Seeing them provides instant relief. The possibility that childbirth pain might be manageable has arisen. With that, the fear level in the room has just gone down, and the confidence level has just gone up.

Now let's take a closer look at these five most common sensations of childbirth and review when they occur.

Cramping

Cramping sensations are part of early labor. You'll most likely experience these sensations in the lower abdomen, right above the pubic bone, where you feel menstrual cramps, if you've ever felt those. The cramping sensations of early labor are not very strong and usually come irregularly. Sometimes the cramping radiates around into your lower back. Some women don't experience the cramping sensations of early labor at all because their body just skips this stage. Remember, we just don't know. Early labor may be uncomfortable, but it can also be exciting; it means that the process that will bring your baby out of your body and into your arms has finally begun.

Stretching and Tightening

Stretching is the primary sensation of the first stage of labor; you feel these sensations because the cervix is *stretching* open. But make no mistake about it: this stretching has an intensity like none other. Simultaneously you feel sensations of *tightening;* when the cells of your uterus are contracting, your uterus gets very, very tight. This tightening is usually not experienced as painful. In labor, I can gently press my fingers on a woman's belly during a contraction, and while it may feel slightly bothersome to her, it doesn't cause pain.

To understand these stretching and tightening sensations, where they come from and what is happening, we need to understand a little bit more about the structure of the uterus. In the classroom I draw a uterus on the whiteboard and begin to describe it. When I've finished, we're all looking at an image that looks something like you see in Diagram A.

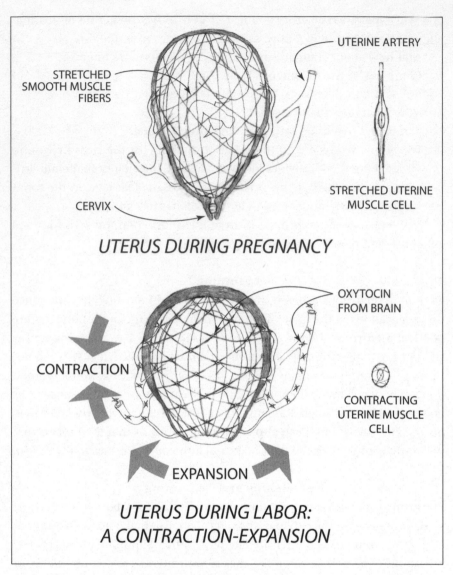

Diagram A: The Uterus During Pregnancy and Childbirth

While every system in your body is transformed by pregnancy, the change is most profound in your uterus. When you are not pregnant your uterus is actually quite small, measuring only three to four inches (around 9 cm) in length. Its walls are fairly thick, and it can hold only about 2 teaspoons (10 ml) of fluid or less. Once you become pregnant, your uterus gradually enlarges, becoming a thin-walled muscular organ that holds an average of 1.3 gallons (5 liters). If need be, it can hold as much as 5.28

gallons or 20 liters—remember, some women grow several babies at the same time, two or three or even more!

While your uterus is certainly getting bigger, the number of cells is exactly the same as it was before you were pregnant. Your uterus is becoming bigger because the muscle cells are stretching as the baby grows. What is also growing is a remarkably strong fibrous network of connective tissue around it; in one of the many wonders of the pregnant uterus, it actually becomes stronger as it gets thinner and bigger.

With each labor contraction, the muscle cells of your uterus tighten and shorten. When the contraction is over they release and lengthen again. Over time, as a result of the continual contracting and releasing during labor, the actual cells of your uterus change; they become shorter and thicker again. This stretches the cervix open, and that is what you experience in the first stage of labor—intense sensations of stretching, mostly in your lower pelvic region, right above your pubic bone. Your uterus knows that its work of lengthening its cells to hold your baby is finished. It's now time for your baby to be born, so it proceeds to do the work it knows how to do: tightening, contracting, and shortening its cells, stretching the cervix open, and releasing and sending forth your baby.

Pressure

Pressure is the fourth sensation of labor. It usually makes its appearance somewhere toward the end of the first stage of labor or at the beginning of the second stage. Remember, while your uterus has been tightening and your cervix has been stretching open with each contraction, your baby has been moving down on his or her journey through the bones of your pelvis. When your baby's head has moved down low enough through your pelvic bones, it stimulates *stretch receptors* in muscles deep inside your vagina and around your rectum, causing sensations of pressure. The result is an urge to push your baby out.

One reason transition, the time between the first stage and the second stage of labor, can be so challenging is sometimes you not only experience labor contractions at maximum frequency and duration, but you may also feel the sensations of pressure from the baby moving downward. All of these sensations coming at once can mean maximum intensity and maximum challenge—but it also means that there is a minimum amount of time until the next stage, second stage, begins. But whether the pressure and the urge to bear down arise gradually or suddenly, at some point you will experience pressure on a grand scale. How could it be otherwise? Your uterus is engaged in the process of releasing a baby who weighs somewhere between six and nine pounds, more or less. And so at this point you help the process along by enlisting some of your voluntary muscles. We're talking big-time pressure and big-time effort here.

Some women find great pleasure, even exhilaration, in working with their body to actively push their baby out. Others find that once they figure out how to push "into" the pain, it lessens considerably or even disappears altogether. Other women find the sensations of second stage even *more* challenging than the sensations of stretching and tightening of the first stage. Sometimes the pressure becomes so intense that fear arises. It may take the form of a fearful question: Can I really expand enough for the baby to come through? The vast majority of time the unequivocal answer to this question is *yes*. Your body and its capacity for giving birth are utterly remarkable. And from a mindfulness perspective, your task in labor is to use your inner skills to work with the powerful physical sensations as well as any thoughts, emotions, or mind states—especially fear—that may arise at any moment during the process.

Burning

Burning is one of the last of the sensations you will be working with in labor. As I mentioned earlier, burning sensations come from your baby's head stretching the muscles and tissues around your vagina so the baby's head and body can slowly ease out. These burning sensations are very intense and usually quite brief, typically lasting for ten minutes or so at the very end of labor. In birth time, that's about three contractions. You're almost done!

Lisa's description of her birth experience using mindfulness practice is a wonderful illustration of the power of staying in the moment. "I remember the sensations so well. I could feel the baby's head moving down through my pelvic bones. I could feel all these little pops. It was very intense, but it wasn't overwhelming. And I knew it wasn't going to be like this forever. So I just stayed with the sensations and took it one little push at a time. I could hear the nurses saying to me, 'Just think about your baby. Your baby is about to be born.' And I remember thinking to myself, 'I can't even think that far. All I can think about is this moment, this push.' And that really worked for me—not thinking about the next contraction or the next push. Just being in this moment was all I needed to do. And Olivia was born really easily. Perfectly healthy. It was all perfect in every way."

Remember that the body is guiding this process. You didn't have to *do* anything to grow your baby (except of course participate in getting sperm and egg together), and you don't have to *do* anything to make the uterus tighten and the cervix stretch. You also don't have to do anything to feel the pressure from the baby's head urging you to bear down or to feel the sensations of burning as your baby's head is being born. Your work is to *drop into mindful presence and just be with the sensations and any thoughts and emotions that arise.* Nothing needs to be different than it is.

Allowing, accepting, opening to, even welcoming this powerful physiological change as best you can, you embrace the process even if it is painful. Using the breath as an anchor, you can let the information from your body to your mind arise and pass, moment by moment. The uterus is opening, and with it the entire mind-body entity that you are is opening too. As best you can, you say yes to the sensations, yes to this change. You remind yourself that this is normal, transformational pain. All is well.

I remember Julia delightedly sharing the story of her labor. Julia had been committed to not using drugs during childbirth. "At one point in the labor, I think I was about eight centimeters dilated, I thought to myself, 'This can't be right. It's not supposed to hurt *this* much.' So I opened my eyes. The lights in the room were dim. Tim was sitting beside the bed holding my hand. My sister was taking a nap in a chair across the room. My mom was calmly sitting on the end of the bed, her hand gently holding my foot. A nurse stood at a table in the corner of the room writing some notes. The room was peaceful, and everyone looked relaxed. I thought to myself, 'Well, if they aren't freaking out, I guess this much pain is normal.' I closed my eyes again. When I felt another contraction beginning, I went back to work, focusing on my breath like I had learned to in our pain practice, observing the sensations of tightening and stretching rise in intensity, reach their peak, and slowly pass like a wave. When the time came for pushing, I experienced other sensations, like the pressure and the burning from the baby's head, but I just kept at it, one contraction at a time. I think Christopher was born about two hours later. It was far and away the most amazing experience of my life."

CONTRACTIONS, EXPANSIONS, OR BOTH?

During the labor process it can be helpful to have some reference points about your body and about your baby, such as how dilated your cervix is, how far your baby's head has descended through your pelvic bones, and what position your baby's head is in. To gather this information, someone—a midwife, doctor, or labor and delivery nurse—does a vaginal exam, which entails putting their index and middle fingers inside your vagina. To get as much information as possible, this exam is often done during a contraction.

Performing a vaginal exam on a laboring woman during a contraction, which of course as a midwife I have done many times, is quite an extraordinary experience because what I feel beneath my fingers during what we call a contraction is actually *an expansion*—an expansion of the cervix. By naming the sensations of labor as "contractions," we're really only telling half the story. Yes, the powerful muscle called the uterus is powerfully contracting, but *in those very same moments the cervix is expanding*. We could just as accurately say that what we are experiencing during labor are *expansions*.

How does it feel when you think of the sensations of labor as expansions rather than contractions? More spacious? More open? Easier? Spaciousness, openness, and ease are what you want in both the body and the mind as you move toward birthing your baby. Women often report a dramatic shift in their mind-set—and body-set—when they fully embrace the notion that during the intense sensations of labor a glorious expansion is taking place!

FINDING EASE AND PEACE IN THE BIRTH PROCESS

Now let's look at the labor process again, this time intentionally paying close attention to the moment-to-moment experience of labor, just as you intentionally pay attention to your moment-to-moment experience in meditation practice. If you apply your mindfulness practice to labor in this way, paying attention in the present moment without judgment, opening to and allowing the physical sensations of the contractions *and* expansions to come and go, you will make an amazing discovery: right in the midst of the process of childbirth there are profound moments of ease and peace.

Yes, you read that last sentence correctly. *Right in the midst of the process of childbirth there are profound moments of ease and peace.*

How is this possible?

In the third class, as part of the whiteboard presentation I mentioned, I draw a diagram to illustrate how this is so. The diagram looks like what you see in Diagram B.

The large wave pattern represents the contraction-expansions of the uterus and the cervix or transformational pain as it comes and goes during the first stage of labor. The smaller wave pattern represents the inhalations and exhalations of the breath, which you are using to anchor your attention in the present moment, giving your mind a place to rest in the here and now. During the first stage of labor, when the process is in full gear, a wave of contraction-expansion arises and passes about every five minutes. One wave lasts about sixty seconds. This means that if we measure from the beginning of one contraction-expansion to the beginning of the

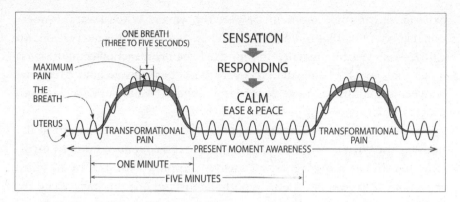

ONE BREATH
(THREE TO FIVE SECONDS)

SENSATION

RESPONDING

CALM
EASE & PEACE

MAXIMUM
PAIN

THE
BREATH

UTERUS

TRANSFORMATIONAL
PAIN

TRANSFORMATIONAL
PAIN

PRESENT MOMENT AWARENESS

ONE MINUTE

FIVE MINUTES

Diagram B: Contraction-Expansions with Mindfulness

next, *in one hour of the first stage of labor, there will be only about twelve minutes of intermittent transformational pain.* Can you handle that to get your baby born? Of course you can.

And there's more good news. Like an ocean wave, the sensations of a labor contraction-expansion begin, build in intensity moment by moment, come to a crest or peak, then break and begin to ebb. And just like an ocean wave, when the contraction-expansion disappears, it's gone forever, back into the vastness from which it came.

The crest of the wave is the point of maximum pain. And how long does this last? About three to five seconds. And how long is a breath? About three to five seconds. So again, let's do the math. In one hour of active labor, when the contraction-expansions that last about sixty seconds are approximately five minutes apart, *there are only about twelve breaths, or sixty seconds, of maximum pain.* That's sixty seconds in one hour. Definitely doable, don't you think? Especially when you know how to pay attention to the breath and let the process carry you, moment by moment.

And there's even more news. Remember that as labor progresses these sixty-second contraction-expansions get stronger and closer together. The closest they ever get is about two to three minutes apart. This happens during transition, the shortest and most intense time of labor. Now how long does transition last? Usually about an hour, more or less. So let's do the math again: during the most intense part of labor, when the contraction-expansions are coming about every two to three minutes and lasting approximately sixty seconds, *you will have only about twenty to thirty minutes of intermittent transformational pain.* Not bad for the most challenging time of labor.

Now here's a very important question. If the pain comes and goes in waves, builds to a crest before easing and disappearing, then what are you experiencing in those moments *between* the waves? When I ask this question, expectant parents often say, tentatively, "Rest?" or "Recovery?" or "No pain?" Well, yes, but actually, the time between contraction-expansions is better than rest. It's better than recovery. It's better than no pain. That time between the contraction-expansions is *pleasurable*. A time of deep ease and peace.

How is it possible to find ease, peace—and even pleasure—right in the midst of the birth process? Since long before the advent of modern medicine, nature has provided us with ways of coping with intense physical sensations. At these times our hypothalamus and our pituitary gland release endorphins, naturally occurring opiates, which you may have heard about in relation to "runner's high." Endorphins produce analgesic effects as well as feelings of wellbeing that counteract intense physical pain. During labor, endorphins go straight to the appropriate receptors in your brain. And do you know what endorphins are chemically similar to? Morphine. And Demerol. And heroin. Some people will do whatever it takes—legal or illegal—to get the euphoria of this chemical high. And you get it for free, just by giving birth!

During labor, your body is also producing very high levels of oxytocin, the hormone of calm and connection that reduces pain and fosters courage. (You'll read more about oxytocin in Part 2 of this chapter.) Eminent physician Michel Odent calls this state "going to another planet." Pam England, midwife and pioneering childbirth educator, calls it "being in labor land." I'd say that you are in a state of utter calm, ease, and peace. But whatever you call it, during labor your inner pharmacy is flooding your mind-body with unbelievably high levels of not just one but *two* of the most powerful pleasure-inducing chemicals known to science.

If this is true (which it is), why does childbirth have such a terrible reputation? Why are the pleasurable moments, the moments of ease and peace, that are right there in the birth process rarely, if ever, talked about? Mostly because in this time of stillness and peace, in the period *between* the waves of intense physical sensations, the *untrained* mind—the mind that does not know how to be in the present moment—is reacting, reacting with fearful thoughts like, "Oh, my god, that last contraction was so bad!" or "How am I going to handle the next one?" or "When is this going to be over?"

Caught up in a stream of distressing thoughts about the past or the future, our mind stimulates adrenaline, putting us into the stress reaction of fight or flight. Not only are we missing the moments of pleasure, ease, and peace that are right there to be found in the birth process itself, the mind is adding a layer of suffering; we are

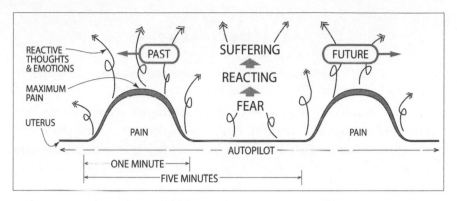

Diagram C: Contraction-Expansions Without Mindfulness

working directly against the very process that is bringing our baby to us. In this agitated state, labor looks something like what you see in Diagram C. We will learn more about how this happens in Part 2 of this chapter.

Cara, the daughter of my dear friend Deborah, didn't miss this pleasure during her birthing process. About midway through the MBCP course, Cara and Luis honored me with an invitation to attend their labor. I was of course thrilled to be sharing the birthing experience of this young woman who had been birthed into my hands thirty-two years ago, an event that would be all the sweeter for knowing it would make my friend a grandmother for the first time.

Cara's labor was short—only about six hours—and very intense. Most of that time we were at Cara and Luis's home, until it became clear that it was time to go to the birth center where she had chosen to give birth. When we arrived, the midwife had a birthing tub filled with hot water waiting for her. Cara climbed in just as she felt the first urge to push. Comfortably submerged in the water, she did the work of bearing down with each contraction-expansion. At one point Cara opened one eye, looked at me, smiled, and said in a dreamy voice, "Nancy, you were right. The time between the contractions is awesome. Glad I'm not missing it."

"I'm glad you're not missing it too, sweetheart," I replied. Deborah and I exchanged knowing smiles as Cara went back to work breathing with the next contraction-expansion. Luna, Cara and Luis's daughter (and Deborah's granddaughter), was born forty-five minutes later.

PART TWO: FEAR

When fear is abandoned, all that remains is sensation.
—Robert Brower

Having deconstructed the experience of pain during childbirth, we can now apply the same approach to the other half of childbirth's dynamic duo: fear. Let's set the stage for that discussion by exploring how mindfulness can make an important contribution to the normal physiology of childbirth.

EXPANDING OUR VIEW OF CHILDBIRTH: THE MIND-BODY CONNECTION

I'm standing in the classroom at the whiteboard, a blue marker in my hand. As part of our exploration of the sensations of labor, we have been looking at the diagram of the uterus (Diagram A). Now it's time to expand our view of childbirth, moving from the body to the mind and focusing on how, from a mind-body perspective, they work together. Giving birth entails a lot more than a powerful muscle contracting to expel its contents.

"The uterus isn't a voluntary muscle we can control, like our bicep or quadriceps," I tell the class. "So what actually causes the uterus to contract?"

A bit timidly someone volunteers, "Hormones?"

"Yes, that's right. Hormones. And what hormone in particular?"

After a pause someone says, "Oxytocin."

"Right again. And where does this oxytocin come from?" I ask, knowing this is a more difficult question.

"The pituitary?"

"Exactly. And where is the pituitary located?"

"In the brain."

"Yep. Your pituitary gland is in your brain, right behind your eyes, and it's closely connected to the hypothalamus, the body's master gland. It's your hypothalamus that actually makes the oxytocin, which it then sends to your posterior pituitary, where it's stored and then released during labor. You'll see in a few moments why knowing this is at least as important as knowing the stages of labor."

We visited the brain briefly in relation to pain and perception, but now let's look at it more closely. For, as unlikely as it may seem, childbirth occurs not only in your uterus. From the broader mind-body perspective, the conductor of the symphony of labor is actually the brain. Our brain, this incredibly complex tofu-like organ with its billions of neurons and trillions of neuronal connections is the body's central headquarters, sending and receiving electrical impulses via an elaborate network of nerve fibers throughout your body. According to Stephen J. Smith, PhD, professor of molecular and cellular physiology at the Stanford University School of Medicine, "In a human, there are more than 125 trillion synapses just in the cerebral cortex alone. That's roughly equal to the number of stars in 1,500 Milky Way galaxies. . . ."

Some of these electrical impulses stimulate the release of chemical messengers called hormones, which circulate through the bloodstream, causing profound effects on essentially every organ in the body. This means that although what goes on inside your head may seem separate from what's happening in the rest of your body, the brain and its partner, the mind, are in fact distributed throughout the body in one interconnected whole.

Thanks in part to remarkable new brain imaging technologies like functional magnetic resonance imaging (fMRI), which show us real-time changes in blood flow to different parts of the brain, the frontiers of neuroscience have advanced dramatically over the past several decades. In fact, an entirely new paradigm of who we are as living, evolving beings and how our mind and body work together is emerging. As mentioned in Chapter 4, one of the more fascinating aspects of this new research confirms that meditative disciplines can actually change the neural wiring in our brain, thereby contributing to happier, healthier lives.

It can be helpful to remember that this organ each of us carries inside our skull is the product of 650 million years of evolution. In the 1950s neurologist Paul MacLean proposed a theoretical model for how the brain worked that he called the "triune brain." His theory was based on the idea that our brain evolved in three stages so that we essentially have not one but three brains inside our head: the reptilian brain, the limbic brain, and the neocortex. Contemporary neuroscience has replaced many specifics of MacLean's theory, but his triune brain is still a helpful way to understand the structures of the brain and how they influence human behavior.

The *reptilian brain* is the oldest part of the brain. It is responsible for muscle movement, balance, and basic autonomic functions like heart rate, blood pressure, and respiration. It includes the brain stem and the cerebellum, which tend to dominate in reptiles. In terms of behavior, this part of the brain is aggressive, territorial, compulsive, and doesn't learn from mistakes. The limbic or *mammalian brain* is the primary seat of emotions, attention, and emotionally charged memories, and it tends to be predominant in mammals. Instincts such as feeding, fighting, fleeing, and sexual behavior are rooted here, as well as our instinctual, social, and emotional needs to feel connected, calm, and cared for.

Structurally, the limbic brain includes the hypothalamus, the master gland, which manufactures both oxytocin and CRH, the precursor to the cascade of hormones that eventually results in adrenaline production; the hippocampus, which compares external images to stored memories; and the amygdala, which sends the signal to flood the body with the chemicals of fight or flight when the hippocampus senses danger.

The third part of the brain, *the neocortex*, and especially the prefrontal cortex or neomammalian brain, is the newest of the three. It's responsible for what we think of as our higher cognitive functions, such as abstract reasoning, language, enhanced learning and memory, introspection, and insight. This is the part of our brain that rehearses and worries about the future, rehashes and analyzes the past, makes plans and reasoned arguments, and attempts to solve problems.

All three parts of our brain are interconnected by a vast network of neurons. Though we might like to believe that the newest part of our brain, the more rational, "thinking" neocortex, is in charge, in fact it seems that the limbic system, the seat of our emotions, can all too easily dominate our behavior. (Road rage is a perfect example of this.) Together the three areas of the brain shape our experience from the bottom up as we go about daily life, learning from and attuning to each other and our surroundings according to the patterns of our culture, our language, our unique personal and emotional history, and our temperament, all of which contribute to our view of ourselves and the world in which we live.

THE AUTONOMIC NERVOUS SYSTEM

The Parasympathetic Branch: Calm and Connection

Your brain has several systems that coordinate your body's activities. The autonomic nervous system (ANS), the part that directs your involuntary body processes, has the most relevance for understanding the mind-body connection and the value of mindfulness training for childbirth. The ANS has two branches: *the parasympathetic nervous system* (PNS) and *the sympathetic nervous system* (SNS). The parasympathetic nervous system, in which the hormone oxytocin is the key player, is what world authority Dr. Kerstin Uvnäs Moberg calls the "calm-and-connection" system.[1] This oxytocin-based system is associated with trust and curiosity, growth and healing, contentment, and positive social interactions and emotions. (Some call this the "approach" system.)

The other branch, the *sympathetic nervous system*, regulates the fight-or-flight reaction using the stress hormones adrenaline and noradrenaline (sometimes called epinephrine and norepinephrine) and cortisol. We commonly refer to this collection of hormones simply as adrenaline. Triggered by fear, the fight-or-flight reaction helps us defend ourselves or flee from anything we perceive as a threat to our survival.

Our bodies are constantly shifting between the parasympathetic and sympathetic nervous systems in a complex and ever-changing dance of balancing and rebalancing according to how we perceive both our inner and outer conditions. Both systems are mediated through the hypothalamus, and both are essential to our continued existence: we need to be able to marshal our defenses, *and* we need to rebalance, rest, recover, reconnect, and heal, or we won't last very long. During childbirth it is most important that the calm-and-connection system be the predominant mode of being—although, as you will see, the fight-or-flight system also has an essential role to play. Ideally, the territory of calm and connection would also be the baseline of our life, the place where we live most of the time.

As we've seen, when the parasympathetic calm-and-connection system predominates, we feel peaceful, content, calm, happy, open, friendly, at ease, relaxed, generous, contemplative, safe, trusting, and in balance. (When I think of the calm-and-connection system, I often visualize a troop of baboons on the savannah just hanging out, calmly grooming each other, at peace as gazelles and wildebeest graze nearby.) When the levels of oxytocin, of calm and connection, are high, we have a higher pain threshold, feel more courageous, and are more open to learning. Oxytocin contributes to orgasm in females and males and makes you feel cuddly and affectionate after making love or relaxed after a massage. It encourages us to form lasting social bonds, to fall in love (and stay in love) with our babies and our partners. It triggers breast milk to let down during breastfeeding, and most important for our purposes, oxytocin is what makes the cells of the uterus contract and gradually shorten during labor.

Oxytocin comes into full play during the first stage of labor.[2] Released in little pulses from the posterior part of your pituitary gland, oxytocin flows through your bloodstream to every part of your body. Traveling through your uterine arteries to your uterus (see Diagram A again), the oxytocin-rich blood reaches receptors on the surface of your uterine muscle cells, and when it does, it stimulates those muscle cells to shorten and contract. When you create the optimal conditions for oxytocin to flow during labor, all the muscle fibers in your uterus will contract strongly and in a well-coordinated, regular pattern.

This is exactly what we want even if it hurts: a strong uterine muscle contracting regularly, frequently, and effectively, because this is what will bring your baby into your arms as efficiently and quickly as possible. The conditions that encourage your body to produce lots of oxytocin include both the external birthing environment (we'll look at these in Chapter 16) *and* your inner birthing environment, which is deeply influenced by the state of your mind. As you will see, this is where mindfulness practice for childbirth is key.

The Sympathetic Branch: Fight or Flight

The other part of your autonomic nervous system is your sympathetic nervous system, which is responsible for fight or flight, or the "stress reaction." Stress gets a lot of attention these days, certainly much more than calm and connection, in part because there is so much stress in everyday modern life that it has become a significant factor in less-than-optimal physical and mental health. Stress can be triggered by an external event, such as an unexpected job layoff or an illness in the family, or by an internal event, such as pain in the body, including the pain of childbirth.

Stress is a normal part of life, and whether its source is external or internal, *how we view a stressor makes all the difference in the world.* For example, if I am laid off from my job, that is highly stressful. However, if I see this event as a complete and total threat to my very existence, I can become so despondent that I fall into depression or so anxious that I'm unable to function. Caught in these afflictive mental states of anxiety or depression, I am so out of balance that I am unable to see clearly and decide on a wise course of action.

But if I'm laid off from my job and, after a brief period of confusion that perhaps includes anger and fear, I can use mindfulness practice to come back into balance, I may be able to see this unfortunate experience as a challenge to be met rather than as a threat to my total existence. Perhaps I'll find a new job, maybe even one I like better than my old one. Or maybe I'll use the layoff as an opportunity to return to school or to change careers or start a business of my own. This is the *internal resilience* that mindfulness practice makes available to us in response to the unwanted. I didn't have a choice about being laid off from my job; that is how it is. But I absolutely have a choice about my perception, about the way I view this stressful event in my life.

In some sense, it's a matter of degree. Multiple studies have shown that when stress or worry is chronic, it becomes a contributing factor to heart disease, high blood pressure, asthma, insomnia, migraine headaches, digestive difficulties such as irritable bowel syndrome, weight problems, neck and back pain, and decreased immune system function. And of course stress also has very real effects on our psychological wellbeing, leading us to feel anxious, apprehensive, or tense much of the time, sometimes spilling over into panic attacks or angry outbursts. Stress can also push us into depression and despair.

Stress in pregnancy has been associated not only with preterm labor but with a decrease in the quality of the childbirth experience, an increase in postpartum depression, decreased quality of attachment between a mother and her infant, postpartum couple conflict, and less-than-optimal neurocognitive development of the child. In short, an overabundance of stress in our daily lives, whether we are pregnant or not, can lead to our not being very happy—or healthy—campers.

This is where mindfulness practice comes in. Studies show that mindfulness practice helps us cope more effectively with stress, chronic pain, illness, depression, anxiety, and many other adverse conditions. It also improves brain and immune function. A small pilot study published by my colleague Larissa Duncan and me in 2010 showed that pregnant women who took the MBCP course experienced decreases in anxiety and depression and more positive emotions after completing the course.[3] Though there is still much to be learned about how mindfulness practice can affect our health and wellbeing during pregnancy, childbirth, and the postpartum period, it seems clear that something measurably beneficial is happening for many people who take up a mindfulness meditation practice, including pregnant women.

Like physical pain, the fight-or-flight system is not a bad thing. It's just that as we evolved, the stress reaction was meant to take care of an immediate threat, like the proverbial tiger. When monkeys spy a tiger, you'd better believe they flee—and real quick too. Stress was meant to be discharged through activity; we chased after and attacked our lunch (fight), or we ran away to keep from becoming someone else's lunch (flight). That's why exercise helps us reduce stress.

This fight-or-flight reaction needs to be *fast*. When the hippocampus perceives something that might be a threat, the amygdala immediately sounds the alarm, causing the master gland, the hypothalamus, to signal the pituitary, which sends neurochemical signals through the bloodstream to the adrenal glands above our kidneys, flooding our body with adrenaline and profoundly altering our entire physiology. (If that's not a mind-body event, I'm hard-pressed to think of one that is.) Our heart rate and blood pressure increase; breathing gets faster; our palms get sweaty; blood flow is redistributed to big skeletal muscles to prepare us to fight or flee; our pupils dilate so we can see if there is more threat on the horizon; and our shoulders and legs tense in preparation for action. We are on high alert, and we call this decidedly uncomfortable mind-body state "fear." This neurochemical cascade happens in milliseconds deep inside our older mammalian brain, the limbic system, long before our newer and slower neocortex, the more rational, thinking part of the brain, can get into the act.

In modern life, stress is mostly triggered by the tigers in our mind—a deadline at work, being late for a meeting, traffic, or a disagreement with a loved one. When I talk with expectant couples about why they want to take the MBCP course, they often say that in addition to preparing for childbirth, they want to be able to handle stress better, and they have heard that meditation practice can help with that. These expectant parents realize that they need tools for destressing now *and* for childbirth; they also know that a stressed-out parent is not so great for a child. Getting a handle on stress now, before your baby arrives, is a very smart move.

MORE CALM AND CONNECTION, LESS FIGHT OR FLIGHT

Due to our evolutionary history—our need to be on alert to danger—we humans actually have a bias toward negativity. As neuropsychologist and meditation teacher Rick Hanson puts it, "Your brain preferentially scans for, registers, stores, recalls, and reacts to unpleasant experiences. . . . It's like Velcro for negative experiences and Teflon for positive ones."[4]

The good news is that we have a way to influence this tendency of the mind to put us—and keep us—on high alert, and that way is quite literally right under our nose. The breath, our anchor to the present moment, is actually the link between the parasympathetic and sympathetic nervous systems. When we breathe in we energize the sympathetic system—we're ready to act—and when we breathe out we are inviting the calm and ease of the parasympathetic system. And when we breathe in *and are aware that we are breathing in,* and when we breathe out *and are aware that we are breathing out,* we have introduced mindfulness—an entirely new element—into our

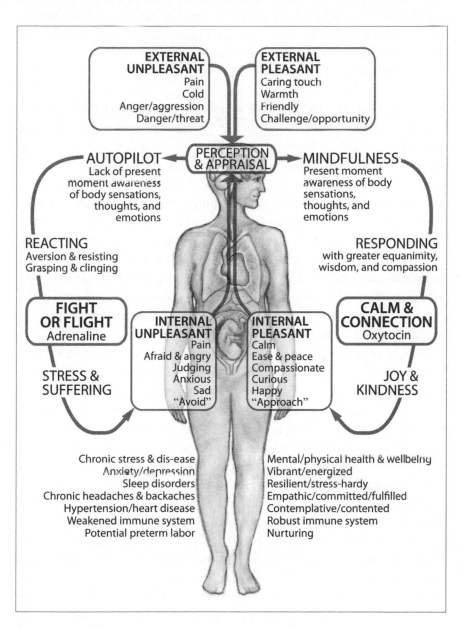

The Power of Mindfulness[5]

limbic brain's cycle of fight-or-flight reactivity. *Being aware* of what we are feeling in our body, our emotions, and the thoughts running through our mind, we are choosing to be mindful. By bringing awareness to the breath, we may find a degree of equilibrium, equanimity, and inner peace—the territory of "just being," which is always available to us—even under the most challenging of circumstances, like birthing a baby.

FIGHT OR FLIGHT DURING CHILDBIRTH

So what happens if the stress reaction gets triggered during childbirth? Well, a few things. First and foremost, the adrenaline from fight or flight *inhibits the oxytocin-producing neurons in your hypothalamus,* reducing the amount of oxytocin available to your uterus, just when you need it most. Second, as part of the redistribution of blood flow during the fight-or-flight reaction, the uterine arteries narrow, and the blood that could be carrying oxytocin to your uterus is shunted away to the large muscles of the body in preparation to fight or flee. And what is the result? Labor contractions become weaker, farther apart, and more irregular. This decreased blood flow to the uterus results in a buildup of lactic acid, the waste product of muscle cell activity, thereby making labor longer and more painful and increasing the possibility that medication and technology will be needed.

Millions of years of evolution have beautifully hardwired us and all other female mammals to react in just this way if disturbed during the labor process. If you're in labor and have to run away from a tiger, it's a very good thing that the fight-or-flight mechanism kicks in to slow down or even stop the process. Survival through the power of adrenaline definitely trumps the oxytocin-engendered calm-and-connection system needed to give birth.

Those of us who work with birthing women know quite well how fear disrupts the normal labor process. It is not at all unusual for a laboring woman to call the Labor and Delivery unit to report that her contractions are regular, strong, and frequent and that she is on her way to the hospital, only to arrive with her labor slowed to a virtual standstill. Unless a woman is well into the first stage of labor, the anxiety that results from a car ride to the hospital and the unfamiliar hospital environment can and sometimes does actually stop labor, at least for a time. The advice to "stay home as long as possible" is partly an attempt to mitigate this kind of disruption. Whether you're birthing at home, in a hospital, or in a birthing center, it's important that you perceive your birthing environment as safe.

Although there are usually no real tigers hanging out in Labor and Delivery, there are some very real conditions in modern maternity care that are a bit tiger-like, and we must be aware of them if we are to navigate this life-changing journey with some degree of calm and wisdom. As sad and disturbing as it may be, much of maternity care in the United States today is not as attuned to the normal healthy laboring woman as it could be, and in Chapter 16 we'll look at ways to use your mindfulness practice to maintain the best possible relationship to these external conditions during your birthing experience.

However, the other conditions we need to pay attention to during childbirth are the internal ones—the tigers we may be carrying in our mind. Though of course there are no guarantees that labor will go the way you hope or expect, when you develop your mindfulness practice during pregnancy, you are taking a very important step toward taming your internal tigers and keeping your normal physiology on track. Through mindfulness practice we are learning how to let go of the thinking mind, the mind that generates all those imaginary tigers, and to allow our deeper, limbic brain to fully do what it knows how to do: produce and release into our bloodstream the essential hormone oxytocin we need to birth our baby. In this way, mindfulness helps us learn how to get out of our own way.

Sarah's experience is a wonderful example of how mindfulness practice can help untangle pain and fear. Pregnant with her first baby, Sarah was having lots of back pain. One night in class she said, "You know, I'm beginning to realize how amazingly creative my mind is. The other night I got up to pee, and I just started worrying about *everything.* I worried that my labor pain would be worse because of the back pain. I worried that I would have to use drugs during labor, and you all know how much I don't want to do that. I worried that my back pain wouldn't go away after the birth and that my mom would have to come to live with us because I wouldn't be able to take care of the baby. I worried that I would have to take pain medication for my back pain after the birth and I wouldn't be able to breastfeed. All these fantasies about the future—it was really amazing. My mind was a nonstop fear-making machine!"

Sarah continued, "And then I remembered my breath, and I started practicing. I just lay there, and every time I became aware of thinking, I let go of the thought and came back to my breath. I could see that *my thoughts were just thoughts,* something my mind was doing, and that I didn't have to take them all so seriously! Then I just fell asleep. It was very cool."

Besides discovering that she could use mindfulness practice to work with fearful thoughts, Sarah found she could use it to work with her back pain. By paying closer attention to her moment-to-moment experiences in everyday life, she found that there were times during the day when her back pain was quite tolerable and that there were even stretches when she didn't have any pain at all. By using her back pain as an opportunity for mindfulness practice, Sarah found a way to offer acceptance and kindness to her pain. It would be fair to say that by the time Sarah went into labor she had found some inner peace with things as they were.

Kim's birth experience is another example of mindfulness at work. While attending a friend's labor at the same hospital where she intended to deliver, Kim came to distinctly dislike the obstetrician-in-training assigned to her friend. During the MBCP course Kim often mentioned that she was worried that this particular doctor would be on call when she went into labor. All the sensations associated with the stress reaction coursed through her body whenever Kim thought about her imaginary tiger, the doctor. Over time Kim came to see her fear as an emotional contraction, one that she could work with in the same way she was learning to work with the physical pain of a labor contraction—breathing with it, observing it, accepting it, and allowing it to just be. As her mindfulness practice grew stronger, Kim was able to keep her fear about the doctor manageable.

About a week after her due date Kim went into labor. By the time she got to the hospital, she was already nine centimeters dilated. The hospital was very busy that evening, and the only room available for Kim to birth in was the triage room. The nurse deposited her there and quickly went to fetch the doctor. Within a few minutes the door opened, and who do you think walked in? Of course, it was none other than the doctor she had worried about for months.

Kim described her inner experience this way: "It was amazing how my mindfulness practice just kicked in when I needed it. He walked in, I took one look at him, and I said quite calmly to myself, 'Oh, it's you. Well, I'm too busy having a baby to get all worked up about it. I'm just not going there.' I just kept pushing, and Miriam was born less than an hour later. And you know what's really funny? It turned out that he wasn't such a bad guy after all."

THE FETAL EJECTION REFLEX

While the adrenaline rush generated by the stress reaction is not optimal during the first stage of labor (assuming the tiger isn't real), a jolt of adrenaline at the end of the second stage of labor, just before birthing, may be just what is needed. As your body moves toward the crescendo of the birth process, something remarkable happens. As if sensing our vulnerability at this time, nature can release an intense burst of adrenaline, increasing your blood sugar and giving your voluntary muscles, the ones you are using for pushing, more energy and blood flow, which adds greater power to the work your uterus is already doing. It makes evolutionary sense: being this close to giving birth, the safest course for an animal in labor is to get her baby born as quickly as possible. Like the marathon runner who has a burst of energy to sprint across the finish line, the birthing mother may feel a surge of strength and power beyond anything she has ever known. French physician Michel Odent has named this phenomenon the Fetal Ejection Reflex.

I remember attending Nicole as she labored to birth her first baby. Nicole was working hard to push her baby out, and the baby was descending, but slowly. Over the course of three and a half hours we tried various positions for birthing—squatting, sitting on the birthing ball and on the birthing stool, standing in the shower, hands and knees on the bed—all intended to help her uterus contract strongly and her pelvis expand maximally so her baby could be born. Even though Nicole was pushing well and there were no signs of distress from the baby, I knew Nicole's strength was not limitless. My job as a midwife is to facilitate a safe and healthy passage for mother and baby, and while patience and watchful waiting are usually the best course, this must be balanced with wise action. Although I knew Nicole wanted a drug-free birthing experience, waiting does have consequences. More out of caution than concern, I felt it was time to check in with her.

"Nicole, there's no problem here, but this is taking a while and I want to know how you're doing. I'm fine with continuing, but tell me, how's your energy? Do you want to keep on pushing like you are?"

Nicole replied, "I'm getting pretty tired. And discouraged. What are my options?" Her question was a very good one.

"Well, we could try giving you a little Pitocin [synthetic oxytocin] to increase the strength of your contractions just a little bit. To do that safely, we would have to start an IV and use the fetal monitor. Or I could call the backup doctor, and she might be able to try a vacuum or forceps delivery."

"And if those don't work?" Nicole asked.

"Well," I replied softly, "there's always a cesarean. . . ."

As I spoke those words, Nicole sat bolt upright. Seeing a future scenario she really didn't want, she exclaimed in a voice of fierce determination, "I just want this f–ing baby out!" With adrenaline coursing through her body in support of her intensely focused mind, Nicole gave birth to her beautiful daughter Liza in three powerful pushes, less than ten minutes later.

CHILDBIRTH: A THREAT OR A CHALLENGE?

For most women, though certainly not all, having a baby come into their life is a happy life event. However, it would be fair to say that childbirth—*the process* of getting that baby into your life—often has some degree of fear or anxiety associated with it.

This is not necessarily a bad thing. For, like pain, fear or anxiety can help us focus our attention. It's a rare woman who at some point during pregnancy doesn't have a worried thought about her baby's health or some anxious rumination about how she will manage the process of giving birth. Partners can get pretty worried too—about the health of their partner, the health of the baby, or whether they will know what to do when the time comes. This is just part of the normal emotional package of pregnancy for both a woman and her partner.

While the degree of our fears, and the reasons for them, may vary widely, the *physiological* manifestation of fear in the body is universal. Fear is fear, and when we are anxious or frightened it is adrenaline, not oxytocin, that flows through our bodies. We don't need to make the fear of childbirth completely go away; we probably couldn't even if we tried. But we can develop mindfulness skills to work with fear when or if it arises. Since fear begins with our mind perceiving and interpreting something in a particular way, we can prepare for childbirth by paying attention to our mind. As the saying goes, "We see things not as they are but as *we* are."

A folktale about a man and a snake illustrates this point nicely. A man is walking down a country road on a dark, rainy night when suddenly he sees a long curvy object on the ground. Immediately he thinks: "Snake!" Convinced that the snake is poisonous, his mind fills with fearful scenarios: he will be bitten; he will be writhing in pain all alone on this country road; perhaps he will even die. The man feels his heart pounding as his breathing becomes shallow, his palms get sweaty, and his shoulders tense. He is in a full-fledged fight-or-flight reaction.

Grabbing a flashlight out of his pocket, the man quickly turns it on the snake—and lo and behold, what he sees is nothing more than an old piece of rope! There never was a snake at all, but his hippocampus, his brain's sentinel, compared the image of the long curvy object on the ground to the stored memory of other long curvy objects, decided the long curvy object was a snake, and took appropriate action. His sympathetic nervous system did its job, which was to ensure his survival: it produced all the physiological manifestations of fear in the body *just as if the snake was real.* But after shining the flashlight on the snake, the man sees that in fact it is just a rope.

As his mind comprehends what is real, he calms down. His heart rate and breathing return to baseline levels, his body rebalances, and his feelings of fear subside. Feeling safe once again, he actually becomes curious about the rope and investigates it more closely.

In childbirth and in our lives, mindfulness is the flashlight; *knowing* that the powerful sensations of childbirth are a rope (intense physical sensations) and not a snake (pain from true injury or illness) helps us make the all-important shift to seeing childbirth as a challenge rather than a threat. Even when you are in the midst of very intense physical sensations, you can turn the light of awareness toward them. Holding the unpleasant sensations in awareness, you anchor yourself in the breath and mindfully observe them. Shining the flashlight of awareness on the thoughts arising in relation to the body sensations, you can be aware of, observe, and accept them too. Like the contraction-expansions of labor, this contraction of the mind, fear, will not last (because nothing does), and thanks to your mindfulness practice your fear is less intense and of shorter duration. Like the man with the rope, you can take a step back, see reality more clearly, and cope more effectively with things as they are.

TURNING THREAT INTO CHALLENGE: A STORY OF TRANSFORMATION

During a weekend workshop called "The Mind in Labor" that I teach at the Osher Center, I witnessed a dramatic example of mindfulness practice transforming the fear of childbirth. The expectant parents were taking turns introducing themselves and sharing what they hoped to get from our weekend together. When Mei-Li's turn came, she confessed to the group that she was absolutely terrified of the pain of childbirth. She expressed the hope that over the weekend she might learn something, anything, to help her be less afraid.

"All my life my mother has been telling me how painful childbirth is. Now that I'm pregnant, I just don't know what to do. I've taken lots of childbirth classes—I've even seen a therapist—and I'm still terrified. In fact, I'm so terrified that even though my baby and I are completely healthy, I've convinced my doctor to let me have a cesarean." It was clear to everyone that this was not what Mei-Li wanted, but she just couldn't see any other way.

Throughout the weekend Mei-Li and her partner, John, actively participated in the various mindfulness practices for working with pain (practices you will learn in the next chapter). By Sunday afternoon, when I invited everyone to practice the most intense pain exercises—mindfully putting both hands into bowls of ice water—Mei-Li had found enough confidence that she didn't hesitate to take up the challenge.

After the workshop, Mei-Li approached me to say good-bye. Her face was softer and more open than it had been at our first meeting Friday evening, and her voice was much firmer. "I don't know how to thank you, Nancy," she said. "I've finally learned that I can deal with pain. I'm stronger than I thought. I am not my mother. I can do this."

THE BOTTOM LINE

Coming full circle, we now return to the original question, "What do we need to learn in order to prepare for childbirth?" We certainly need to learn about creating the optimal external circumstances so we feel safe in order to maximize the oxytocin calm-and-connection system and minimize fight or flight. There are many ways to do this, as you will see in Chapter 16. However, knowing that we cannot completely control the external conditions, more is needed: *we need to strengthen, through mindfulness practice, our internal calm-and-connection system.* And that is exactly what you are doing by practicing mindfulness meditation during pregnancy.

MINDFULNESS PRACTICE: A SPEAKING AND LISTENING INQUIRY ON FEAR AND HAPPINESS

During the MBCP course, expectant parents learn a practice called the Speaking and Listening Inquiry.[6] This multilayered meditation of discovery enhances the capacity for self-reflection and promotes intimacy. It is a meditation practice, not an ordinary conversation where two people are trying to fix something or figure something out. Through this way of speaking and listening to one another, couples explore and often come to a deeper understanding of the nature of fear and happiness—and of communication itself.

The form of the Speaking and Listening Inquiry is deceptively simple. A series of requests relating to fear is asked three times and responded to three times by each partner. Then the requests are repeated in relation to happiness. If you decide to try this practice, please remember, *this is a meditative inquiry, not a conversation, and it is important to follow the form.* The form itself has wisdom embedded in it.

Most likely you will notice how different this way of speaking and listening is from the way you and your partner usually communicate. Just observe your habit of wanting to discuss, analyze, ask questions to satisfy your own curiosity, or fix or change how your partner is thinking or feeling. Experience as best you can what it is like to be present with affectionate attention during speaking and listening. You might learn something quite interesting—about yourself and about each other.

Set aside at least forty-five minutes for the Speaking and Listening Inquiry. Sit facing your partner. Decide who will make the request first and who will respond in the first round. Between each round of requests and responses, pause, close your eyes, and come back to the breath for fifteen to thirty seconds, or three or four breaths, noticing any sensations in the body and any thoughts or emotions arising in those moments. It's fine to hold hands or in some way be in physical contact during this practice.

➤ SPEAKING AND LISTENING INQUIRY: FEAR ➤

Person 1: Please tell me one thing you notice in your body when you feel fear.
Person 2: (Answers.)
Person 1: Thank you. (Pause.) Please tell me one thing you notice in your body when you feel fear.
Person 2: (Answers. This can be the same answer given the first time or a different one.)
Person 1: Thank you. (Pause.) Please tell me one thing you notice in your body when you feel fear.
Person 2: (Answers.)
Person 1: Thank you.

Now changing roles with your partner, go through another round, making the same request three times.

After each of you has had a turn to both request and respond, you are invited to close your eyes and come back into silence, back to the breath for fifteen to thirty seconds, or three or four breaths. Notice any sensations in your body, any emotions, or any thoughts present in the mind. Then, opening your eyes, begin the next inquiry. As you practice, you will most likely find a certain rhythm to the experience.

The next request gives you the opportunity to investigate *thoughts* that may be generating sensations of fear in the body. Remember, fearful thoughts are *always* about the future. The thoughts you choose to explore may be thoughts you have about the coming birth experience, about the baby, about your relationship with each other, about finances, work, parenting, or anything else. To begin with, however, you might want to take this opportunity to explore fearful thoughts about your upcoming birth experience.

Person 1: Please tell me one *thought* that causes fear to arise when you think about the future.

Person 2: (Answers.)

Person 1: Thank you. (Pause.) Please tell me one *thought* that causes fear to arise when you think about the future.

Person 2: (Answers.)

Person 1: Thank you. (Pause.) Please tell me one *thought* that causes fear to arise when you think about the future.

Person 2: (Answers.)

Person 1: Thank you.

Switching roles, do another round with this request. When you have each requested and responded three times, close your eyes and come back to silence, back to the breath for fifteen to thirty seconds, or three or four breaths, as you did before. Notice any sensations in your body, any emotions, or any thoughts present in the mind. Now opening your eyes, begin the next inquiry.

This next inquiry allows you to go deeper into *one* of the fearful thoughts you named. Tell your partner which fearful thought you would like to explore more deeply now. You needn't choose the most fearful or challenging one; just choose what you are ready to explore right now. The choice is yours.

Person 1: Please tell me one way you would cope if what you feared actually came to pass in your life. What resources—both externally, such as family, friends, professionals, books, or organizations, and internally, such as mindfulness practice, prayer, or confidence in your inner strength—would you draw on if what you feared actually manifested?

Person 2: (Answers.)

Person 1: Thank you. (Pause.) Please tell me one way you would cope if what you feared actually came to pass in your life.

Person 2: (Answers.)

Person 1: Thank you. (Pause.) Please tell me one way you would cope if what you feared actually came to pass in your life.

Person 2: (Answers.)

Person 1: Thank you.

Switching roles, continue for another round with this request. After each of you has had a turn to request and respond, you are invited once again to close your eyes and come back into silence, back to the breath for fifteen to thirty seconds, or three or four breaths. Notice any sensations in your body, any emotions, or any thoughts present in the mind. Now opening your eyes, begin the next inquiry.

Sometimes we may have uncomfortable feelings about a particular situation that we would rather not look at. Like the saying goes, denial is more than a river in Egypt. Or perhaps we aren't in denial, we just haven't learned a way to slow down enough and name what we fear.

While we can't control the future, we are not passive recipients of the future either. We are part of its unfolding. The future is, at least in part, a result of our intentions and the choices we make in the present moment. This next inquiry is an opportunity to take time to see if there is anything you can do, or need to do, *now* to decrease the likelihood of what you fear actually manifesting.

For example, if you are having your baby in the hospital, have you learned about the hospital's guidelines and protocols with regard to certain procedures and its use of technology in certain situations? (See Chapter 16.) If you are having your baby at home, do you and your midwife have a clear understanding of a backup plan in case things don't unfold as you hope and a transfer to the hospital becomes a wise course of action? Do you need to talk with someone on your support team to clarify any concerns you may have regarding their role at the birth? Has your healthcare provider said something that has raised questions in your mind but you have been hesitant to ask for clarification? Using a problem-focused strategy, you look directly at your discomfort and set your intention to engage, discover, and explore.

However, you may find that you have a fear, for example about the health of your baby, and there is absolutely nothing you can do about it that you are not already doing—eating well, exercising, reducing stress. This is when you can turn to mindfulness for an emotion-coping strategy to reduce the suffering caused by your worrying mind. Recognizing that your fear about your baby's health can end only by giving birth and seeing your healthy baby, you can use your practice to acknowledge your fearful thoughts. Practice continually recognizing them as just thoughts and simply return to the breath over and over again. After all, what else is there to do?

So let's continue the inquiry.

Person 1: Is there anything you can do *now* to decrease the possibility of what you fear happening in the future?

Person 2: (Answers.)

Person 1: Thank you. (Pause.) Is there anything you can do *now* to decrease the possibility of what you fear happening in the future?

Person 2: (Answers.)

Person 1: Thank you. (Pause.) Is there anything you can do *now* to decrease the possibility of what you fear happening in the future?

Person 2: (Answers.)

Person 1: Thank you.

Switching roles, continue for another round with this question. When each of you has asked and answered the question three times, once again you are invited to close your eyes and come back to silence, back to the breath for fifteen to thirty seconds, or three or four breaths. Notice any sensations in your body, any emotions, or any thoughts present in the mind.

This is the end of the inquiry about fear. As you sit with the breath, let yourself fall back into stillness as best you can. Notice if there are more questions arising. Notice if you have energy for another inquiry practice or if this is enough for now. If you decide to end your inquiry practice, thank your partner and perhaps exchange a hug.

If you do have the time and energy for another practice, it is recommended to do the following inquiry on happiness. This inquiry helps balance the negative tendency of the mind that we just stimulated with our inquiry into fear. If you are not able to practice this inquiry now, do make a commitment to yourself and each other to come back to the happiness inquiry at a later time. If you are following the MBCP program outlined in Chapter 21, this inquiry practice is given as a home assignment in Week 6.

If you want to explore in regular conversation something your partner shared during the inquiry, please ask if it is okay with your partner first. Being respectful of each other will serve you both well.

⟶ SPEAKING AND LISTENING INQUIRY: HAPPINESS ⟵

As we saw in the description of the autonomic nervous system, the calm-and-connection dimension of life is the quieter but no less important complement to the more dramatic fight or flight, and it is essential to nurture this softer, calmer aspect of our selves as well, for it is here where we promote happiness, health, balance, and ease of being. The calm-and-connection system is also a key consideration as we make choices about the kind of family we want to create. How much stress will we generate for our children by overscheduling our own lives, surrounding them with a sense of endless urgency, just as we perhaps are doing now before the baby is born? Or how much time will we find to just be with each other as a family, at ease, connected—cooking and sharing a meal, taking a walk, playing a game, gardening, or going to the library? This kind of peaceful, ordinary life feeds both ourselves and our children—and it might just be where happiness resides.

In this next Speaking and Listening Inquiry, you can explore this dimension of living. Using the same form as you did with fear, ask the following:

Person 1: Please tell me one thing you notice in your body when you feel happiness.
Person 2: (Answers.)
Person 1: Thank you. (Pause.) Please tell me one thing you notice in your body when you feel happiness.
Person 2: (Answers.)
Person 1: Thank you. (Pause.) Please tell me one thing you notice in your body when you feel happiness.
Person 2: (Answers.)
Person 1: Thank you.

Switching roles, continue for another round with this request. When each of you has requested and responded three times, allow your eyes to close and come back to silence, and back to the breath for fifteen to thirty seconds, or three or four breaths. Notice sensations in your body, emotions, and thoughts present in the mind. Now opening your eyes, begin the next inquiry.

Person 1: Please tell me one *thought* that causes happiness to arise when you think about the future.
Person 2: (Answers.)
Person 1: Thank you. (Pause.) Please tell me one *thought* that causes happiness to arise when you think about the future.
Person 2: (Answers.)
Person 1: Thank you. (Pause.) Please tell me one *thought* that causes happiness to arise when you think about the future.
Person 2: (Answers.)
Person 1: Thank you.

Changing roles, do another round with this request. When you have finished, each of you having requested and responded three times, allow your eyes to close and come back into silence, back to the breath for fifteen to thirty seconds, or three or four breaths. Notice sensations in your body, emotions, and thoughts present in the mind. Notice how inclining your thoughts toward happiness perhaps changes your mood, or brings a certain lightness to the body. Now you can open your eyes and begin the next inquiry.

Person 1: Please tell me one way you can bring more happiness into your
   life as you are living it *now*.
Person 2: (Answers.)
Person 1: Thank you. (Pause.) Please tell me one way you can bring more
   happiness into your life as you are living it *now*.
Person 2: (Answers.)
Person 1: Thank you. (Pause.) Please tell me one way you can bring more
   happiness into your life as you are living it *now*.
Person 2: (Answers.)
Person 1: Thank you.

And changing roles once again, continue for another round with this inquiry. When each of you has requested and responded three times, close your eyes and come back into silence, back to the breath for fifteen to thirty seconds, or three or four breaths as you have before. Notice sensations in your body, emotions, and thoughts present in the mind. Notice how it feels to even consider bringing more joy into your life right now. Now, opening your eyes, begin the next inquiry.

Person 1: Please tell me one thing you see as an obstacle, either inner or
   outer, to bringing more moments of happiness into your life.
Person 2: (Answers.)
Person 1: Thank you. (Pause.) Please tell me one thing you see as an ob-
   stacle, either inner or outer, to bringing more moments of happiness into
   your life.
Person 2: (Answers.)
Person 1: Thank you. (Pause.) Please tell me one thing you see as an ob-
   stacle, either inner or outer, to bringing more moments of happiness into
   your life.
Person 2: (Answers.)
Person 1: Thank you.

Switching roles, continue with another round of requests. And again, when each of you has requested and responded three times, close your eyes and come back into silence, back to the breath for fifteen to thirty seconds, or three or four breaths. Noticing sensations in your body, emotions, and thoughts present in the mind, and now opening your eyes once again.

While each of us needs to take responsibility for our own happiness, it is also true that most of us can use a little encouragement or practical help in that direction. Our happiness is intimately intertwined with the happiness of others, especially those near and dear to us, and when we nurture the happiness of others, it impacts us in a positive way. With this in mind, we request and respond in this final inquiry.

> Person 1: Please tell me one way I might support you to bring more moments of happiness into your life.
> Person 2: (Answers.)
> Person 1: Thank you. (Pause.) Please tell me one way I might support you to bring more moments of happiness into your life.
> Person 2: (Answers.)
> Person 1: Thank you. (Pause.) Please tell me one way I might support you to bring more moments of happiness into your life.
> Person 2: (Answers.)
> Person 1: Thank you.

Switching roles, continue for another cycle of inquiry. When each of you has requested and responded three times, you are invited to close your eyes and come back into silence, back to the breath for fifteen to thirty seconds, or three or four breaths. Notice what it feels like to offer support to your partner to be happier. Notice how your body feels right now and any emotions or thoughts that are present in the mind.

COMMON EXPERIENCES DURING THE SPEAKING AND LISTENING INQUIRY

During the Speaking and Listening Inquiry it's quite common for tears to flow. In fact, I often find myself walking quietly around the room with a box of tissues in my hand, offering them where needed. When we feel safe, when we are truly paid attention to, especially by a trusted loved one in the spaciousness of mindful presence, it seems that we connect not only with our mind but also with our heart. Why this opening of the heart brings tears is unimportant. It happens.

If you find that one or both of you begins to cry or feel a new sense of openness, perhaps in the chest, take this opportunity to be mindful, and deeply experience whatever emotion you are feeling in the moment, even in the presence of the other person. Feel the sensations of tears rolling down your cheeks, notice whatever emotion is arising. Bring awareness to any thoughts that might be present, perhaps judging thoughts that you shouldn't cry or worried thoughts about how your partner may be feeling. Notice the expression on your partner's face as you cry; hear the sounds you make from blowing your nose, feel the tissue as you wipe your nose. See what it might be like to just accept the experience of crying with an open heart. After all, once your baby is born, you are going to be with someone who will be experiencing powerful emotions accompanied by crying quite frequently. It's not a bad idea to explore the territory of crying for ourselves before birth; it's more preparation for parenting.

As a culture we have very strong injunctions against crying; some of us may have received this message very powerfully when we were children, particularly if we are male. This childhood conditioning may have led to a denial or repression of certain emotions, thereby narrowing our own ability to fully feel our emotions or be able to tolerate strong emotions in others. This may not serve you well in your own life and as the parent of a very small person who passionately feels emotions without filtering them. Becoming familiar with and allowing the full range of human emotions within yourself may help you bring greater understanding, empathy, and compassion to parenting—and to your own experience of what it means to be fully human and alive.

The opposite of crying may also happen in this Speaking and Listening Inquiry: uncontrollable laughter. Once again, there's no need to suppress the underlying emotion or to get caught up in judging or analyzing. Observe how the new and unexpected can stimulate mirth, and allow the waves of laughter to move through your body. Notice where you feel the laughter—in the belly, in the chest—and notice how contagious laughter can be. It is sometimes said that the shortest distance between two people is laughter. Enjoy yourself if this particular experience arises.

Because of time constraints in the MBCP course, we ask the questions of each other only three times, but you are certainly not limited to that. Many couples find that they want to explore the questions more fully, and they find it useful to continue this practice at home for longer periods of time. You may find that your answers deepen as you continue to inquire. If you do decide to ask the questions more than three times, decide together beforehand how many times the two of you will ask and answer the question. Be sure to ask and answer the questions of each other an equal number of times.

As important as the topics of fear and happiness are in this inquiry, it is the *experience* of mindful speaking and listening that is ultimately most important. Notice how it feels to be truly listened to. Notice how it feels to truly listen to another person. Notice how it feels to receive the repeated "thank you." It's a crucial part of the inquiry, a wonderful acknowledgment that one has been seen and deeply heard, and that speaking the truth from one's heart has been received as a gift. Remember to give the gift of this kind of listening to your children. You'll be glad you did.

CHAPTER 7

Mindfulness Practices for Being with Pain

Hokusai says . . .
He says don't be afraid.
Don't be afraid.
Look, feel, let life take you by the hand.
Let life live through you.
—Roger Keyes

IT'S SNACK TIME in Class 4. Small groups of expectant parents are scattered throughout the room, animatedly chatting about an online resource they just found or a meet-the-doula night at a local birthing resource center. We've just had a lively discussion about working with pain if it arises during any of our formal practices—moving into the sensations, being with them for as long as we can, investigating unpleasant sensations with interest and curiosity, breathing into the sensations on the in-breath, softening and letting go on the out-breath, and gently and intentionally changing position during the stillness of the Body Scan or easing up during yoga practice. (You will learn about yoga practice in the next chapter.) We have explored working with pain and discomfort in everyday life, and how the common discomforts of pregnancy provide an opportunity to prepare for labor. We have also reviewed the Pleasant Events Calendar, which was given as part of the home assignment for this past week (see Appendix C).

We are now ready to take another step of discovery in relation to the intense physical sensations we call pain: seeing how with mindfulness practice we might maintain ourselves in a state of calm and connection, the one that promotes the optimal physiology of labor, even in the face of strong physical discomfort. To do this we will practice with the real thing, sensations of discomfort generated by holding ice cubes.[1] Since you may find it helpful to see how other people have experienced the formal pain practices before learning them yourself, I invite you to briefly join an MBCP class to see how our learning begins.

"Folks, please get yourself a floor chair from the closet, and take a seat," I say, laying out clean sheets on the floor. "Help yourself to a towel from this stack over here, and put it on the floor in front of you. We're going to set ourselves up for some pain practice."

Once people settle, I continue. "As I come around, please take a nice big handful of pain from this ice cooler and put it on the towel in front of you." I begin slowly walking around the circle, pausing to let each person take a handful of ice.

"Okay, now I'd like to invite everyone to please pick up the ice. And when it starts to hurt, whine and complain. Really let each other hear how much you don't like this experience. Whining and complaining is the assignment now."

I push the start button on my stopwatch, as each person picks up a handful of ice. Before long the room fills with sound.

"Owwww." It's Vicki.

"This really hurts!" adds Greg.

"I don't like this!"

"The pain is moving up my arm!"

"When is this going to be over?"

I sit quietly during the chorus of complaints. Tightly furrowed brows, hunched shoulders, and rocking body movements indicate that many are having a hard time. Others are coping with laughter. And still others have adopted a stoic "this isn't going to get the best of me" approach; despite my invitation to complain, they set their mouths tightly in fierce determination and don't utter a sound.

At the one-minute mark, I click my stopwatch and say loudly enough to be heard above the din, "Okay, you're done." Hands drop the ice in relief, and the complaints quickly turn into questions. "How long was that? How does this compare to labor pain? Is it going to hurt this much?"

I smile. It's not time for answers.

"Okay," I say. "That's ordinary mind, our typical way of relating to pain. We react. We want to stop it, to get away from it as quickly as possible. Nothing wrong with that; it's human. However, it's just not that helpful as a way to go through childbirth. Adding reactivity to an already challenging experience uses up an awful lot of energy, and there are other choices.

"So now let's do this exercise again," I continue. "Only this time let's see how we can use our mindfulness practice to work with these physical sensations. Please pick up the ice again, in the other hand. And this time pay full and complete attention to the breath. As if your life depended on it."

Save for the sounds of melting ice dripping onto clean sheets, the room is completely quiet. Most people have closed their eyes and are concentrating on the breath. Some have kept their eyes open, focusing softly on the floor in front of them. The visible tension in faces and bodies is much less now. Shifting my gaze between the couples practicing and the stopwatch, I follow my own breath.

When the time is up, I say quietly, "Now take a rest."

Ice cubes drop, and eyes pop open in amazement. "Wow! That was so much easier! Was that the same amount of time?"

"What was your experience?"

"It seemed so much shorter!" Many heads nod in agreement.

I smile and point to my stopwatch. "The amount of ice time was *identical* to the first round—one minute, the average duration of one contraction. Isn't that interesting? Absolutely nothing changed—except how you used your mind to relate to the unpleasant sensations in your hand. Instead of reacting and adding a layer of suffering to your experience, you were responding with mindfulness, being with things as they are. Perhaps we are beginning to discover the power of awareness."

⚊ PRACTICES DURING SENSATIONS ⚊

Each of the formal pain practices taught in MBCP classes is built on one of the two aspects of mindful awareness: focused concentration or open awareness. As we learned in our Raisin Meditation, mindfulness is like a lens with an aperture that can vary according to what is most appropriate at any given moment. Sometimes a laser beam of concentrated focus is most skillful, as we saw when we studied the raisin as if it were under a microscope. At other times we can choose a more open and spacious quality of attention, taking in the larger view, as we did when we saw the vast web of interconnectedness in the second meditation on the raisin.

When you first practice these pain coping skills, try them in succession, one after another, noticing which ones are most effective for your particular mind-body. You will see that there are many ways to hold ice cubes mindfully. Once you learn these various practices, when you are actually in labor you will have lots of tools to choose from.

I recommend that you not interrupt the flow of your experience to talk with your partner about what just happened. Let every moment be a practice moment, a time of sustained, quiet meditation and concentrated inner learning. If the mind wanders, gently bring it back to the breath or to the particular object of attention you are working with.

When working with ice, hold it for sixty seconds; then put it down and bring awareness to the breath for ninety seconds. *It is important to come back to the breath, or to whatever object of attention you are using, during this time between intense sensations as this is what you will do between the intense sensations of a contraction-expansion during labor.*

If you and your partner are learning these pain practices together, I suggest that first you go through the full series of practices that follow while your partner keeps track of the time. It should take about twenty to thirty minutes to go through the full series. Then have your partner go through the same series of practices while you take over the stopwatch. Enjoy learning how similar or different your mind and nervous system may be from your partner's when it comes to working with challenging physical sensations. Remember, we are all different, and there is no one right way.

If your partner can't be with you for pain practice, or if you are having your baby on your own, perhaps you can practice with a doula or a friend. It can also be interesting and confidence building to practice all by yourself. After all, no matter what happens, *you* are the one giving birth. While support, suggestions, and encouragement from other people can be extremely valuable, having a baby takes inner work, and like meditation practice, no one can do it for you.

In the beginning you can use one hand to pick up the ice. As you practice and your confidence grows, see if you can gradually increase the intensity of the sensations by holding the ice in two hands or by putting the ice on a more sensitive part of your body, like your inner wrists or behind your ears. Eventually, when and if you feel ready, you can practice "Bringing It All Together" as described later in this chapter, immersing first one hand and then both hands into a bowl of ice water for one minute. It's intense, but so are the powerful sensations of childbirth. And with practice, mindfulness will help you find an expansion of what is possible.

While there is no doubt that ice practice is really helpful, the sensations we intentionally create with ice do not come and go in a wavelike pattern. When you stop holding the ice cubes, the unpleasant sensations in your hand (or hands) diminish, but they do still continue for a time. This is very different from the contraction-expansions of labor. In labor, when the sensations of a contraction-expansion are over, they're over. *There is no pain in the moments between contraction-expansions*, just lovely moments of pleasure, calm, ease, peace, and renewal.[2]

During ice practice, it's absolutely fine to bring pleasant sensations of warmth to your hand during the rest intervals. Hold your own hand, or bring your hand to the warmth of your cheek, or have your partner warm it. Notice how it feels, both physically and emotionally, to be the recipient of a warm, caring touch.

Each of the practices described here has been useful to some women at some point during their labor. Try them all to discover which ones serve you. But remember, what you are really learning here is how to hold ice cubes. While this training will transfer to your labor, we don't know now which of these practices will most serve you at that time. So if you practice them all, you will have many tools to choose from when the time comes.

Remember, there is no goal here. We're certainly not trying to get rid of pain. We are working at expanding our capacity to be with the unpleasant—turning toward, accepting, and embracing our experience (our physical sensations, our thoughts, and our emotions)—however it may be, moment by moment.

Awareness of Breathing

You already learned the foundational Awareness of Breathing practice in Chapter 4, so see what it's like to apply it in this context. Picking up the ice, bring your full attention to the sensations of breathing as you hold the ice in your hand. Each time the mind wanders—to the sensations in your hand or to thoughts or feelings—gently bring your attention back to the breath. After one minute, set the ice down. Then return your awareness to the breath for one and a half minutes.

Breathing Into and Letting Go of Sensations

As you pick up the ice, become aware of the sensations of breathing, as in the practice above. After a few breaths, experiment with breathing directly into the sensations in your hand on the in-breath. Then as you breathe out, see if you can let go of some of the intensity of the sensations in your hand, softening, releasing, and letting go. This is one of the ways you learned to work with discomfort when you practiced the Body Scan. Experiment with applying this learning now to the sensations created by holding ice in your hand.

Awareness of Sensation

Picking up the ice, move your attention directly into the sensations in your hand. Just as you did in the Body Scan, see if you can carefully and precisely notice the sensations that are present—aching, numbness, burning, cold—whatever they may be. Notice where the sensations are most intense.

And least intense. Notice how the sensations generated by the contact of ice with your hand are not fixed but are changing, moment by moment. Find the edges of the sensations, where other sensations might be present. Notice any thoughts or emotions—perhaps negative, resistant, contracting thoughts or any expressions of *no*. See if you can bring an attitude of kindness and open curiosity to these sensations in your hand. After all, how many moments in your life do you get to learn how to hold ice cubes? Or experience the powerful sensations of transformational pain that result in the birth of your baby?

After one minute, set the ice down and practice breath awareness for one and a half minutes.

Playing with Sensations

Picking up the ice, gently move your attention back and forth between the breath and the sensations in your hand or hands. Let your awareness lightly rest on the sensations for a second or two. Then move it back to the breath. Play with the sensations you are experiencing in your hand or hands. Dance with them. Learn from them.

After one minute, set the ice down and practice breath awareness for one and a half minutes.

Counting the Breaths

Picking up the ice, silently and very gently count to yourself: one on the inhalation, two on the exhalation, three on the inhalation, four on the exhalation, and so on. If you get lost or forget what number you are on, not to worry. You were just momentarily distracted. Kindly and without judgment, simply start over again with the number one. You can also try quietly saying to yourself "in" on the in-breath and "one" on the out-breath, "in" on the in-breath and "two" on the out-breath, and so on.[3]

After one minute, set the ice down and practice breath awareness for one and a half minutes.

Many women report that counting breaths during labor is extremely effective for maintaining concentration during a contraction-expansion. Knowing the sensations last for only a certain number of breaths—usually between seven and ten—can help keep you grounded and present. Counting can also serve to keep your curiosity engaged. One contraction-expansion may last to the count of seven, another to the count of nine or even eleven. Curiosity and interest, even about powerfully intense physical sensations, can support and sustain a helpful state of mind, diminishing suffering in challenging times.

Expanding Awareness

Experiment with expanding awareness to your body as a whole, as you learned to do at the end of the Body Scan. When you pick up the ice, keep your awareness open to the whole body. Notice how much of your body is *not* in pain. Notice how large the body is, and how the unpleasant sensations are concentrated only in a very small location—in your hand. Keep your awareness as spacious and expanded as you can for your minute of ice-holding practice. You may come to see that mindful awareness is bigger than physical pain. Much, much bigger. Mindfulness is big enough to hold anything and everything.

After one minute, set the ice down and practice breath awareness for one and a half minutes.

The Half-Smile

If you haven't already done so, perhaps you are ready to challenge yourself by picking up ice in both hands. (Remember, labor increases in intensity.) Bringing awareness to the muscles at the corners of your mouth, ever so gently tighten those muscles so that the corners of your mouth turn upward slightly. Do this for one minute and then release the ice from your hand(s). Did this slight half-smile make a difference in your experience?

Research shows that when we smile, endorphins—those feel-good neuropeptides we learned about in Chapter 6—are released throughout the body. This is why humans like to smile and laugh and be around others who are happy and make us laugh. When you are in labor, take advantage of all the wisdom and assistance your mind-body has to offer! Turn up the corners of your mouth, and notice what it does to the mind.

If you choose to practice the half-smile and you are birthing in a hospital, there is a good chance that the nurses will be fighting over who gets to take care of you. I can hear them now. "Did you see the woman in Room 352? She's *smiling* during her contractions! I want to take care of her!" Mindful awareness has an effect not just on you but on everyone around you.

Gathas

Gathas are a type of metered, rhythmic, poetic verse. Gathas can be repeated silently to oneself in rhythm with the breath, like the counting practice, as a way to focus the mind and evoke certain feelings. Like mantra practice, this is an age-old technique for calming the mind and maintaining concentration in the present moment. Thich Nhat Hanh, the inspiring Vietnamese Buddhist monk and meditation teacher, often instructs his students to use gathas during meditation practice. In the late 1980s my family and

I attended several family retreats with him. One of the gathas he taught us went like this:

In, Out
Deep, Slow
Calm, Ease
Smile, Release
Present Moment
Wonderful Moment

The first word, *In*, is said on the in-breath, the second word, *Out*, is said on the out-breath, and so on. Experiment with this gatha while holding ice. See if it increases calm, concentration, and ease for you, right in the midst of the strong sensations in your hand(s). Feel free to say fewer words or to change them to ones that especially resonate for you.

Experiment with making up a labor gatha of your own. Some women have found that words like *open, yes, baby,* and *out* are particularly helpful. Or you might encourage an attitude of curiosity by saying "What's this?" on the in-breath and "Don't know" on the out-breath. Be sure to coordinate the words with the in-breath and the out-breath as you practice.

If you already know words or phrases that are comforting for you, such as words from a prayer or a song, see if silently repeating those words in rhythm with the breath has a positive effect on your mind-body during ice practice. If so, explore repeating those words to yourself when you are in labor. Tell your partner, and your doula if you decide to have one, to remind you of the words in case you forget this practice during labor.

Loving-Kindness Practice

In Chapter 14 you will learn a meditation called Loving-kindness. In the MBCP course it is taught in Week 7, and participants are encouraged to begin folding it into both their formal and informal daily practice. Women have told me that they have used phrases from Loving-kindness practice during labor and found them very helpful. After you have learned it, experiment with repeating some phrases from the Loving-kindness meditation during ice practice.

Making It Up Practice

During ice practice or during labor, a spontaneous thought may arise about how to be with these challenging physical sensations. Honor your intuition and creativity by experimenting with the gift that has been sent to you from this deep place. See what happens. You may discover something totally new, useful, and wonderful.

⌐ PRACTICES BETWEEN SENSATIONS ⌐

When you are first learning these practices, use the moments between sensations to come back to the breath and just be. Remember, this is where the moments of calm and ease are found. Don't miss them. As you become more comfortable with the rhythm of work and rest, work and rest, you might want to see if you can move deeper into those peaceful in-between moments in various ways. Remember, anything that keeps your awareness in the present moment, whether during a contraction-expansion or in the time between, will serve you well.

The Body Scan

Practicing a brief Body Scan between sensations may help you maintain a state of calm and ease throughout your labor. Beginning at the top of the head, as we learned to do in Chapter 5, move your attention down through your body to your feet. If you find an area of tension—for example, between the eyebrows, at the jaw muscles, the tops of the shoulders, or around your hips—bring your attention directly into that area. Breathe into the sensations. As you breathe out, see if the tightness softens or releases just a bit. Practicing in this way between contraction-expansions, you may find that you are able to welcome the next ice contraction with a bit more equanimity and ease. You may also be able to do the same during labor itself.

The Body as a Whole

Earlier you used the expanded sense of the body as a whole for working with the physical sensations of ice in your hand or hands. This sense of the body as a whole, a body that is opening and allowing another human being to leave the world inside your body and enter another world, can also be a place to rest between contraction-expansions. Try it. Notice your experience.

Choiceless Awareness

In Chapter 9 we will learn Choiceless Awareness, the skill of holding whatever is most predominant in your immediate experience—the breath, body sensations, sounds, thoughts, emotions—in mindful awareness, moment by moment. You can practice Choiceless Awareness in labor both during and between contraction-expansions.

The Image of a Baby

We all have the capacity to visualize—to create images in our mind's eye. For some, this capacity is very well-developed and easier to access than it is for others. Conjuring up an image of a baby during labor may help you remember what these powerful sensations in your body are all about: they're helping to bring your baby out of your body and into your arms.

Between ice sensations, experiment with allowing an image of a baby to arise in your mind's eye. See the color and texture of the baby's hair and the miraculously tiny fingers and toes. Imagine the softness and smell of the baby's skin and the warmth and weight of the baby as you hold him or her close to your body. Continue to hold that image of a baby in your mind as you pick up some ice and hold it through a minute of ice practice. If you'd like, experiment with adding the half-smile during this time. What is your experience of the sensations from the ice in your hand(s) as you visualize a baby? As you visualize a baby *and* gently smile?

In class we have been practicing ice-pain practices for about half an hour, mimicking the rhythm of labor as I lead participants through the many options for being with pain that you have just read. Time has passed, and it is getting late.

"We have to stop for now, but before we say good-night, I'd like to invite each of you to share how your labor is going. Just a word or a short phrase will do." I turn to Ted, who is sitting to my left. "How's your labor going, Ted?"

"It's peaceful," he says, smiling at my request. "Fine," says Monica. "Calm," adds Tomiko. "Manageable." "Surprising." "It still hurts," to which I reply, "No one said mindfulness was going to take away the pain."

"Curious." "Wanting more." "Relaxed." "Doable." "Empowered." And so it goes around the room as each person shares her or his experience of working mindfully with pain.

"It's time to wrap up, but before we go, I want to leave you with a question to ponder this week. When you are practicing, ask yourself: *"Is that which is observing the pain, in pain?"*

Some people look puzzled.

"No," says Emily with certainty. "That which is observing the pain is not in pain."

"Well, then, you have found a place within yourself that is not in pain. Perhaps you can choose to live there more often."

PAIN PRACTICE AND PARTNERS

In the MBCP class it's a given that partners do the pain practices too, even though they're obviously not going to be giving birth. However, not many of us go through this life, or leave it, without having some sort of physical pain. And by participating in the pain practices, partners are learning a valuable life skill for themselves as well.

Pain practice is also an opportunity for partners to open the heart, to cultivate empathy and compassion. Empathy is the ability to resonate with someone else's feelings or difficulties. Its close cousin, compassion, is the ability to identify with the difficulties of another along with the desire to take action to help alleviate those difficulties. The qualities of empathy and compassion in a partner can prove to be invaluable for a woman in labor. They can also be invaluable qualities in the work of parenting—and all dimensions of life.

This permeable envelope that we live in, our skin, is the largest sensory organ of our body, and studies show that warm, pleasurable touch activates the calm-and-connection system. Gentle touching and stroking seems to decrease the fight-or-flight stress hormones, lower blood pressure, and increase oxytocin levels, pain tolerance, and feelings of wellbeing. By using the modality of touch during labor, we can enhance the wisdom already present in our body to help us birth our baby[4]

Although being touched or massaged during labor is welcomed by many women, others don't find it helpful. There is nothing wrong with this, and if this is true for you, your partner needn't take it personally. (Not taking *anything* personally is a profound mindfulness practice in and of itself.) It is not rejection; it's just that being touched at particular moments during labor may not be helpful for a particular laboring woman—nothing more and nothing less. If you find that utter and complete focus on your breath or the body sensations you are experiencing during pain practice is more helpful than touch, so be it.

➤ TOUCH PRACTICES WITH PARTNERS ➤

In the fifth session of the MBCP class, partners learn some simple mindful touch practices for childbirth. They are given below, and you and your partner may want to devote one full pain practice session specifically to experiment with them. They are intended to be used by your partner while you, the pregnant woman, are holding ice, so you can explore how touch works for you in relation to pain.

However, it can also be instructive for partners to experience the touch practices while holding ice and receiving touch from you, the pregnant woman. Though the experience of what is helpful (or not helpful) for them may well be different from yours, their experience of being touched while holding ice will inform how they touch you. And who knows, someday your partner may be experiencing physical pain and be very appreciative that you know something about what brings him or her comfort.

Touch practices involve giving and receiving. For you, the laboring woman, receiving the warmth of loving touch may provide a comforting anchor for your attention during the intense sensations of childbirth. If you're the partner, the one who is giving touch, it can be helpful if you bring the focus of awareness to the warm point of contact between your hand and your partner's body. You might ask yourself this: In the realm of touch, who is giving and who is receiving? Where do I end, and where does the other person begin?

The following seven touch practices are done while you, the pregnant woman, are holding ice in the rhythm of work and rest that you have been practicing. After a minute of touch practice, you can let your partner know what is working for you or what would be more helpful. Partners, adjust your touch according to the feedback, and then practice again. Once you've learned how to work together with some ease while holding ice, practice a series of ice contraction-expansions together in silence, bringing awareness to the breath between ice sensations.

Holding a Hand

Sometimes conveying love and support through touch is very simple, as simple as holding someone's hand. Some partners have told me that their laboring partner was coping so well during the birth process that there really wasn't much for them to do except to be present and hold her hand. That said, there is hand-holding and there is hand-holding. A loosely held hand, a light, tentative touch, or agitated stroking does not convey presence; a firm, confident touch does. Go toward that.

Holding the Head

Place one hand on your partner's forehead and the other at the base of her head, where her skull meets her neck. Let your hands be relaxed as they mold to the shape of her head, yet let the pressure be firm enough so she can totally let go and allow you to hold her head. This can be extremely relaxing; perhaps it evokes a body memory of trust from a time when your partner's head was held as an infant.

Connecting with the Heart

Place one hand on your pregnant partner's breastbone and the other hand on her back, between her shoulder blades. Let your hands make full contact with her body. Imagine how it might feel to be receiving your touch. Do you sense that your partner finds it comforting? If not, ask what she needs, and adjust accordingly.

Connecting with the Uterus

This touch may help focus awareness of the breath at the abdomen, the breathing we do when we are most at ease. Placing one hand on the top of the uterus, place the other hand at the lower back. Keep your hands in this position for one minute while your partner holds ice. Another option is to place one hand directly above the pubic bone and the other hand at the low back.

Holding the Feet

In many places in the world, women labor and give birth with their feet on the ground, either standing or squatting. If your partner is laboring in bed, holding her feet during a contraction-expansion may feel very grounding. Try it. See what her experience is.

Stroking

Some women find that stroking is helpful. See if this is true for your partner. Our nervous system is hardwired so that stroking downward is relaxing while stroking upward is energizing. (This dates way back to when hair covered our bodies.) Experiment with stroking her head, or down her arm, or perhaps down her spine or her legs (especially her inner thighs), or any part of the body she finds comforting. Stroke only one part of her body—her arm or legs or down her spine—during a contraction-expansion, coordinating the downward stroke with her out-breath: she breathes in, your hand is at rest, she breathes out, you stroke down. A slow, steady rhythm is important. For partners, it takes true concentration to do this.

You might also experiment with deeper strokes, massaging her head or her feet or putting pressure on her lower back when she is in Child's Pose, a yoga pose you will learn in Chapter 8. This can be particularly helpful if your partner has back labor.

Making It Up Practice

Just as a laboring woman is encouraged to respond creatively to the messages coming from inside her body during labor, you too can use your senses to respond mindfully and creatively to your partner in the moments of labor. If, for example, you observe that her shoulders appear to be tense, a caring touch there might bring her awareness to that part of her body and allow her to release some tension. Or if you observe her tightening her facial muscles, especially between the eyebrows, during contraction-expansions, your touch there might bring ease as well. Or perhaps you know a way that your partner enjoys being touched when she is not in labor, such as having her hair stroked or her back rubbed in a particular way. By all means, use all that you already know about her and her body to give comfort during labor. Look, listen, feel, and respond in whatever way seems most appropriate in the moment, given who she is, what you already know about her, and who you are.

⟶ THE PRACTICE OF SOUNDING ⟶

One of the most effective, nonpharmacological methods for being with labor pain is sounding. Sounding is an ancient way of sustaining concentration in the present moment. Sometimes it's called chanting and is performed in a ritual or religious context. Gregorian chants of Christian monks, Buddhist chants practiced by monks throughout Asia, and the ceremonial chants of Native Americans are all used to focus the mind in service of a deeper purpose. In labor, we can intentionally use this capacity for sounding in wonderfully helpful ways.

You may feel self-conscious when you do this practice, telling yourself, "I'll never do that in labor" or "This isn't me." Self-consciousness is nothing more than a strongly held idea about who you think you are. If you notice feelings of self-consciousness arising when you do this practice, see if you can just accept those feelings and practice sounding anyway. The truth is that the vast majority of women become so engrossed in the labor process that they report feeling little or no sense of self-consciousness during labor itself.

Meredith, who took the MBCP class because she was terrified of the pain of childbirth, confessed to me on the evening we learned sounding practice that she felt very self-conscious while doing it. A quiet, somewhat shy woman, Meredith worked as a ward clerk in the postpartum unit at the local hospital. After giving birth, she shared this experience in an email to the class.

"That night when we learned sounding in class, I thought to myself, 'I'll never make sounds like this in labor'—especially since I was going to be giving birth around the people I work with. I was worried about what they would think of me. I had some image of myself that I thought I had to uphold.

"But when I was actually in labor, I surprised myself and Shawn by spontaneously making sounds. They were sounds I'd never heard myself make before and will probably never make again—unless of course we have another baby! They just came from a place deep inside. I think that because we had practiced them in class, I knew it was an okay thing to do, so I just let them come. It was so basic—primal even. I just heard the sounds and felt their vibration in my body. I kind of watched myself doing it. It felt really comforting. If I had to pick one thing, I'd say it was sounding that got me through labor."

Some sounds are more effective in labor than others. A high-pitched sound made with a tight throat and a tight mouth is a sound we make when we are afraid or in some kind of distress: we shriek; we scream. However, when the mouth is relaxed, the jaw is soft, and the throat is open, we can have a very different sounding experience, one that contributes to a sense of relaxation or wellbeing.

See what happens when you allow an open vowel sound such as "ahhhh" or "ohhhh" or even the universal sound of "aum" to come from deep within as you breathe out. Remember, the in-breath, with its life-giving oxygen, energizes. The out-breath lets go of that which is no longer needed. Elongating the out-breath may help you let go even more fully into the parasympathetic calm-and-connection system. Feel the energy coming into your body on the in-breath. Feel the sound originating from your diaphragm and belly, vibrating through your rib cage, throat, and vocal cords on the out-breath. Listen to the sounds you are creating as you let go. Sounding can be deeply calming.

Experiment with having your partner sound with you, following the lead of your breathing. Let the pitch of your partner's sounding be slightly lower and just a tad softer than the sounds you are making. This is a time for you to lead and your partner to follow.

See what it might be like to have your partner move in close to you, perhaps putting your head against your partner's chest or letting your heads touch each other as you sound together. You may find the familiar sound of your partner's voice quite soothing. It may remind you that although you are the one birthing your baby, you are not alone.

Sounding and the Fear of Losing Control

Some women have fear of "losing control" during labor. When I ask women who have this particular fear what their image of losing control looks like, they often describe a laboring woman lying in bed, screaming and writhing in pain. Although it may seem paradoxical, sounding can be especially helpful for women who have this particular fear.

When a woman in labor appears to be out of control, what is really happening is that she has gotten lost in her reactions to pain and is very far from the present moment. My midwife strategy for helping a woman who is lost is always the same: bring her back to the present moment, and keep her there. Touch, focused eye contact, and sounding on the out-breath are often key. Moving in close, I place my hand in hers, and with our eyes locked we sound and breathe together, sounding in the moments of contraction-expansion, quietly breathing together when she is not. Usually it takes only a few contraction-expansions for her to find her way back to the rhythm of her breath and her body: working and resting, working and resting. By being fully present with her, I temporarily become her anchor to the present moment. Reconnected with her breath, she can settle into the rhythm of her breath and body once again and manages on her own. She is no longer lost. She is back in the here and now.

EYES OPEN OR EYES CLOSED?

As we know, the pain of labor increases in intensity as the contraction-expansions increase their power for you to birth your baby. For some women, keeping their eyes open during the more intense contraction-expansions in the later stage of labor (transition) can bring balance and decrease the possibility of feeling overwhelmed. Try keeping your eyes open, even looking directly into your partner's eyes during a minute of holding ice. Is it helpful for you? If so, do it. If not, don't do it. You're in charge. It's your labor. You decide.

A WORD ABOUT SILENCE

Once labor is in full gear, most women naturally turn inward. This inward state is to be encouraged, respected, and protected. As much as possible, stimulating the thinking mind (the prefrontal cortex) of a laboring woman is to be avoided, as it may stimulate mental chatter or induce worrying thoughts, which, as we learned earlier, are counterproductive to the normal physiology of the labor process.

Ideally, whoever is with you during labor can encourage you to fully inhabit an inward state of undisturbed, quiet concentration rather than draw you into the thinking mind by asking lots of questions or engaging you in conversation. Even with the best of intentions, asking you to make small choices (Do you want a sip of water? Shall I put a cold cloth on your fore-head?) can be counterproductive. Remember, you are practicing just being, and that takes concentration. Hopefully you and your partner will have done enough mindfulness practice so that the two of you will feel comfort-able in silence together, trying the various practices you've learned without needing to speak with each other. If your partner's guess of what you might need turns out not to be your preference of the moment, most likely he or she will be able to accept this gracefully rather than taking it personally.

The degree to which you will be able to maintain a quiet, peaceful envi-ronment during labor may vary, depending on where you intend to deliver. Monitoring this is something your partner or other members of your birth-ing team can do for you. However, after making known your preference for quiet in your birthing environment, you may be given another opportunity to let go. Sometimes the environment for birthing is wild, noisy, and some-what chaotic, and you may need to maintain focus and concentration any-way. We just don't know how it will be for you, but your friend the breath will be there for you no matter what.

MINDFUL MOVEMENT DURING LABOR

Before giving birth, you may imagine yourself lying in bed during labor. However, your body may tell you otherwise when you are actually in labor. Being upright can be very comfortable during childbirth, often more comfortable than lying down. And research shows that the uterus works most efficiently when the body is upright. Standing or walking during labor can help you feel more comfortable, help your baby move down through your pelvic bones, and keep the whole process moving along. And moving along is definitely what we want!

During pregnancy mindfulness practice helps you become more sensi-tive to the messages of your body so that during labor you will be more attuned to it and do as it asks. In the more active stages of labor, your body may tell you to change positions frequently; standing, sitting, kneeling, squatting, or being on your hands and knees can all be quite comfortable. As mentioned earlier, Child's Pose, a position you will learn in the yoga se-quence in Chapter 8, can also be very comfortable during labor, especially for back labor. Changing positions often (maybe every twenty minutes or so) not only helps you work with the sensations of labor, it may help bring your baby into an optimal position for delivery.

While changing positions can be useful, some women become very still during the labor process. They find a spot—in the corner of a couch, on a bed, in the shower or tub—and just want to stay put, like a mother cat birthing her kittens in a nest of clothes on the floor of a dark closet. If the birthing process is moving along, then staying put is just fine.

Sometimes, however, women resist moving about in labor because they fear that the movement will intensify the sensations of the contraction-expansion. In cases like this, if a woman's labor isn't progressing, I adopt a "midwife knows best" stance, kindly yet firmly encouraging her to get up out of bed, change positions, and move about. Sometimes this means the laboring woman has to confront a new layer of resistance or fear. She may not want to move because she thinks she is handling all she possibly can handle.

This then becomes the time for courage. Courage is not the absence of fear but the inner strength to feel the fear and do what needs to be done anyway. Most often, courageously changing positions and opening to the powerful sensations of transformational pain leads to the change that is needed.

Sometimes a laboring woman discovers that rhythmically rocking or gently swaying back and forth or side to side can also bring comfort. This makes sense; we were rocked inside our mother's womb before we were born, and we were probably rocked for comfort when we were babies. Experiment with rhythmic rocking and gentle swaying during ice practice. Notice your experience. Learn what might be helpful for you when you are actually in labor.

WATER INSIDE AND OUT

Our evolutionary history of moving from sea to land is carried within our bodies—in the composition of our blood and in the fluid inside and around our cells. From our primal beginnings to the complex creatures we are now, water has been foundational. Over half of our body is liquid, and during pregnancy that proportion increases considerably. Pregnancy is a very fluid state.

Water can be a powerful ally during the labor process, facilitating relaxation and ease of mind and body. From actually giving birth in a birthing tub to using a shower or tub at some point during labor, the skillful use of warm water may help you a lot. I often tell class participants that the cry "I don't think I can do this anymore" uttered by a laboring woman can be decoded to mean "I need to be in warm water." It's lovely if that option is available.

However, it's important to remember to keep a conditional attitude toward the use of water—and everything else—about childbirth. You may or may not have time to use a tub; or despite what you expect before labor, water may not be what you want when you are actually in labor. Being in water may not be appropriate, safe, or possible for you or the baby; nonattachment and letting go continue to be key.

BRINGING IT ALL TOGETHER

In the MBCP course we learn all of these mind-body pain practices over a three-week time period. Couples also include them as part of their weekly home practice. By the time we have learned all these practices, the expectant woman and her partner are able to immerse both hands into a bowl of ice water. Mixing and matching what they have discovered works for them, they have built a strong inner capacity to be with the intense physical sensations. After you have worked your way through these experiences, I suggest that you, or you and your partner, do the same—immersing first one hand then two hands into a bowl of ice water as you do the pain practices you have found helpful. Notice the inner strength, resiliency, and courage that have grown within you. You may discover that you are stronger than you ever imagined.

A NOTE ON INFORMAL PAIN PRACTICE

Practicing the exercises above with ice—in a class or at home—is a type of formal practice, a time set aside to specifically practice mindfulness with pain. However, each and every day, especially during pregnancy, you are presented with many opportunities for *informal* pain practice. The common discomforts of pregnancy—heartburn, swollen feet, an aching back—are all opportunities for such practice. Of course this doesn't mean that you shouldn't take something to alleviate heartburn or that you can't ask someone to massage your aching back or feet. Practicing mindfulness with pain is not about purposefully living in pain; it's about working with things as they are, seeing clearly, and taking wise action.

⤙ THE SECOND STAGE OF LABOR:
A PRACTICE FOR PUSHING ⤚

The practices I've shared up to now are intended to help you work with the powerful sensations of the contraction-expansions primarily during the first stage of labor, when your cervix is opening to ten centimeters. In the usual course of things, once ten centimeters is reached, and perhaps after a lull when the contraction-expansions may slow down and you can rest for a bit, you will begin to feel sensations that call you to bear down and push your baby out into this world. The urge to push comes and goes several times during the wave of a single contraction-expansion and it is usually next to impossible to resist.

As surprising as it may be to hear, the best practice I know of to prepare for working with the sensations of the second stage is the informal practice of mindful pooping. Becoming more mindful of pooping sensations during pregnancy can help you become more attuned to your body during the second stage of labor. Sometimes, if a birthing mother is unable to get in harmony with her body during the pushing phase, or if little progress is being made, I will encourage her to go sit on the toilet and push for a while; often this results in progress toward birthing. (Don't worry—it's a rare baby that is delivered with a woman sitting on the toilet.)

Here is how mindful pooping practice works: When you feel the sensations arising in your intestines that signal your mind that you have to poop, bring your full awareness to those sensations. Notice if they feel like cramping or, perhaps sharp or dull. Notice if there are moments of more intensity or less. Notice how that particular body sensation is a message to your brain to take action, to get yourself to a designated place, usually a bathroom, to sit down on a specially designed piece of equipment called a toilet so that a normal process, the body's removal of that which it no longer needs, can occur. See if you can be aware of the moment you form the intention to go to the toilet. Notice if there is a sense of urgency surrounding the sensations.

Once settled onto the designated seat, notice how you actually engage with this basic bodily function (or perhaps more accurately, how this basic bodily function engages you). Notice how you take in a deep breath, hold it, and, using your diaphragm and abdominal muscles, bear down. In harmony with your body's urges to move something from inside your body down and outward, you work with this process. Notice how a small amount of air might escape from your lungs through your tightened throat as you bear down. Notice if any sound, such as grunting, accompanies (or is suppressed) during this event. Notice any odor coming to your nostrils. Be aware of any thoughts or feelings triggered by the odor or any other aspect of this experience of pooping mindfully. Feel your rectum expanding and stretching as the poop emerges. Notice any thoughts or feelings associated with this entire activity—embarrassment, disgust, fascination, whatever. Notice perhaps relief or a sense of ease or even pleasure as the cramping in your intestines subsides with each bearing-down effort and poop is released.

When you are birthing, the pressure from your baby's head coming through the bones of your pelvis and stretching your vagina are very intense and not unlike the sensations of pooping. Becoming more at ease with pooping sensations can take you a long way toward being able to work with the sensations of the baby emerging from your body.

Pooping practice is helpful not only as preparation for birthing; it's an important awareness practice for parenting. You are going to be spending quite a number of years relating to your baby's, and then your toddler's and your child's, poop. You will guide your child's response to pooping sensations (a process otherwise known as toilet training). Becoming aware of your own thoughts and emotions about poop can help you be a more effective teacher and coach during potty training. Though ultimately it depends on the individual child, your mind-set about pooping will influence how your child eventually comes to view this normal bodily function.

With these mind-body practices you now have a wonderful array of options for responding rather than reacting to the multitude of sensations arising and passing during the labor process. Perhaps the caption on the poster of the wise yoga teacher Satchidananda playfully riding ocean waves on a surfboard best captures the spirit of birthing mindfully: "You can't stop the waves, but you can learn to surf." The pain practices we have learned here will be enormously helpful in doing just that.

CHAPTER 8

The Yoga of Childbirth

Stillness is what creates love. Movement is what creates life.
To be still and still moving—this is everything.
—Do Hyun Choe

THE PRACTICE OF yoga is a superb doorway to deep physical and mental relaxation, and the strength, flexibility, and stamina of body and mind cultivated during yoga practice provide wonderful preparation for the challenges of childbirth that lie ahead. Some expectant women come to the MBCP class because they have already found yoga practice helpful in their lives before pregnancy. Others who have never practiced yoga are curious about it and are glad that yoga is included in their birth preparation class. Partners also welcome the opportunity to begin, or strengthen, a yoga practice.

Tonight we will begin learning the yoga sequence offered in the MBCP course. We will start with our yoga practice, the one that is on the CDs I've already given out to all the participants. Then we will practice our Sitting Meditation. The body is usually wonderfully at ease after yoga practice, which makes it an excellent time for Sitting Meditation.

Because yoga practice creates more vivid sensations in the body than the Body Scan we've been practicing for the past several weeks. I know that some people will find it a welcome change. Truth is, the body loves to be stretched, and for most people yoga just feels good. Our next step is learning how to practice yoga mindfully.

The word *yoga* means "to yoke" or "union," and in yoga we yoke or bring into union the body and mind. Practiced mindfully, yoga *is* meditation. Mindful yoga practice gives you the opportunity to observe all sorts of states that might arise in both your body and mind. You may see striving as you move the body into a particular pose. You may notice the judging mind as you observe thoughts about your body ("I'm so big and heavy") or envy as the comparing mind gets going ("I wish I looked as thin and radiant as she does"). With mindfulness you can observe these thoughts, know that they are just thought patterns arising and passing in the mind, and practice kindness and acceptance as you let them go, gently coming back to the breath or to the sensations in your body in the moment.

EXPANSIONS, CONTRACTIONS, AND MINDFULNESS

Sometimes the physical sensations in yoga practice are wonderfully pleasant, like the moment when tightness in the back or shoulders or hips releases and you feel the body let go and become more open. At other times you may experience some not-so-comfortable physical sensations, when you're intensely contracting or stretching your muscles in a challenging pose. During yoga practice you can notice this discomfort, breathe with it, and watch it change into other sensations. When you repeatedly observe how discomfort changes moment by moment during yoga practice and notice how it can be replaced with ease as you go deeper into or let go of a particular posture, you are learning concentration of the mind, inner strength, and confidence in your body—and yourself. This is what happened to Jeri.

Jeri was eight months pregnant. She had been active and healthy throughout her pregnancy, but now she was beginning to feel physically uncomfortable. In class one evening, Jeri described an experience that helped her wake up.

"One of the poses, the Warrior Pose, was really hard for me. My arms would hurt, my legs felt weak, and I just didn't like doing it! I found myself in the future a lot, really dreading the time when I'd have to do that particular pose. But the last time I practiced I decided to see if I could just do it without all the drama my mind was getting into. When I noticed I was worrying about the pose coming up, I just brought my attention back to the breath and to the sensations of whatever pose I was doing in the moment. And when I finally came to the Warrior Pose instructions, somehow it wasn't such a big deal. I still didn't like the sensations in my arms and my legs, but I think my mind let go of some of the expectations about how bad it was going to be, so my body wasn't as tense when I was actually doing it. And of course I totally see how I can use this for labor. I really surprised myself when I had the thought that maybe labor might not be such a big deal too! Yeah, I should be so lucky!" She laughed.

Like Jeri, you can use yoga practice as an opportunity to work with the mind's resistance to unpleasant or intense sensations in the body and perhaps move through them. You can notice the exact moment your mind generates resistance in the form of a contracting thought of "not liking" certain poses, and you can choose how to relate to those sensations. If the mind says, "I don't like this" or "this is too hard" or "I can't do this," you can notice and let go of these resisting, contracting thoughts, just like Jeri did, and return to the breath or the body sensations themselves.

In your yoga practice you can also experiment with breathing into the uncomfortable sensations of a pose and perhaps softening around them on an out-breath, just as you might during labor. Or you can move your attention directly into the sensations and explore them with focused concentration and curiosity.

GOING TO YOUR EDGE

With yoga you have a special opportunity to cultivate the attitude of non-striving, one of the qualities of mindfulness you learned about in Chapter 2. This non-striving attitude may be different from the way you have practiced yoga in the past or the way you have approached other forms of physical activity. Yoga is sometimes viewed through the lens of physical exercise, particularly by those new to yoga, bringing the same habit of striving to reach a goal that can characterize the attitude you bring to, say, working out at the gym. Though yoga is certainly a tremendously beneficial form of physical activity, it's also helpful to see it as a meditative discipline. This way we can use yoga as a chance to practice not trying to be anywhere other than exactly where we are.

Practicing yoga mindfully, you go to the edge of discomfort, listening to what your body is telling you, respecting its limits, and taking care not to push beyond them. Being pregnant, you need to take special care not to overstretch. Relaxin, a hormone released at ten times its normal concentration during pregnancy, is softening the ligaments and joints in your pelvis, preparing for the expansion that occurs when your baby passes through it. While this is wonderful for the pelvis, relaxin also softens the joints throughout your entire body, making you particularly susceptible to overstretching. So while it's important during yoga to challenge yourself and explore your limits, it's also important not to overstretch. In general, this is sound advice for partners too. Listening to the body and responding to its sensations with respect, intelligence, kindness, and care, you practice yoga mindfully.

I sometimes hear pregnant women say that one reason they are afraid of childbirth is because they've never done any demanding physical work or faced any kind of challenging pain. This makes it especially interesting to notice what the mind does in a yoga pose that brings intense sensations. Does it go to a fearful place, like, "I don't think I can do this" or "I'm afraid if I hold this pose any longer I'll hurt myself"? Watch what thoughts or images arise when you're close to your physical edge. Is this a time when you might want to explore courage and inner strength a bit more? Perhaps you have more of both of them than you imagined. Or is this the time to back off with the grace and kindness of non-judging? Only by listening to your body can you know what is best for you in any particular moment.

Remember, with mindfulness there is no success and no failure. There is only what is.

STANDING, SITTING, LYING DOWN, AND WALKING: BEING IN THE BODY MINDFULLY DURING CHILDBIRTH

Sensations are the only language the body can use to speak to us, and we are wise to listen to their messages. During labor, the body often asks us to be in many different positions—standing, walking, sitting on a birthing ball, or leaning forward onto a bed or chair. All of these postures can bring greater ease to labor. Being upright in labor often feels good, and this is the position where the uterus contracts most efficiently. Alternating periods of walking or standing with periods of rest can definitely help in the process of labor.

If you are giving birth in a hospital, it's helpful to know what the hospital's guidelines are for being upright and out of bed during labor and what their guidelines are for continuous fetal monitoring for a laboring woman who has had a normal, healthy pregnancy. For many women, it's not necessary to be tethered to a machine throughout labor. (You will learn more about this in Chapter 16.) However, even if the use of a fetal monitor machine becomes necessary, you needn't stay in bed just because you have a monitor belt around your belly. Stand up. Move. You're not sick. You are in labor, working to birth your baby!

It has been said that there are at least sixty-five thousand yoga postures and that if you are moving and stretching the body, you are most likely using a yoga posture—or a variation of one. A friend and midwife who for decades assisted birthing families at home, where women were free to assume any position during labor, kept a journal of the positions women used both for labor and birthing. She stopped counting when her count was well over two hundred. I wonder, had she had kept counting, if she eventually would have come up with sixty-five thousand postures for giving birth!

Remember, there are as many ways to give birth as there are women who are pregnant. There is no one right way. There is only you, in your body, finding your way, moment by moment. Through yoga practice you can cultivate the attentiveness, strength, flexibility, freedom, and courage to move and adapt to the changing conditions of the labor process, practicing the yoga of childbirth during labor and birthing itself.

THE REST BETWEEN TWO NOTES

While we obviously focus on the various postures during our yoga practice, it's important to know that *sustaining awareness between poses* is as important as the poses themselves. In these moments between poses the mind often flies away, just as it does in the space between inhaling and exhaling. Maintaining our attention between poses by coming to the breath gives us a sense of how we can sustain awareness in those precious moments between contractions, as the childbirthing rhythm of work and rest, work and rest, unfolds.

In addition to the breath, the prenatal yoga sequence in the MBCP course often uses the Mountain Pose, which is essentially Standing Meditation, as a place of rest. Like the breath, the Mountain Pose can become a kind of home, a stable, grounded posture between the more fluid, active standing postures and a familiar place of refuge during labor itself when you are upright.

MINDFUL MOVEMENT

While everyone in the MBCP course, expectant women and their partners, practices yoga, some people already have an established exercise routine, such as walking or swimming. While yoga is explicitly a meditative discipline, *any* physical activity done mindfully can become a mindfulness practice. My point is this: yoga is a fabulous mind-body preparation for childbirth, but you don't have to practice yoga in order to prepare for childbirth. By practicing *any* physical activity mindfully, you will be training your mind and body for giving birth.

A competitive swimmer in high school and college, Sue delightedly reported to the class one evening how she was applying mindfulness practice to her favorite exercise. "Now I'm practicing mindful swimming. I'm really paying attention to the sounds and the sensations as I breathe out in the water, and really paying attention as I turn my head to take a breath.

Sometimes I concentrate on the sensations in my arms or sometimes on the sensations in my legs kicking in the water. It's weird to say this, but I've been swimming for most of my life, and I'm just realizing how much of the time I haven't really been swimming!"

Walking, dancing, using machines at the gym—and birthing a baby—all can be opportunities to practice yoking the body and mind and to be more awake and present in our lives.

THE YOGA OF EVERYDAY LIFE

We can extend the mindfulness we cultivate in our formal yoga practice to all our movements throughout the day: the yoga of balancing as we mindfully stand on one leg to put on our pants; the yoga of reaching and stretching as we mindfully put away clean dishes from the dish drainer; the yoga of mindfully lifting a baby from a car seat. These are the blessings of fully living the yoga of everyday life.

⇀ A SIMPLE YOGA SEQUENCE ⇀

The yoga sequence outlined in the following figures works well for anyone, pregnant or not. Here are some general guidelines to keep in mind as you practice yoga mindfully:

1. Though these yoga poses are relatively simple, don't underestimate their power. If you practice consistently, as participants in the MBCP class do, you will notice that your body will develop greater musculoskeletal strength and flexibility all on its own.

2. Do the postures slowly and deliberately, paying careful attention to the sensations in your body as they change moment by moment. When the mind wanders, notice where it has gone, and bring it back to either the sensations in the body at that moment or to the breath.

3. A general guideline about breathing is to inhale when you bring the arms upward or outward and to exhale when you release the arms or go down into a pose. No need to worry about coordinating the breath with the movements once you are in a pose; just use the breath as an anchor for the mind. As it does during labor, the breath will take care of itself.

4. As mentioned earlier, the time *between* poses is as important as the poses themselves. Do your best to sustain present-moment awareness between the postures by staying with the breath and body sensations after a particular pose. In

this way you may be able to become familiar with the rhythm of work and rest that you will also experience in labor. The Mountain Pose can be used as a resting pose between the standing postures in this particular sequence.

5. If you are new to yoga, you might begin by holding a pose for three to five breaths or about fifteen to twenty seconds. As you practice you may find that you can gradually increase the time you are in a pose. Finding what is appropriate for you and your body in any particular moment on any particular day is part of finding your own way.

6. Do your best to go toward your edge without going beyond it. Maintaining an attitude of non-striving is key. If you ever wonder about whether to expend more effort or less, err on the side of caution. Take care not to overstretch the ligaments, especially at the joints in the pelvis—the symphysis pubis, or sacroiliac, joints. Honoring and respecting the limits of your particular body at any moment in time cultivates self-compassion and acceptance.

7. While maintaining an attitude of non-striving, see if you can turn toward rather than away from sensations of discomfort, softening or relaxing into the sensations gently, with openness and goodwill.

8. From time to time you might like to experiment with closing your eyes during yoga practice. It may help you bring more focus to the sensations of contractions and expansions you are experiencing as well as to the time between yoga poses.

9. When your attention is going back and forth between looking at an illustration in this book and coming back to the body, it's difficult to drop deeply into the present moment. Unless you are familiar with the poses and this way of practicing, you may find it easier, at least in the beginning, to practice with the audio guided meditations. You can order them from the MBCP website listed in Appendix B.

10. Adapt any given posture to suit the needs of your particular body by adjusting a pose so that it is either more strenuous or less. If you are using the audio guides, do come out of a pose sooner than is being suggested there if you need to. If there is a pose you are unable to do, just imagine yourself doing it in your mind's eye, or replace it with another pose you are able to do.

11. If your body is asking for more stretching and a longer practice session, feel free to practice a pose more than once, add some poses, or make up a pose of your own.

12. If you are attending a prenatal yoga class in addition to this home yoga practice, see if you can set an intention to bring more mindful awareness into your prenatal class time.

A SIMPLE YOGA SEQUENCE

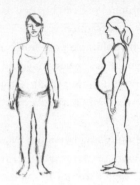

Figures 1 and 2

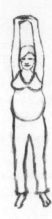

Figure 3

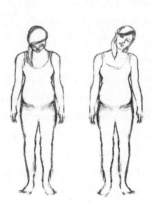

Figures 4 and 5

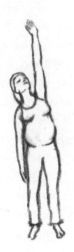

Figure 6

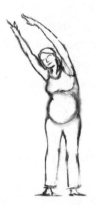

Figure 7

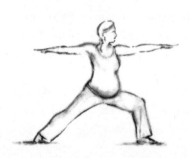

Figure 8

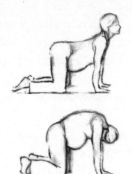

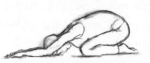

Figure 11

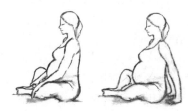

Figures 9 and 10

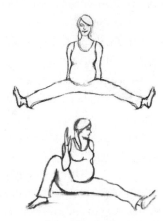

Figures 12 and 13

Figures 14 and 15

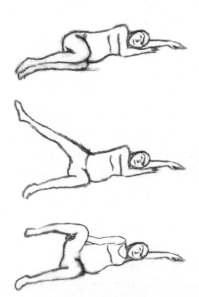

Figures 16, 17, and 18

NOTES FOR INDIVIDUAL YOGA POSES

In addition to the general guidelines, you may find it helpful to review the following notes about the individual yoga poses shown in the diagrams, especially if you are not using the audio guided instructions. This sequence of poses should take about twenty-five to thirty minutes, depending on your pace and whether you repeat any poses or add some of your own.

Mountain Pose (Figs. 1 and 2)

The Mountain Pose is essentially Standing Meditation. With your feet body width apart, bring your awareness to the places where your feet make contact with the floor. Let your knees soften slightly, and let your sacrum drop toward the floor so that your pelvis holds your pregnant belly like a basket. Let your spine lift upward, relaxed but not rigid, as your arms hang gently at your sides. Let your head be balanced, rising toward the ceiling so that you become a stable, standing, breathing mountain, feet grounded below you as your head reaches upward toward the sky.

Deep Breath Chest Opener x 3 (Fig. 3)

Standing in Mountain Pose, interlace your fingers and turn your palms outward. As you inhale deeply, sweep your arms up over your head. Align your arms alongside your ears as best you can. Feel the expansion in your rib cage created by inhaling—in the chest, along your sides, and in your back. As you breathe out, let go of your interlaced fingers and rotate your arms back and down, feeling the movements in the shoulder joints. Let your arms come to rest at your sides. Repeat two more times.

Return to Mountain Pose, standing, breathing, balanced, and fully present.

Neck Rolls x 3 (Figs. 4 and 5)

While in Mountain Pose, inhale deeply. As you exhale, drop your head forward, letting your chin fall toward the center of your chest. Inhaling, and then on the exhale, rolling your head diagonally to the right. Let the head hang so that your right ear is over the right shoulder, pausing here for a breath or two, feeling the stretch on the left side of your neck. And when you are ready, breathing in, and on the out-breath, slowly rolling your head diagonally down and over to the left side, being aware of sensations in your neck as they change, moment by moment as you move. Let your head hang with your left ear over the left shoulder, feeling the stretch on the right side of your neck. Repeat rolling your head from side to side at least two more times, paying particular attention to the sensations of stretching. Return to the stillness of Mountain Pose. Notice sensations in the neck.

Picking Fruit (Fig. 6)

Letting your weight shift to your right leg and foot, inhale as you lift your right arm slowly above your head, letting your right palm face inward. Raise your left heel slightly off the floor. Exhale, and on the next in-breath, stretch upward as if you're picking a piece of fruit that's just barely out of reach. Dropping your head back and looking up at this imaginary fruit, feel the stretch all along the right side of your body, expanding as you breathe in, softening and releasing as you breathe out.

Notice if your left shoulder has lifted up toward your left ear. If so, release it. Hold the stretch for several breaths, or as long as is comfortable or appropriate for you. On an out-breath, slowly lower your right arm and left heel, bringing your awareness to the sensation of your arm lowering moment by moment until it comes to rest at your side and both feet are flat on the ground once again.

Repeat as above on the left side, then return to Mountain Pose—standing, resting, being present, right here, right now.

Side Stretch (Fig. 7)

Breathing in, bring your arms overhead, palms toward each other. As you breathe out, bend to the left. Become aware of the expanding, opening sensations on the right side of the chest, ribs, and back as the breath comes into the lungs and is released. Reaching the arms outward, keeping the head centered between the arms, being in this posture, just breathing and observing, for several breaths. And when you are ready, slowly return to standing upright on an in-breath. On the next out-breath, bending slowly to the right side. Notice the sensations on the left side of the body—between the ribs on the side, front, and back. Stay in this posture, breathing and observing, for several breaths. And when you are ready, inhale and come up to standing once again. Sustaining awareness, slowly lower your arms on the out-breath, and return to Mountain Pose once again.

Warrior Pose (Fig. 8)

Placing your feet three or four feet apart, let the toes of the front foot turn outward and the toes of the back foot turn inward about thirty degrees. Make sure that the heel of the front foot is aligned with the arch of the back foot, giving your body a stable base for this pose. Now as you inhale, raise your arms to shoulder height, and as you breathe out, bend the front knee, keeping it aligned with the front ankle. If the knee moves beyond the ankle, move your feet so that they are a little farther apart. Sitting down into the pose, hips facing forward, look out over the front arm and its outstretched hand and fingers.

Feel the warrior energy in this pose. Notice the sensations of contraction in the front quadriceps and perhaps some stretching, expanding sensations in the opposite groin. Keeping your arms parallel to the floor, let your shoulders drop away from the ears, your shoulder blades sliding down your back, opening and lifting the chest at the breastbone. Breathing, being present with sensations just as they are. And when you are ready, inhale, and on the exhale let your arms come down and legs straighten. Bringing your feet together, return to Mountain Pose—and rest there.

Repeat as above on the opposite side.

Cat-Cow (Figs. 9 and 10)

This pose is basic for back health, whether you are pregnant or not.

Coming to your hands and knees, place your arms directly under your shoulders and your knees directly under your hips. If you feel any wrist pain in this pose, you can make fists instead of placing your hands flat on the floor. Now on an in-breath, lift your head and look up toward the ceiling as you extend the front of your body from the pubic to the breastbone. Keeping your arms straight, slide your shoulder blades down your back. Taking care not to strain your lower back, let your pelvis stay over your knees as you gently extend your lower back and buttocks toward the wall behind you so that the low back remains flat.

Now on the out-breath, allowing the head to drop, looking toward your pubic bone and letting the back arch upward, like a Halloween cat. Feeling the stretch in your lower back as you hold the pose. And on an in-breath, raise your head so that once again you're looking toward the ceiling, taking care to bring the lower back into a neutral position. Continue moving back and forth between these positions as many times as feels comfortable. And when you are ready, move into the next pose, Child's Pose (fig. 11), and rest.

If you find yourself getting up several times during the night to pee, you might experiment with doing the Cat-Cow on your bed ten to fifteen times, then roll onto your side to sleep. The movement of the Cat-Cow lifts the uterus off the bladder, giving it more room to expand, so you may find that you don't have to get up to use the bathroom quite as often.

Child's Pose (Fig. 11)

Moving your knees slightly outward from the Cat-Cow position, lower your buttocks onto your lower legs, and let your forehead come down to the floor. Your arms can either extend forward as you see in the illustration or be along your sides with your palms facing upward. You can also stack your hands or fists underneath your forehead if that's more comfortable. Rest here in Child's Pose, bringing full awareness to the breath and sensations in the body. This can be a wonderfully relaxing pose now and during labor, especially if you are feeling a lot of intense sensations in your back.

Sitting Pose (Figs. 12 and 13)

(Fig. 12) Maintaining awareness as you shift out of Child's Pose, come to a sitting position. Bringing the soles of your feet together, let your knees fall to the sides, as shown. If you have pillows or blankets available, you may wish to sit on them, so that the pelvis tilts forward slightly (not shown). You could also put something under your knees for support. Allowing your spine to be upright but not rigid, with the head balanced on the neck, shoulders dropping away from the ears. Sitting in stillness, feeling the breath; noticing any thoughts and emotions; maintaining your awareness of body sensations; dwelling in the here and now.

(Fig. 13) This is a variation on the Sitting Pose. With your arms behind you, your hands resting on the floor, fingers turned toward the buttocks, lift the breastbone slightly upward, opening the chest. This can be a very restful pose, one that allows for a full expansion of the chest, which can bring both renewed energy and ease.

Gentle Seated Twist (Figs. 14 and 15)

(Fig. 14) Supporting the upper body as in Fig. 13, place the legs in a V, letting the pelvis tilt slightly forward. Let the legs be straight, feet flexed with toes pointing up toward the ceiling. Feeling the stretch in the backs of the legs and perhaps in the inner groin and hips, rest in an awareness of sensations of contraction and expansion, just being with things as they are.

(Fig. 15) And when you are ready, bend one of your legs, placing your foot on the floor as you see in the illustration. Inhaling, and as you exhale gently turn toward the outstretched leg, placing the elbow and arm in front of the bent knee, letting the opposite arm provide support behind you as you twist gently toward the outstretched leg, moving first from the lower back, then the midback, the upper back and shoulders, and finally turning the head so that it looks out over the back shoulder. Take care to go only as far as is appropriate for your body right now, not pushing beyond your limit. Stay with the sensations of expansion and contraction for several breaths, and when you are ready, slowly unwind on an out-breath—first the head, then the shoulders, the midback, and the lower back—until you return to the starting position.

Straighten the bent leg, and bend the other knee as you place that foot on the floor. Repeat as above, this time turning toward the other out-stretched leg.

Side-Lying Birthing Squat (Figs. 16, 17, and 18)

(Fig. 16) Lying on your side with your knees bent so that they are at right angles to your pelvis, let your head be supported by your arm, with your hand placed above the ear, elbow bent, or rest your head on your arm lying flat on the floor, as you see illustrated.

(Fig. 17) Now straightening the top leg, very slowly raise it toward the ceiling, feeling the contraction in the leg and hip muscles as you do so. Raise the leg as high as is appropriate for you today.

(Fig. 18) Now, bending the knee, bring the bent leg up and out in the direction of the armpit, feeling the pelvis open as you do so. This side-lying squat can be very restful. It opens the pelvis quite wide and therefore can be a wonderful posture for giving birth.

Straightening the leg so that the foot is toward the ceiling, rotate the foot a few times in one direction, then the other. This can be very helpful if you have swelling in the lower legs and ankles as it helps pump blood and other fluid back from your legs where it may be pooling. After rotating the foot several times in each direction, breathe in, and then on the out-breath very, very slowly lower the leg down to the floor, noticing the contraction in the muscles of the leg and the sense of ease and release as that leg comes to rest against your other leg at the end of the pose.

Turn to the other side and repeat the movements above.

Lying Down/Resting Pose

If you are early in your pregnancy or are a partner, come to rest on your back in the same posture you used for practicing the Body Scan. Allowing your attention to come to the breath at the belly—to the rising of the belly on the inhalation and the release of the belly on the exhalation. Expand your awareness to the body as a whole, lying here, just breathing, dwelling in stillness.

If your pregnancy is further along, lie on your side as you did in Fig. 16 above. Consider putting a pillow under your head, under your belly, between your knees, and underneath the top arm. Once again, become aware of the breath at the belly as you lie here. If you care to, you can widen your awareness to the body as a whole, dwelling in stillness, and perhaps in peace.

And when you are ready, opening your eyes and slowly rolling onto your side if you have been lying on your back. Gently push yourself up to a sitting or standing position, noticing any sense of relaxation or ease. Allowing this inner ease and calm to become a part of the next moments of your life—and the next, and then the next.

CHAPTER 9

Deepening and Expanding Your Practice
Sitting Meditation

We study the mind because we want the harmony of peace to
prevail, because we need the joy of love in our hearts, because we
care about the quality of life our children will inherit. . . . To be
attentive requires tremendous love of living.
—Vimala Thakar

IN THE MBCP course we begin our Sitting Meditation practice on the very first evening using Awareness of Breathing, as you learned in Chapter 4. As we practice week by week and our concentration becomes steadier, we gradually expand sitting practice to include other objects of awareness, such as body sensations and the body as a whole (as we learned in the Body Scan), as well as awareness of sound, thoughts, and emotions, until finally we sit in Choiceless Awareness: just sitting, just noticing whatever is arising and passing in our mind-body, moment by moment. Though the breath remains our anchor and our refuge, this gradual scaffolding of other elements within our formal sitting practice allows us to strengthen awareness of the ever-changing nature of experience and to connect more deeply with the many-faceted ways of being human.

The majority of expectant parents who take the MBCP course are new to meditation practice and in the early weeks when they first begin paying attention to the breath, they find that their moments of awareness are few and far between. If you are new to meditation practice, this may be true for you as well. But through weeks of practice, gently bringing the mind back every time it wanders, you may discover that a certain continuity of attention begins to emerge. If you commit to a daily mindfulness practice like the course participants do, you too may find that gradually you are here, in this moment, more often. Like muscles being developed through weight training, your capacity to be mindful gets stronger with practice, and you may find that you have more concentration, calm, and presence in your daily life.

The well-known meditation teacher Thich Nhat Hanh sometimes uses the analogy of unfiltered apple juice when he talks about the mind. When a bottle of unfiltered apple juice sits on a shelf for a while, the sediment settles to the bottom of the bottle and the juice itself becomes clear. However, if the bottle is shaken it becomes cloudy and opaque. With mindfulness practice, if the apple juice of our mind gets shaken a little, or even a lot, we have a way to settle it down again.

Life being what it is, there will always be times when the mind becomes agitated. And that can certainly be true when we are pregnant, giving birth, or parenting. But we can always come back to the breath and let the sediment settle once again. Apple juice doesn't judge itself—it isn't bad or wrong for having sediment or for becoming agitated, and neither is our mind. With practice we may find we get agitated less frequently, or when agitation does arise it isn't as strong or doesn't last as long as it did in the past. Able to see both our inner experience and our relationship to the outer world with more clarity and accuracy, we open the way to greater equanimity, clarity, and contentment.

It's a little before 7:00 P.M. on a Friday evening, and I am standing at the door of my home, greeting the expectant parents who have signed up for an intensive mindfulness-skills weekend workshop that I call the Mind in Labor. One of the couples looks vaguely familiar. The woman greets me with a broad smile and says, "Hi, Nancy! My name is Marjorie, and this is Neal. You might not remember us, but five years ago Neal and I spent two hours with you when I was pregnant with our first baby, Coby. What you taught us was truly life-changing and definitely got me through the labor. So when I was looking for a refresher class and saw that you were teaching this weekend, I said to Neal, 'We've got to do this!' It's really great to see you again!"

Sometime during the workshop on Saturday I used the analogy of the untrained mind and the apple juice, and on Sunday morning Marjorie arrived bursting with excitement.

"Nancy, you won't believe what happened! When we got home from the workshop yesterday, Neal and I found this big gallon jar of muddy water on the kitchen counter. The mud in the water had almost all settled to the bottom, but still, it was pretty gross to have this dirty jar on the kitchen counter. So I said, 'Hey, Coby. What's this?' And he says to me 'Oh, Mom, that's something Allison showed me today.' (Allison is the college student who takes care of Coby sometimes.) 'Look, Mom, this is your mind if you don't meditate.' And with that he goes over and gives the jar a big shake. And then he says, 'Allison showed me how to meditate today. Bye, Mom, I'm going to settle down my mind.' And with that, he skips off to his room and closes the door. Wow! I wish I had known about meditation when I was five years old!"

⟶ FORMAL SITTING PRACTICE ⟵

Before you begin any of the meditation practices that follow, take some time to find a position that is comfortable, stable, and balanced. If you are far along in your pregnancy, you may find it helpful to put a pillow at your lower back. Sit however you need to, but do see if you can bring some openness to the chest and front of the body. It's helpful to sit with your spine upright but not rigid. Being pregnant, you may find that lying on your side is best; however, if you do practice lying down, take care not to fall asleep; use the remedies you learned for working with sleepiness in the chapter on the Body Scan.

As you have already learned, if at any time you feel the baby move while you are practicing, just let your attention be with those particular sensations and the breath at the belly; then, when the baby has quieted, return your attention once again to whatever practice you are working with. If you ever feel lost or unsure what to do during any of the practices, return home to your friend, the breath.

Mindfulness of Breathing

Now, if you are ready, allow your attention to come to the sensations of breathing, wherever you experience the breath most vividly as a physical sensation—perhaps at the belly, perhaps at the nostrils, or perhaps at the chest. And just rest in the awareness of the changing sensations of breathing. Breathing in and *knowing* that you are breathing in, breathing out and *knowing* that you are breathing out, bring your attention as best you can to the moment-to-moment changing sensations of this process we call breathing. When thoughts carry you away from the breath, after noticing what is on your mind, let go of the thought, and kindly and gently return your attention to the breath.

This basic Awareness of Breathing practice is profound, and if you learn to do nothing more than to come to the breath when the mind wanders or when you feel distress, you—and everyone around you—will reap great benefits for the rest of your life.

And when we sit it is possible to learn so much more.

Mindfulness of Body Sensations

Once your attention has become somewhat settled on the breath, open your awareness to other sensations in the body. You have already become familiar with this while practicing the Body Scan. This time, instead of systematically moving awareness through your body as you did during the Body Scan, just allow your attention to focus on whatever sensation in the body is predominant at any particular moment.

You may feel some tightness in your lower back or warmth or tingling in your hands. Simply turn your attention to the sensation or sensations, whatever and wherever they might be, whether they are pleasant, unpleasant, or neutral. Letting the breath be in the background, hold the sensations in your awareness in the foreground, moment by moment, as long as it is your predominant experience. See if you can observe how the sensation or sensations are changing.

If there is no particular sensation calling your attention, turn your awareness to a place where the body is in contact with a surface, such as your back against the chair, your buttocks and backs of your legs against whatever you are sitting on, the soles of your feet against the floor, or the weight of your hands on your thighs or your lap. Wherever you place your attention, see if you can bring a sense of curiosity to your experience.

Mindfulness of the Body as a Whole

After bringing awareness to specific sensations in your body, let your awareness expand to a sense of the body as a whole, just sitting, breathing, alive, perhaps having a sense of entirely inhabiting the porous, flexible envelope we call our skin. Notice if, when you're expanding your awareness to the body as a whole, you can sense your baby cradled within.

Notice how your mind, like your body, has the innate capacity to expand *and* that you can make a choice to do that. If you are pregnant, an extraordinary expansion of your body is already taking place within your expanding uterus and abdomen, within your expanding breasts as the structures that will provide milk for your baby grow and mature, and in all the expansion that comes from the increased blood and other fluids that are a part of this life-giving process. Remember that you are learning a skill here, a way to expand your mind to be in harmony with this expansion taking place in your body.

Mindfulness of Sound

Your ability to receive sound through your ears is quite amazing, and when you stop to really pay attention to sound, your appreciation for this capacity may grow. When sound waves are set in motion by vibrations in the air within hearing distance—a car engine starting, the strings of a guitar being strummed, the enthusiastic shouts of children on the playground, rain drumming on the roof—they are received into your body through your ears. Incredibly sensitive mechanisms—membranes, bones, and fluids—pick up these vibrations, transform them into neural impulses, and send the information we call sound to your brain. We may think we hear with our ears, but actually we hear with our brain. What an extraordinary ability this is, and how infrequently we acknowledge this astounding capacity of ours!

During your sitting practice, allow your attention to turn toward sound. Notice that there is nothing you need to *do* to receive sound. You can just turn your awareness toward sound and allow it to be received, just as you can allow and receive the breath. And as you will be able to allow and receive the contraction-expansions of labor.

Notice that some sounds are near, perhaps so close by that they're coming from your own body or the room you are sitting in—the sounds of your own breathing, the furnace turning on or off, a clock ticking, or the refrigerator motor humming. Other sounds may be farther away—a songbird in full voice in a neighbor's tree, a car or sounds of traffic from a nearby street, or a dog barking in an apartment across the way. Notice how sound travels to you from a particular direction. Notice that sound arises out of silence, is present for some moments, changes, and passes away. Notice if within a sound that may seem constant you can detect variation within the sound.

Notice too if you have a preference for some sounds over others. Sound is a wonderful vehicle for noticing our reactivity and for learning how to work with "not-liking" in the present moment. When we hear a sound that we don't like we call it noise and do our best to change it, stop it, or get away from it. Forgetting that the label *noise* is a personal interpretation, and forgetting that we have the option of acknowledging, allowing, being with, and accepting sound in the present moment as it is, we can generate a huge reactive story in response to what we call noise, complete with lots of unpleasant emotions, including anger. Loud music from a neighbor's sound system can easily become a drama of our own making: "I don't know how those people can stand that music! Why can't they turn it down!" Like throwing kindling on an already burning fire, our reaction adds a layer of suffering to the unpleasant experience of hearing loud sounds not of our choosing.

While you're practicing with sound, notice if the mind gets busy creating a story. You're practicing being with this moment however it is right now— there's no need to evaluate, judge, fix, or figure anything out. Of course if sounds are present indicating that action needs to be taken, by all means do so. But if that's not the case, see if you can just be aware of sound as sound, holding the impermanent vibrations you are receiving through your ears in mindful awareness. Simply hearing. Nothing more.

You may have the expectation or hope that during your labor you will be surrounded by silence or by the pleasant sounds of favorite, soothing music. This may indeed happen, but it may not. Like Marie, who found herself laboring to the sounds of city workers repairing a broken sewer pipe outside the window of the only available labor room, you may find the situation in which you give birth unexpectedly noisy. Yet with your practice, you may still be able to stay balanced, focused, and centered regardless of what is going on around you. Practicing being with sound, even when it is unpleasant or unwanted, is excellent preparation for "being with what is" during childbirth.

Mindfulness of Thoughts and Emotions

After being with the breath, then being with sensations in the body and the body as a whole, then being with sound, observing all these experiences as they arise, change, and pass away, we are now ready to turn our attention to thoughts and emotions. In this meditation we notice thoughts as discrete events that arise and pass through the mind. We practice noticing thoughts and emotions much the same way we observed the breath. We notice the exact moment a thought arises in the mind, and then, sustaining our attention, we observe the thought as it moves through the mind, until finally that particular thought ends. It's done. Over. Gone. And then another thought arises. And again we place our attention on the arising and passing thought and watch it pass.

When we practice being aware of thoughts as just thoughts, it can be helpful to imagine the mind as a vast blue sky and thoughts as clouds that appear, float through the mind, and then disappear. Some thoughts can be like storm clouds, densely charged with the energy of emotion. Other thoughts are like light, wispy clouds that float gently through the mind without much charge. But whether the thoughts are heavy ("She should never have said that to me!"), or light ("I wonder what we'll have for dinner"), the vast blue sky of the mind remains unaffected. See if you can just sit with your awareness as spacious as the vast blue sky, observing the interplay of thoughts and emotions, moment by moment.

Another image that can be helpful when trying to become aware of the thinking process itself is to imagine your mind as a blank movie screen and thoughts as insubstantial images flashing onto the screen and then disappearing. Or imagine the mind as an empty stage, with thoughts appearing from one wing, dancing across the stage, and then disappearing on the other side. Whatever image you use, if any, see if you can just notice thoughts as temporary, effervescent, fleeting events in the mind.

Sitting and observing thoughts gives us the opportunity to disengage from the *content* of our thoughts and to take a closer look at the thinking process itself. Because of this amazing capacity of ours to observe our own thoughts, over time we can learn to disengage from the endless content of our thinking, at least to some degree. And with this learning we may come to an insight that is as profound as it is simple: *our thoughts are just thoughts*. Realizing that thoughts are just thoughts, neurobiological events coming and going, can be enormously liberating. Realizing that *we are not our thoughts* can certainly open up a way to become more flexible in our thinking and perhaps stop taking our thoughts—and ourselves—quite so seriously.

Fiona, who took the MBCP course, was talking with a friend who also practiced meditation. She was describing how frequently her mind wandered and how upset she got when that happened, when her friend said with a wave of her hand, "Oh, that rascal mind!" and they shared a laugh. And with the laugh came a moment of realization: "I had just been taking *everything* so seriously—my meditation practice, Justin and I having a baby, everything at work. I was thinking I had to do everything right—that I had to read all the books, that the birth had to be a certain way, that we have to be perfect parents: this was serious business. I was forgetting all about having fun! That 'rascal mind' phrase unlocked something in me, this tightness that I had been carrying around. Now when I meditate and watch my thoughts jump all over the place, I just say to myself, 'Oh, that rascal mind,' and smile. It has helped me lighten up about everything!"

As we've come to see, a great many of our thoughts are about the future or the past. And the main character in so many of our thoughts is this person we call "I." We give the "I" a starring role—making up story after story about ourselves and all the reasons why we are the way we are. Often the story we tell ourselves about ourselves is incredibly unkind: judging, critical, and self-limiting. Sometimes the story gets positively boring! How liberating it can be when we see that this story is just a string of insubstantial thoughts that arise and pass rather than some unshakable truth about who we are! We are always changing and growing, and we always have choices, even about this entity that we think of as "me." And then we might ask ourselves the delicious question, "If I'm not my thoughts, who am I?" Now *that's* a question that can keep us in don't-know mind for a very long time!

More on Mindfulness of Thoughts and Emotions

An important aspect of observing our thoughts is becoming aware of the interplay between thoughts and emotions. If we pay careful attention to thinking, we can come to see that certain thoughts trigger certain emotions, and other thoughts trigger other emotions. This is something that happens not only in our mind: like those charged storm clouds, thoughts release chemicals in our brain that stimulate changes throughout the body. We saw in Chapter 6 that the body is affected by adrenaline generated by fearful thoughts and that having the stress reaction turned on most of the time is detrimental to our health. It's interesting to note that after years of studying how the mind creates suffering like anxiety or depression, some scientists are now turning their attention to how positive thoughts generate *health* for our mind-body. And over and over again many are landing in the same place: that meditation practice can open a door to real happiness.

While you are sitting, if a thought arises that triggers a difficult emotion, such as fear or anger, see if you can locate exactly where in your body you are feeling the particular emotion. Is it in your chest or your throat or your belly or perhaps in the area right under your breastbone called the solar plexus? If your body feels contracted and tight, notice exactly where you feel the tightness. Work with this emotional contraction in the body triggered by thoughts in the mind *in exactly the same way* that you have been learning to work with the physical sensations of birthing contractions. Breathe with it. Be with it. Become curious about it. Be kind to yourself. And know that it won't last.

Conversely, as you sit you can notice thoughts that trigger positive emotions, such as happiness, joy, gratitude, generosity, or contentment. Notice where in the body you feel ease or joy or peace or a sense of expansion and openness. You may notice that these feelings often center in the chest, around the heart. Ever wonder why the heart is a symbol for love? Maybe it's because this is the place in the body that is activated when we feel love.

Choiceless Awareness

Once you have practiced paying attention to the breath, body sensations, sound, thoughts, and emotions, you can experiment with practicing Choiceless Awareness. In Choiceless Awareness you pay attention to whatever is predominant in your experience in each moment. In this moment. And in this moment. And in this moment. Letting go of any particular object of awareness, you just sit in open awareness. The experience of the present moment becomes your practice.

If a pain or ache somewhere in the body calls your attention, notice—aching, pulsing, tightness—and observe it. After a few seconds perhaps a thought arises about the discomfort. Then you notice the thought, the succession of words in the mind that make up the thought as it arises and passes. Then notice with curiosity an attendant emotion if it arises—perhaps fear triggered by a worrying thought that the unpleasant sensation will increase. Then notice where in the body that sensation of fear is located. As the momentary fear passes, you may become more aware of your breath. So you sit, noticing your breath. After you notice several breaths, a sound may call your attention, perhaps from a fire engine passing by. If the sound moves to the fore of your experience, let your attention turn to that, moment by moment, noticing the sound—how it arises and changes. If the sound is far away, you might let the sound be in the background of your awareness, or you might investigate the sensations of agitation in the body that were perhaps triggered by the sound of the fire engine. Or you may stay with the breath. And then you may have another thought. We watch that. And then another thought. We watch that too.

Sitting in awareness, we don't look for anything to happen. We don't hold onto anything. We just sit: still, open, receptive, letting whatever comes come. Dwelling in being, we are in the here and now.

CHILDBIRTH AS PROCESS

As our meditation practice deepens, as we turn our attention inward to all the elements of experience—the breath, body sensations, hearing, thoughts, and emotions—we may come to realize *from our direct experience* that no one moment is like any other and that absolutely nothing stays the same. Really experiencing the impermanent nature of all phenomena on an unmistakable, experiential level can deeply inform your attitudes, your decisions, and the way you live your life.

Knowing unshakably that everything is in constant transformation can be extremely helpful during childbirth. No matter how long your labor takes—hours or days—or how challenging or easy the experience is, it *will* end. Like each meditation and each moment of our lives, each labor lasts only a certain number of breaths. Then it's over. We don't know how many breaths we will take in and release during labor or how many intense physical sensations we call contraction-expansions will arise and pass, but however it goes, it goes. That much we do know.

This awareness of impermanence seems to be invaluable to the expectant parents who learn mindfulness in preparation for childbirth. Over and over again I hear new mothers saying such things as, "Knowing that this wouldn't last was so helpful" or "All I had to do was be in this moment, right now, one contraction at a time, one breath at a time, and I knew I could do this." This isn't ideology; it's wisdom that comes from a true knowing place, a place born from a commitment to cultivate something important—mindfulness—and from the diligence needed to sustain the practice of it over time.

CHAPTER 10

When You're Walking, Just Walk; When You're Birthing, Just Birth

Walking meditation is not a means to an end; it is an end.
Each step is life; each step is peace and joy.
—Thich Nhat Hanh

WALKING MEDITATION is another formal meditation practice we learn in the MBCP course, after the Body Scan, yoga, and Sitting Meditation practices. It is taught during the all-day session that you will read about in Chapter 12. Many expectant parents report how much they enjoy Walking Meditation, which can become an informal practice that is easily incorporated into everyday life. Women commonly mention how helpful Walking Meditation was for them during labor, especially in the early phase, and both parents describe how helpful it can be for comforting a crying baby.

In the formal practice of Walking Meditation, we deliberately bring awareness to this activity we have performed so automatically for most of our lives. Unless we have had some sort of difficulty walking, we generally take it pretty much for granted. If we think about walking at all, we probably think of it as an activity that gets us somewhere other than where we are. Rarely do we think of walking as an activity that can anchor awareness in the present moment.

By bringing mindful awareness to walking, we can begin to appreciate this extraordinary capacity of the human body to move about on two legs. We are the only mammals on earth who do so exclusively, and our evolutionary shift to walking upright changed everything for our species—and for the planet. Having their hands freed from locomotion opened up a world of new possibilities for our primate ancestors, which in turn influenced the development and structure of the brain, especially the prefrontal cortex, the area of the brain associated with problem solving, reasoning capabilities, creativity, complex social interaction, self-awareness, and the modulation of intense emotion—all of which make us culturally complex and distinctively human.

This change to bipedalism also changed the structure of the human pelvis. Human newborns are unique in the animal kingdom for their extreme immaturity and long dependency, in part because of a necessary compromise between physics and the timing of human birth: our human babies need to be born before the skull, which houses this large brain of ours, gets too big to fit through the mother's pelvis. In short, walking on two legs is a very big deal.

Just stop for a moment and take a look at the bottoms of your feet. It's pretty remarkable that such a small surface area can support a body your size. It's quite a feat to be able to shift your weight onto one foot, lift the other foot off the ground, move your raised foot forward, plant it on the ground again, shift your weight onto it, and make the same forward motion with the other foot. Yet we do this over and over again without thinking about it at all. As you may notice while practicing Walking Meditation, the moments when we actually have two feet on the ground as we walk are very few; much of the time while walking we are actually engaged in a kind of controlled forward falling.

Like life itself, walking is a dynamic, fluid process. And like giving birth, walking is an inborn capacity of the body. Scrapes and bruises are inevitable parts of both of these enterprises, yet we keep on keeping on anyway. Eventually we all learn to walk, and eventually birth happens.

During the day of silent meditation practice, Kelly reported a particularly powerful insight. "I had never done Walking Meditation before, and I was curious about it. Well, after walking back and forth maybe eight or ten times, paying attention to lifting my foot, then moving it, then setting it down, followed by the other one, my legs started getting tired. Then I suddenly had this thought: 'I have absolutely no idea how long we will be doing this!' At home, when I was practicing with the CDs, I knew exactly how long the practice would be—thirty minutes. I think of myself as a relatively in-charge person, especially when it comes to my schedule, so this was really a new experience—being asked to do something without knowing when it would end.

"And then I had another thought: 'Maybe she'll have us doing this for the entire day!' And I started to worry. And then I said to myself, 'Wait a minute, Kelly. This is a lot like labor. You won't have any idea how long that will last either. So just accept it as it is and keep walking. If she has us walk for the entire day, so be it.' And then I just really let go and let myself sink into walking. And I felt like I could walk forever."

Some people absolutely fall in love with Walking Meditation practice. Serena, who had a high-powered marketing job, was one of them. "My job is pretty stressful, especially now, when I'm training someone to take over my work while I'm on maternity leave. So by the time the day is over my mind is racing a mile a minute about all the things that happened during the day and what I need to do tomorrow.

"On my way home from work I've started to use Walking Meditation to calm me down. I walk fast but still mindfully. It's like I'm walking off the stress of the day in my mind and body at the same time. My feet remind me to come back to the moment and to just pay attention to them as I walk. Now by the time I get home I'm pretty calm and centered, ready to start dinner or help Kevin cook."

Kevin agrees that Walking Meditation has really helped Serena—and, by extension, him. "She used to come home all stressed out. It could take her most of the evening to unwind but that just isn't happening anymore. It's pretty amazing."

When Serena came to the reunion class and reported that she had used Walking Meditation during much of her labor, no one was surprised. "I had intended to labor at home as long as possible before going to the hospital, so when labor began Kevin and I went to the playground just across the street from our house. It was a really lovely day, and we walked quietly and intentionally. It was so sweet, being in labor and watching all the parents with their kids—pushing the swings and helping them up and down the climbing structures—knowing that this would be us pretty soon."

Kevin and Serena returned to the house and kept on walking mindfully. "When I had a contraction," Serena says, "I would stop and just lean on Kevin and notice my breath. Then when the contraction was over, we'd start the Walking Meditation again. Sometimes during a contraction I experimented with the breathing we learned at the end of the Body Scan, where you actually send the out-breath all the way down and out your feet. It was great because it felt like I was breathing the pain down into the earth. It made me feel grounded, especially when things got pretty intense.

"When I felt tired I would just lie down on the couch and rest for a little bit—I don't know for how long, maybe about twenty or thirty minutes—and then I would get up and start walking again. It actually felt so much better to be walking. It wasn't like we'd planned to do all this walking or anything; it was just what I wanted to do in the moment. Like you said so many times in class, 'Just pay attention to your body, and you'll know what you need to do when you're in labor!'"

Gradually Serena's contractions grew stronger, and they decided it was time to go to the hospital. "The car ride was tough, but I got through it by remembering it wasn't always going to be like this. I was lying on my side in the backseat while Kevin drove, and I remember pushing my feet against the car door so I could still do my 'down to the feet breathing out the pain' thing.

"When we got to the hospital they checked me and I was nine centimeters dilated! The nurses couldn't believe it, and neither could I! I squatted to push, and again, it was great to feel my feet against something. Nathaniel was born about an hour later."

Kevin joins in. "The walking really worked for both of us. And now when Nathaniel cries in the middle of the night, I just take him into the hallway and do Walking Meditation. I figure he liked it when he was being born, so maybe he'll remember that. I don't know if it's true, but it calms *me* down. And when I'm calmer, he seems to be too. Walking Meditation is where it's at for our family!"

⟶ WALKING MEDITATION ⟵

What follows here are instructions for formal Walking Meditation.[1]

1. Find a place, indoors or out, where you can walk back and forth on a path about ten paces long. Walking Meditation looks a bit odd to those who have never seen it before, and their glances (or stares) might make you feel self-conscious, so do your best to find a location for practice that is relatively private.

2. Begin by standing at one end of the walking path with your feet body-width apart and parallel to each other, with your knees slightly bent. Let your arms hang loosely by your sides. (You might recognize this as the Mountain Pose at the beginning of the yoga sequence.) It's fine to clasp your hands in front of you or behind your back if you find that more comfortable. Let your gaze be soft as you look straight ahead.

3. Bring the focus of awareness to the soles of your feet, feeling the physical sensations of your feet in contact with your shoes and the ground underneath them. Feel the weight of your body being transmitted through your legs to your feet and then to the ground. It's fine if you want to practice Walking Meditation barefoot.

4. Now, allowing the left heel to rise slowly from the ground, noticing the sensations in the calf muscles as you do so. Continue allowing the whole of the

left foot to lift gently as your weight shifts onto the right leg. You might notice a small wobble in the right foot, ankle, and leg as they balance the weight of the entire body while your left foot is slowly moving through the air to the ground in front of you. Bring your awareness to the sensations in the left foot and leg as you slowly and carefully move it forward, allowing the left heel to come in contact with the ground. A small, natural step is best. Allow the rest of the left foot to make contact with the ground, experiencing the weight of the body as it shifts forward onto the left leg and the right heel begins to lift off the ground.

5. With your weight fully transferred to the left leg and foot, allow the rest of the right foot to lift. Moving it slowly forward, bring awareness to the changing patterns of sensations in the right foot and leg as you do so. Focus your attention on the right heel as it makes contact with the ground. Being aware of the weight now shifting forward onto the whole of the right foot as you place it gently on the ground and the left heel rises again. You may be quite aware of how different it is to balance your body now, with a belly that has a baby growing inside it, than it was before you were pregnant.

6. In this way, slowly move, step by mindful step, from one end of the walking path to the other, fully aware of the sensations in the bottom of the foot and the heel as they make contact with the ground, as the muscles move each leg forward and your balance shifts as the heel of the back foot begins to lift again.

7. Whenever you care to, if it seems appropriate, you can also expand your awareness to include a sense of what the breath is doing during the various phases of walking. If you find yourself exerting so much effort that you are actually holding your breath, stop walking for a moment and, with both feet on the ground, take a big intentional breath or two, and then begin again. You can also expand your awareness to include a sense of the body as a whole walking and breathing, along with the changing sensations in the feet and legs with each step.

8. When you come to the end of the path, stop for a moment or two and just be aware of standing. Notice where your mind is, and if you need to, gather your attention and gently bring it back to the physical sensations of the feet in contact with the ground. Then slowly turn around, step by step, appreciating the complex movements you are making as the body changes direction. Then mindfully walk back in the reverse direction. You might also notice from time to time what your eyes are taking in as your position changes along the path and you receive whatever view is in front of you.

9. Walking back and forth in this way, sustaining as best you can an awareness of the full range of your experience of walking, moment by moment. Whenever you notice that the mind has wandered away from the sensations of walking, gently escort the focus of attention back to whatever aspect of walking you are attending to in that moment, using it as the anchor to bring your mind back to the body.

10. If the mind is very agitated, stop for a moment or two and just stand in Mountain Pose with your feet shoulder-width apart, in touch with the breath and the body as a whole, until both mind and body stabilize themselves. If the baby is vigorously moving, you can also stop for a few moments and just feel the baby's movements and the breath at the belly. Then resume mindful walking.

11. Continue to walk in this way for ten to fifteen minutes, or longer if you wish.

12. When you begin the meditation, walk at a normal pace. Once you have walked the path two or three times, experiment with slowing down. Walking slower than usual gives you a better chance to be fully aware of the sensations of walking. When you feel comfortable walking slowly with awareness, you can experiment with walking faster, up to and beyond normal walking speed. If you are feeling particularly agitated, it may be helpful to begin your practice by walking quickly with awareness, then slowing down naturally as the mind settles.

13. You can also use what's known as "noting practice" during Walking Meditation. To do this, very softly and gently say to yourself the words *lifting* as the heel and then the entire foot comes off the ground, *moving* as the foot and leg move forward, *placing* as you actually set the heel and then the entire foot on the ground in front of you, and *shifting* as the weight of the body shifts onto the forward foot and leg. *Lifting, moving, placing, shifting; lifting, moving, placing, shifting.* When you come to the end of the path, note *turning, turning, turning*— anchoring your attention on the actions of your body as you turn—and then walk back again. Gently repeating the words in sync with the movements of walking. There's no place to go; just this step, in this moment.

14. You might also experiment with adding the half-smile practice to your Walking Meditation. (We learned the half-smile in Chapter 7.) Adding the half-smile may increase your sense of calm and ease while walking.

15. Remember to take small steps during Walking Meditation, particularly if you are pregnant, as this will help if your balance is unstable. And there is no need to look at your feet. They know where they are, and you know where they are. You can *feel* them.

16. As often as you can, bring the same kind of awareness that you are cultivating in Walking Meditation to your normal, everyday experience of walking. Of course if you are a runner, you can always bring a similar quality of attention to the step-by-step, moment-to-moment, breath-by-breath experience of running.

It's noon in Santa Monica, California. The August sun is high, and despite the occasional ocean breeze, it's hot. At this moment I am standing at the bottom of a steep hill with my three-and-a-half-year-old grandson, Niko, and two bags of groceries. He is hot, tired, and hungry, and in order for us to get home for lunch and his nap, we have to walk up the hill.

"Grandma, I'm tired. Carry me."

My mind's first thought is, "You've got to be kidding," followed by the next thought: "Ah, life presenting me with another opportunity to practice mindful grandparenting."

"Sweetheart, Grandma can't carry you and the groceries all the way up the hill."

"But I'm tired. It's too far. Carry me." His voice borders on a whine, and Niko is not a whiner. I know he is really tired. I look at him, look at the two bags of groceries, and look back up the hill, which somehow just got steeper. How in the world am I going to get him to walk up that hill? Then the insight comes.

"Niko, I wonder how many steps it would take to get up that hill. Fifty? Sixty? A hundred?" His face brightens.

"One hundred," he says definitively.

"No way," I reply. "I bet it's sixty. Wanna see?"

"Yes!" he says with all the enthusiasm of a three-and-a-half-year-old. It always astounds me how kids can find extraordinary reserves of energy when they are engaged. And of course we can too.

"Okay," I reply. "But we've really gotta pay attention to our feet. Every time our foot hits the ground, we'll count a number. And be sure to pay attention to when you are lifting up your foot and moving it forward through the air too. Okay?"

"Okay. Let's go!"

And together we start our marching meditation up the hill, totally absorbed in the moment-to-moment experience of walking and counting. Not thinking about the past, not thinking about the future. Only here, only now, fully engaged in this process of walking that is taking us up the hill. In this way we've cut through the suffering of the mind. And exactly one hundred steps later we arrive triumphantly at the top of the hill.

CHAPTER 11

Mindfulness in Everyday Life

Mindfulness is neither difficult nor easy;
remembering to be mindful is the great challenge.
—Christina Feldman

"SO HOW DID your practice go this week?" I ask of the assembled expectant parents. "What was challenging? What did you learn? Do you have any questions?"

Kristin can barely contain herself. "You know, I think I learned something really important this week. Last week you said something like, 'Mindfulness isn't about becoming a good meditator. It's about being more awake in your life.' Somehow I had the idea that mindfulness and meditation practice were separate from my everyday life, that they were something I would do 'over there' somewhere, and if I did them all these great things would somehow magically happen.

"So last week, I was standing at my bathroom sink, doing my mindful toothbrushing, when all of a sudden I had this thought: 'Oh, my god, Nancy wants us to be mindful *all the time!*' The thought nearly bowled me over. Peter and I discussed it all week. So I want to ask you, is that true? You want us to be mindful *all the time?*"

I heard the incredulity in Kristin's voice. And I remembered asking that very same question to one of my meditation teachers a long time ago.

"Well, what do you think?" I replied.

"Well, food sure tastes better, and I did notice the flowers more when I took our dog for a walk, and I was definitely calmer this week, and Peter and I seem to be laughing more. Maybe you really *do* want us to be mindful all the time."

"Hmm," I said. "Well, not to worry; there's no rush. Waking up is the work of a lifetime."

Paying close attention to the many routine activities that fill our day is known as informal mindfulness practice, and it is every bit as important for preparing for childbirth and parenting as formal meditation practice. When the time comes for labor and birth, you will have the knowledge, pain practice, and communication skills to drop into the present moment and work with the birthing process, however it unfolds. And once the baby has been born, informal practice may predominate, at least for a time. Your new mindfulness teacher—the small one coming soon—is going to keep you pretty busy with informal practice. Nursing and feeding and burping and diaper changing, bathing and playing, comforting and rocking and attuning to cues—these are the informal mindfulness practices of parenting, and why informal practice is such great preparation, not only for childbirth but for parenting as well.

So how do you start your informal practice? In the beginning you just pick one or two activities in your daily life and fully commit to being there as you engage in them: brushing your teeth, making morning coffee or tea, driving to work, greeting a co-worker, turning on the computer, answering the telephone, chopping vegetables, or washing the dishes after dinner. These moments all become part of your informal mindfulness practice, which of course are the very real moments of your life as you live it.

Listed here are a few general guidelines for being more awake and aware in your daily life.

1. *Whenever possible, do just one thing. Then do the next. Then the next. Mindfully, that is.*

Part of the incredible stress of modern life has to do with how much we think we need to get done every day. The result is that we can find ourselves completely absorbed in doing almost all the time. Multitasking becomes the order of the day. However, when we begin to practice paying attention to one thing at a time, fully, and then the next and then the next, we may find that we are less stressed. Paradoxically, we may also find that the quality of whatever we are engaged in improves *and* that we actually accomplish more, with greater joy.

In truth, there is no such thing as multitasking. Research shows that the brain can pay attention to only one thing at a time. We *can* move our attention swiftly back and forth from one task to the next, which gives us the illusion that we're doing more than one thing, but we're not; we're serial processing extremely quickly. When we push ourselves to multitask, we're asking our brain to do something it wasn't really designed to do. We can do it, but it takes a huge amount of energy—and we are certainly asking ourselves to do more than we can do well. The result? We feel frustrated, irritable, overwhelmed, confused, and exhausted. In a word, stressed.

These days technology, as wonderful as it is, has added a huge burden of complexity to our daily lives, so much so that scientists are investigating what we are doing to our brains with all the hours we spend online, text-ing, tweeting, e-chatting, and Skyping. Yet one thing hasn't changed: our children still need our undivided attention, an increasingly difficult thing to get in an overly stimulating world. This is why it's so important to make part of our preparation for parenting the practice, whenever possible, of consciously paying attention to just one thing at a time.

2. Throughout your day, whenever you can remember, bring your attention to your breath.

As we learned in Chapter 6, when we feel anxious, frightened, angry, hurried, or worried, our stress hormones do their fight-or-flight thing and our body changes; breathing rate increases, as does our heart rate and our blood pressure. When we feel at ease and relaxed, we are reregulating back into balance with calm and connection; breathing, heart rate, and blood pressure all decrease. When you can remember to come back to the breath throughout your day, you get a reading on your inner landscape; coming back to the sensations of breathing, you are intentionally helping to calm and rebalance your body and mind. The Three-Minute Breathing Space can be a wonderful practice to enfold into your everyday life.

3. Practice bringing awareness to your moment-to-moment bodily sensations (touching, hearing, seeing, smelling, tasting), as well as your thoughts and emotions, while you are engaged in everyday life.

Bringing mindfulness into your daily activities means doing whatever you are doing and *knowing* that you are doing it. Physical sensations, thoughts, and emotions are all doorways to awareness and the present moment.

4. Practice Being with Baby.

As you learned in Chapter 4, let the sensations from the baby's move-ments call you back into the present moment throughout your day. If cir-cumstances permit, pause from whatever you are doing and bring your full attention directly to the sensations the baby is creating inside your body—the quick little pokes, the rolling movements, the rhythmic pulsings from baby hiccups. In those moments, feel the sensations and *know* you are feeling them.

5. Take time every day to notice the natural world.

While structured activities that put us in direct relationship to nature can be nourishing, like gardening, walking in the park, or going for a hike, the natural world is available to us any time we choose to take notice. This needn't be something we save for the weekend or when we "have time." Whenever we venture outside a building we have an opportunity to be in relationship to the natural world. Even on a rainy or snowy day, when we spend most of our time indoors, we can still use our eyes to be in relationship to nature as we look out the window. The same is true in an urban environment: you can always take a moment to look at the sky. Notice its color, and the clouds or lack of them. Let the infinite vastness of the sky above help put things into perspective, expanding your awareness beyond whatever particular human drama may be temporarily preoccupying your mind.

You may find that if you spend time in nature when you are pregnant, becoming more aware of Horticultural Time—the natural rhythms of the earth, its cycles of beginnings and endings, of the seasons, and of the changing balance between night and day—you may come to feel more connected to your growing baby and the life-giving process taking place within your body, gaining insight into how you are embedded in the larger whole of nature itself.

6. When you do any form of physical activity that you usually think of as exercise—walking, jogging, swimming, or working out at the gym—do it mindfully.

One of the most memorable articles I read in nursing school many years ago was "The Hazards of Bed Rest," which documented how being in bed for any length of time negatively affects every organ of the body. Lungs can't fully inflate because of the pressure of the bed against the back; kidneys can't filter as well as they do when the body is upright; muscles begin to atrophy from lack of use. The take-home lesson for me was that our entire body functions optimally when we are *active.* Our bodies evolved to move.

While we have succeeded in making our lives easier and more convenient in many ways, that ease has come with a decrease in the number of minutes we actually move our bodies each day, which takes a toll on our general health. To make up for our more sedentary ways, we have to find time to exercise. But even while exercising we are often still not fully living in our bodies. Rather than being exactly where we are, feeling our feet moving on the treadmill or the muscles in our arms contracting and releasing as we move a machine or lift weights, we focus on a TV screen or on data from the exercise equipment or on reading a book or a magazine, thereby *increasing* the distance between the mind and body instead of promoting fully embodied presence. So whenever you are doing anything physical (which of course is all the time because you are alive), pay attention to the body. The payoff is huge.

7. *Decrease stimulation of your eyes and ears, and increase your awareness of silence.*

These days we often unthinkingly click on or crank up, subjecting our eyes and ears to a constant barrage of sights and sounds from our first waking moment until the moment we fall asleep. And when we do choose to listen to music, watch TV, get on the computer, or turn to our smartphones, what are we actually taking in, and at what volume? Are we really listening, or are we just turning on our electronic noisemakers out of habit or fear of being alone?

Our nervous systems evolved in a much quieter world than the urban environment many of us live in today. If you haven't yet made silence a friend, you're missing something wonderful. If there is not enough silence in your life, add some in. Mindfulness practice can put us in touch with the simple yet profound pleasures of silence. It is here that we may find peace.

— MINDFULNESS PRACTICES IN EVERYDAY LIFE —

Listed below are some specific activities you might choose to help bring more mindfulness into your everyday life.

1. When you wake up in the morning, become aware of the breath. Take a few moments to appreciate the simple fact that you are breathing and that you have a very small being inside your body who is also being nurtured by your breath. Acknowledge that though you have scheduled plans and tasks you have no idea how the day might actually unfold. See if you can bring a moment of curiosity and wonder to beginning this new day of your life.

2. While you're brushing your teeth, feel how you are holding the toothbrush and how you move it around in your mouth. Feel the sensations of the bristles of the toothbrush against your teeth and gums. Are there certain areas that you habitually don't brush? Taste the toothpaste. Look at the water, if it is running. Take a moment to take in the miraculous—that you have clean, clear running water coming from a tap. Hear the sound of the

water as it runs. If appropriate, be mindful of water usage and turn off the water while brushing your teeth. Notice the moment when you decide you have finished brushing. Hear the quiet that may follow after you rinse your toothbrush and turn off the water.

3. When you are taking a shower, feel where the water falls on your body. Notice its temperature and the sensations in your fingers as you rub soap on your body or on a washcloth. Notice how your fingers and your scalp feel as you wash your hair. Become aware of your body bending and turning to wash and rinse. Notice where your mind is during your shower. Are you rehearsing for an upcoming meeting at the office? Are you rehashing a conversation, planning a phone call, or answering an email? How many people are in the shower with you—in your mind, that is? Notice, and gently and kindly come back to your body in the shower. Feel the towel against your skin as you dry yourself, notice sensations as you apply any cream or lotion to your face or body.

4. If you're a man and you shave, feel the water on your face as you prepare to lather up. Fully experience the contact between the shaving cream on your hand and your face as you apply it. Notice the smell. Notice how the razor feels and the sounds it makes as you move it across the skin of your face. See the water, hear the water, feel its temperature as you rinse.

5. Feel your body move as you dress, arms reaching, body bending, balancing on one leg as you put on pants, or sit to put on shoes. Think of this activity as the yoga of dressing.

6. Eat a meal mindfully. Really look at the food, the shapes, and the colors. Smell it. Pause to consider where the food came from—the sun, the earth, the rain, the soil, and all the people whose activities made it possible for this food to come to be at the table in front of you. Notice any feelings of anticipation before you take a bite of food. Be aware of the fork, spoon, or chopsticks in your hand, your arm reaching for the food, bringing it to your mouth. Be with the taste and texture of the food as you chew it. Notice when and how you swallow. Notice if there is an impulse to rush through this bite to get on to the next one. Notice how the sensations of hunger slowly dissipate. What thoughts and feelings are present? What is your mood? How is your breathing?

7. Bring awareness to all the routine tasks that begin and end your day: making morning coffee or tea, cooking and eating breakfast, washing the dishes (or deciding to leave them in the sink!), packing a lunch. In the evening, pay attention once again to brushing your teeth and flossing, getting undressed, putting on your nightclothes, turning down the bed, setting the

alarm, and reaching to turn out the light. Feel how your body and your partner's body meet under the covers and the warmth that you generate together. The two of you might do Being with Baby practice at this time. You might include some gratitude practice before you go to sleep. Think of three things you are grateful for in your life. Share them with your partner if you like. If your partner is not there, or you don't have a partner, share your gratitude practice with your baby.

8. Many routine tasks around the house offer wonderful opportunities for informal mindfulness practice. In addition to being mindful while cooking and washing dishes, you can practice while folding laundry, making the bed, taking out the garbage, scrubbing the toilet, vacuuming or mopping the floor, dusting, cleaning the stove or refrigerator, and watering a house plant, to name just a few. This is really good practice for your life to come, when in addition to all the activities just mentioned, you will be picking up toys off the floor, sweeping up food from under a high chair, packing a diaper bag, and much more.

9. When you go shopping, become aware of your intention. What do you plan to buy? When you're in the store, notice how your attention is pulled here and there by different objects. Notice if you are feeling any confusion or sense of being overwhelmed. Notice the desire to buy something. See if you can pause and ask yourself if you really need this or that.

10. When you're buying groceries, be aware of the foods that attract you. Before buying something, ask yourself whether you and your baby will truly benefit from eating it. Follow these simple guidelines from renowned author Michael Pollan. Eat food. Mostly plants. Not too much. Whenever possible, eat unprocessed food, or food with five ingredients or less.[1]

11. Drive mindfully. When you get into the car, become aware of your posture, just as you do when you prepare for Sitting Meditation. Feel the pressure of the car seat against your body. Hear the sound of the engine as you turn the key in the ignition; feel the steering wheel in your hands; and be aware of the movements of your leg and foot as you press and release the gas pedal and the brake pedal. Notice if certain parts of your body are relaxed or tense. Experiment with silence while driving by not turning on the radio or CD player. Be aware of your mind planning the route you are going to take. Wake up from the hypnosis of habit, and experiment with driving a new route to a familiar destination. There are many roads to the same place.

Come to the breath throughout your car ride. When you stop at a red light, come to the breath. Notice the sky, trees, people, other cars. Notice if you are worried about being late or frustrated by traffic. Come to the breath again. Being stressed is not going to get you where you want to go any faster. Experiment with driving in the right-hand lane. Drive at fifty-five miles per hour. Drive at fifty miles per hour. Smile. Sing. Enjoy the ride.

Any form of transportation—taking the bus, train, or subway or biking or walking—can provide opportunities for informal mindfulness practice. I find mindfulness practice especially beneficial when traveling by air. It seems the unexpected often arises in airports: the security line is longer than anticipated, a plane is canceled or is late because of a mechanical problem or the weather, a flight connection is missed, a bag is lost, you leave your book or laptop or purse at security, you spill orange juice on your travel outfit, you encounter lots of people who just want to get where they are going rather than be where they are. Travel of any kind is a perfect environment (and metaphor) for preparation for childbirth. Bring all the qualities we have been cultivating—like don't-know mind, patience, kindness, and letting go—into every moment of your travel adventure. Try it. You won't be disappointed.

12. At work, when you greet a co-worker, look that person in the eyes and smile.

13. If you work at a desk, pay attention to how it feels to sit in your chair. Is your workstation ergonomically appropriate for your body, or are you ignoring signals that might over time develop into a repetitive stress injury? Does something need to change? If so, take action.

14. When you're pregnant, it's especially important that you get up out of your chair and walk around for a few minutes every hour. Put your arms above your head, and take some deep breaths. Do some shoulder rolls and hip rotations. Is there a way you can put your feet up while sitting at your desk to diminish the pooling of blood and fluid in your lower legs and ankles? Can you close the door or find a quiet place at work for five or ten minutes of Awareness of Breathing practice? Or how about just a Three-Minute Breathing Space?

The possibilities for bringing mindfulness into everyday life are as numerous as the moments you are living each and every day.

CHAPTER 12

A Day of Mindfulness Practice

*By being with yourself . . . by watching yourself in your daily life with
alert interest, with the intention to understand rather than to judge, in full
acceptance of whatever may emerge, because it is there, you encourage the
deep to come to the surface and enrich your life and consciousness with its
captive energies. This is the great work of awareness; it removes obstacles and
releases energies by understanding the nature of life and mind. Intelligence is
the door to freedom and alert attention is the mother of intelligence.*
—Nisargadatta Maharaj

IT IS THE SIXTH meeting of our class, and we have just come to the end of
our snack break. The expectant parents are so enjoying chatting with each
other that they are slow to reconvene. I begin this second half of the class
by sharing information about the day of mindfulness practice coming up
this weekend. It has been on the calendar since everyone first signed up for
the MBCP course.

"As you know, this Saturday will be our day of mindfulness practice, so
I just want to talk with you a little bit about how we will spend the day
together. Up to now you have been doing the formal practices for a short
period of time each day and bringing mindfulness into your daily life as best
you can. This Saturday will be an opportunity to deepen your practice and
see what it's like to devote an extended length of time turning inward, allowing each moment to arise and pass, just as you will do when you are in
labor. To make the most of the experience, we will be practicing together
almost exclusively in silence."

I pause, allowing this information to sink in.

Cathy bursts out in surprise, "You mean we're not going to talk *all day?*"

"That's right."

"You've got to be kidding. Chatty Cathy quiet for a whole day?"

"How will we know what to do with ourselves all day if no one is talking?" Carlos asks.

"Good question," I say. "Not to worry, *I'll* be doing lots of talking. I'll be guiding you through all of the practices we have learned so far: the Body Scan, yoga, Sitting Meditation, and Mindful Eating. We'll also learn Walking Meditation—that can be really helpful for labor—and another new practice as well. Any other questions?"

I wait. No one speaks up.

"Okay," I continue, "please bring a lunch, and for those of you who are pregnant, some snacks. Wear loose comfortable clothing, and dress in layers. One of your home assignments between now and Saturday is to notice what thoughts arise in the mind in relationship to this coming day. See if there are any worrying thoughts or if you notice any resistance to participating. Or maybe you'll be a little curious about how it will go, or you may even find yourself looking forward to it. All these thoughts and feelings are opportunities to practice, to understand a little more about the patterns of your mind and the stories the mind can make up about the unknown future. And of course they are opportunities to practice letting go of the story and coming back to the present moment, because you really have no idea what the day will be like."

Saturday arrives bright and clear. I'm happy that the famous San Francisco fog is passing us by today and that we will have some warm sun when we practice outdoors. Maddie, the midwifery student who is attending the course as part of her training, meets me at the door of the Osher Center. We're busily arranging chairs in a circle when couples begin to arrive with their gear in tow—a favorite back pillow, a shawl for meditation, and large brown shopping bags filled with food for the day.

As I hug Eileen hello, I feel her hair, still wet from her morning shower, cold against my cheek. Carlos gives me a one-arm hug, holding his cup of hot coffee away from me. Sharon breathes heavily as I lean over her large belly (she's carrying twins) to give her a hug. "A good-morning hug to the three of you," I say, and we both laugh.

I greet Veronica and Ruth, midwives in the community who have shared a ride over the Bay Bridge this morning. They are taking the MBCP course in part to learn mindfulness practice for themselves and in part because they've seen the positive impact mindfulness practice has had on their clients and are curious to find out more. They are what I call participant-observers, making the same commitment to daily formal practice as the couples have made. Ruth is considering training to become an MBCP instructor.

As the couples continue to arrive, they greet each other warmly. The air is filled with chatter and laughter as I gather my meditation bells, a few notes, and the poems I will read at different times throughout the day.

I take my seat and ring the bells. The room becomes quiet.

"Let's begin by just sitting for a few minutes, to help us more fully arrive in this moment," I say.

And so we formally begin our day of silent meditation practice together.

After about ten minutes of sitting, I ring the bells, and people stretch and open their eyes. Then I begin to share some guidelines to help the day go smoothly.

"It's important to know that this is not a day to try to feel a certain way, like peaceful or calm or relaxed. In fact, we're not here to *try* to do or feel anything other than how we are. Like the day you give birth, this will be a day of non-doing—a day of unfolding. If boredom or anxiety or frustration or sadness or fear arises while we are practicing today, we won't turn away from them. We will apply the same approach we have been learning for being with physical discomfort to being with unpleasant emotions: we will look at them closely, explore them, and observe as best we can the relationship between our thoughts and our emotions, just being with them, because this is our life in this moment. And we'll watch them change. So too, if times of peace or calm or joy or curiosity or relaxation are present, we will experience those fully as well. And watch *them* change too."

I offer another guideline for the day: "Besides not speaking, today we will support each other's mindfulness practice by letting go of eye contact. Just as speech can shift us away from direct experience, our eyes can lead us to interacting with others rather than looking inward and staying close to our experience of the present moment. Letting go of eye contact is sometimes called 'cloistering the eyes.' For some of you, this may be one of the more challenging guidelines of the day; for others, you may find it a relief to be in the company of others without the usual pressures to connect. Today we will focus on connecting with ourselves. It is an altogether different way of being together."

I then invite everyone to turn off their cell phones and take off their watches. "About the only thing I can absolutely guarantee about today," I say, "is that the earth will continue to revolve around the sun and this day will pass. I have a watch, and I'll keep track of clock time. For this day at least, you can let go of it.

"Also," I add, "today there are no breaks, for what is there to break from? There are no time-outs from the eternal present. So when you need to use the restroom, see if you can be aware of the moment you choose to go there and of the moments after your decision and before you move. Then, when you do move, do it mindfully. Mindfully stand up, mindfully walk to the restroom, and be mindful of whatever you do while you are there."

I offer one final guideline. "Those who are pregnant are welcome to snack throughout the day, for if you are hungry, your baby is hungry. Those of us who are not pregnant can practice being with the sensations of hunger as they make their appearance in the body. Fully experiencing the discomfort of hunger for a short time can provide us with a valuable doorway into compassion. Soon much of your life will revolve around the body sensations of hunger in another human being's body—your baby's. When we really feel how unpleasant the gnawing sensations of hunger are in our own body, it allows us to cultivate empathy (rather than dismay or anger) toward this small person who may be very unhappy because he or she is hungry. Then we act with compassion to alleviate our baby's hunger.

"Experiencing hunger today may also serve to remind us that there are many, many people in the world who in this very moment are having this same experience of discomfort in their bodies because they do not have enough food to eat. In feeling our own hunger, we may cultivate gratitude for having food to eat in the first place and perhaps a desire to alleviate the suffering of others when and how we can.

"Are there any questions?" I pause. No one speaks.

"Lovely. Then let's have our check-in."

One by one each person takes a turn, briefly describing how they are feeling right now and any expectations they may have about today. This "taking the temperature of the room" is always fascinating. The attitudes are so diverse and I always know that wherever they are now will not be where they will be at the end of the day.

Jeanette begins. "I am so glad not to have to do anything today but be here. I've been so busy running around this past week that I'm just exhausted. I've really been looking forward to today, when I could stop."

Her husband, Joe, follows. "I'm so glad not to have to talk to anyone today. And it will be really fun to talk about what happened with everyone later."

Samir speaks up. "I didn't think about the day at all during the week, and this morning we just got up and came here. I don't think I have any expectations about it. We'll just see what happens."

Sarah says, "I got a phone call this morning from the East Coast that my stepfather is dying. He went into a coma last night." Her voice falters. "So I don't know what this day will be like for me, but I'm glad I'm here."

"I'm so sorry to hear that, Sarah," I say. "If you need to keep your cell phone on today—maybe on vibrate—please do. And if at any time you feel overwhelmed or you want to talk with me, just let me know. We can go off somewhere where we won't disturb anyone and chat for a bit."

"Thank you," Sarah replies. "This has been coming for a while now, so it's not a surprise. I'm okay. The practice has already been helping me deal with it for the last couple of weeks. This is a very good way to spend this day."

Sharon takes her turn. "I was okay about today until you told us that we wouldn't be having any eye contact. Now I'm a little freaked out."

"Just notice where the sense of being freaked out is located in your body," I reply. "Notice what your thoughts are. You might be surprised, and you might learn something about yourself," I say.

After everyone has spoken, it is my turn. "I'm so glad to be here with everyone and have a day of practice. Like many of you, I've had a very busy week, and I'm really happy to have a day to just be."

So many mind-sets in the room. So many perspectives from which to start this day. And we are all perfect, just as we are.

We've spent the better part of an hour getting oriented. "This is a good time for a trip to the restroom, for those who need it. The rest of us can take a few minutes to stand and stretch." Soon we are all assembled once again, sitting in silence.

I guide us through the instructions for Sitting Meditation, ending with Choiceless Awareness, one of the practices you learned in Chapter 9. And then I fall silently into my own practice, observing my thoughts, noticing emotions and the sensations in my body as they arise and pass. At the end of the sitting, I read a poem by Rumi called "The Guest House."

The Guest House

This being human is a guest house.
Every morning a new arrival.

A joy, a depression, a meanness,
some momentary awareness comes
as an unexpected visitor.

Welcome and entertain them all!
Even if they're a crowd of sorrows,
who violently sweep your house
empty of its furniture,

still, treat each guest honorably.
He may be clearing you out
for some new delight.

The dark thought, the shame, the malice,
meet them at the door laughing,
and invite them in.

Be grateful for whoever comes,
because each has been sent
as a guide from beyond.

  Rumi, trans. Coleman Barks

"Now let's move into some yoga practice," I say. "See if you can keep your awareness in the here and now as you walk to the shelves of yoga mats. Feel your arm stretch as you reach out to take a mat. Watch what the mind does as you make a choice about where to put your mat. Notice the sound of the mat as it unrolls. We'll begin with Mountain Pose."

Before long we are all standing on our unfurled yoga mats. After a reminder to approach the practice with an attitude of non-striving, of going to our own edge and exploring it but not pushing beyond it, bringing an attitude of respect to the body and its changing sensations, we begin moving, slowly and mindfully, through a yoga sequence. We finish our yoga practice lying on the floor, pregnant women on their sides, partners and the rest of us on our backs.

I guide us slowly through a Body Scan. We end with expanding our awareness to a sense of the body as a whole and then return to the breath. I ring the bells, announcing the end of our meditation.

"Taking your time, roll onto your side if you are not already on your side, push yourself up to a sitting posture, and just come back to the breath."

Next I give the instructions for Walking Meditation that you read about in Chapter 10 and demonstrate the practice. We each find a walking lane—some in the main room, some in the hallways, some in the clinic waiting area—and for the next thirty minutes or so we silently engage in Walking Meditations. Bodies slowly moving, minds focused, attention directed within: twenty-eight expectant parents, silently walking back and forth, back and forth in preparation for the birth of their baby, while three midwives and a midwife-to-be practice alongside them.

The walking period over, I ring the bells once again, and we silently pull our chairs into a circle for another period of Sitting Meditation. It is nearing lunchtime, and several pregnant women pull a snack from a lunch box or bag. The crackle of an energy bar wrapper, the unmistakable smell of a tangerine, and the crunching sound of an apple being chewed are all part of the early minutes of this sitting. Then utter silence sets in again.

To end our sitting I read aloud a quote from Pema Chödrön:

> The pith instruction is, Stay . . . stay . . . just stay. . . . So whenever we wan-
> der off, we gently encourage ourselves to "stay" and settle down. Are we
> experiencing restlessness? Stay! Discursive mind? Stay! Are fear and loath-
> ing out of control? Stay! Aching knees and throbbing back? Stay! What's
> for lunch? Stay! What am I doing here? Stay! I can't stand this another
> minute! Stay! That is how to cultivate steadfastness.[1]

"I imagine that your body is telling you that lunchtime has arrived, and so it has," I say. "We will be taking our lunches over to the garden across the street, but before we do, I'd like to review the instructions for eating mindfully. When you find the place where you'd like to eat, I suggest that you set the food out in front of you. Take time to really look at the food—its shapes, colors, textures. Smell it, and perhaps reflect for a moment or two on how the food was grown, who prepared it, and how it actually came to be here to nourish you, your partner, and your baby. Perhaps take a mo-ment to acknowledge your good fortune that you have this food to eat. If you are using a fork or a spoon, set it down while you chew your food so you can fully concentrate on chewing, tasting, and swallowing. See if you can bring awareness to the moment when the desire to take another bite arises, when thirst and the desire to drink something arises, and note the sensations in your belly as they change from hunger to satisfaction. There is no hurry. Take as much time to eat your lunch as you care to. Learn what you can.

"A word about being outdoors," I continue. "Remember that mindful-ness is like a lens. Sometimes we make the aperture of the lens very small, concentrating our focus as we did when we ate the raisin weeks ago. At other times we expand our awareness, allowing the mind to take a very wide, open view. Being outdoors in the garden is an excellent opportunity to become aware of how we can shift between these two aspects of mind-fulness. In some moments, we can focus quite intensely on our food, and in other moments we can have a more open, spacious view. Perhaps look up at the sky. When was the last time you really looked at the sky? Maybe not since the last time you went hiking or camping. Maybe not since you were a child. Allow yourself to see that great vastness, which is always there above us.

"Bring your attention to your senses as they interact with the elements.

Feel the warmth of the sun on your shoulder, the breeze against your face; feel the temperature of the air coming into your nostrils; be aware of how you take in odors on an in-breath and how you receive sounds—perhaps there will be sounds from rustling leaves or from birds in the trees. I expect there will be some sounds from cars driving by. Just listen."

I also encourage everyone to honor their commitment to not making eye contact, as best they can, to support each other's inner work. "This can be a little tricky because you'll probably be dividing and sharing your lunch in silence. Not to worry if you forget or accidentally make eye contact. Just smile at each other, enjoy the moment, and begin again.

"So let's get our lunches, put our shoes and jackets on, and gather in front of the elevators. When everyone is ready, we'll walk over to the garden as a group, at a normal pace, in silence."

The air is warm, and the sounds from the cars on the boulevard we have to cross seem louder today. Our senses are more open, our nervous systems calmer and more receptive. The garden is in full bloom—pink roses and yellow pansies in the sun, fuchsia azaleas and white camellias in the shade. The sounds of the water in the fountain greet us as we enter. Each couple finds a place to sit—on a chair or a bench or on the low wall surrounding the fountain. And so we eat, mindfully, in silence. All are absorbed in the activity, following the instructions. After eating, some close their eyes, their bodies drinking in the warmth of the sun, like cats sunning themselves on a warm spot of earth.

When I see everyone has finished, I ring the bells once again. "Let's have a short Walking Meditation through the garden. Really use your eyes, to notice the various plants as we walk by each one of them. Feel the ground beneath your feet, hear the crunch of the gravel with each step, feel the change in temperature as we walk from sun to shade." This time we walk, single file, slowly, snakelike, around and through the garden.

Our Walking Meditation finished, we cross the street again, returning to our meditation space at the Center.

"This morning several of you said how tired you were. So I'd like to invite each of you to get a yoga mat, a blanket, and a pillow or two from the shelves and take a nap, if you'd like. Or if you prefer, you can do more sitting practice." Several faces light up with surprised smiles after this invitation.

Within minutes the floor of our classroom is a sea of sleeping bodies covered in gray woolen blankets. It is so sweet to see how some couples cuddle against each other, a head nestled in the crook of an arm, a hand gently resting against a partner's chest. The intimacy of the moment reminds me once again how when we human beings feel safe and protected, our hearts open too.

When naptime comes to an end, it's time for the Speaking and Listening Inquiry, described in detail in Chapter 6. "Some of you have perhaps heard me say, somewhat humorously, that all we have to do to have a baby is to be able to work with pain and fear," I begin. "Well, we have spent a good deal of time on mindfulness practices for working with physical pain. Now it's time to turn our attention to that profoundly contracting emotion called fear and the balancing positive emotion of happiness. For now, just for the inquiry, we will suspend our guideline of silence and of cloistering the eyes."

The inquiry into fear and happiness takes a little more than an hour, and by the time we finish, there is a good amount of laughter in the room. Each couple has named and explored some of their fears quietly together and may have discovered that they have some of the same fears or have uncovered fears that they never even realized they had. They have explored the truth that some fears may be calls to action, to investigate or change something in the present, and that for other fears nothing needs to be done but to accept their existence, pat them on the head every now and again, and perhaps learn to live with grace in the realm of uncertainty and the unknown.

It's time now for another period of Walking Meditation. I find a place in the hallway for my own walking practice—lifting, moving, placing, shifting, lifting, moving, placing, shifting—pausing before I turn, noticing where my mind is, coming to the breath, then to my feet on the floor, turning, turning, turning, and walking back again.

When I ring the bells, I tell everyone that we just experienced our last practice for our day together. Many seem genuinely surprised by this news—have they really spent an entire day in meditation practice? I invite them to come back into our more usual mode of relating, to look around the room at each other and reconnect. Faces come alive as eye contact is made once again.

"Let's break into groups of threes and fours to share a little bit about what you experienced today. If anyone isn't yet ready to speak, please just let the people in your group know you want to remain in silence. We will spend more time in class next week sharing how the day went for everyone."

The room fills with animated voices as each person has a turn to share. Laughter is common; delight is not far away. All is well.

We gather again in the large circle, and a few people offer to share their experiences. Daniel says, "I was surprised by how much I liked being alone in the company of others." Liana adds, "Everyone knows how anxious I was about today; I was so surprised by how much I enjoyed it." The ice broken, others chime in with their comments. "I loved the Walking Meditation. You have to really balance to walk!" "And it sure does look weird." "I was surprised by how little I ate. I felt full about halfway through lunch and didn't need to eat any more." "I really liked taking a nap as a group. It was like a big slumber party."

I caution everyone that as they return to everyday life, they might not realize the impact a day like this can have. After a day of silent practice, we may be more open and sensitive than we might realize. Given that the world we will be reentering is so fast paced and stimulating, we need to remember to be gentle with ourselves and to honor the experience we just had. Stopping off at the crowded supermarket on the way home or seeing the latest action movie tonight may not be the best idea. I also say that in the time immediately following the baby's birth they may experience this kind of emotional openness, sensitivity, and need for quiet. It will be helpful to honor that sensitive time too.

It's time to formally close our day of practice. Standing together, we acknowledge and thank each other with our eyes and our smiles. This day has indeed been a gift. We can see each of us as whole within this larger interconnected whole, interwoven by our experience together.

I look at the room's participants and offer some words from the Lovingkindness meditation you will learn in Chapter 14. "May the work we have done here together today be of benefit to ourselves, to our babies, to our partners, to the new family that is being birthed, and to all beings everywhere. May each of you be safe, healthy, happy, and at ease until we meet again."

CHAPTER 13

Befriending
Mindfulness in Relationship

Not causing harm requires staying awake. Part of being is slowing down
enough to notice what we say and do. The more we witness our emotional
chain reactions and understand how they work, the easier it is to refrain.
It becomes a way of life to stay awake, slow down, and notice.
—Pema Chödrön

WHEN I FIRST began teaching mindfulness as a way to prepare for childbirth, I felt fairly confident that the practice would ease the stress of this
radical life change, help address the pain and the fear of pain during childbirth, and diminish the fear of the unknown that is inherent in this transition. Though I certainly suspected that practicing mindfulness together as
a couple would have a positive impact on a couple's relationship, I didn't
know what that would look like. Once again it was the students who taught
the teacher—and for that I am deeply grateful.

As the weeks unfold and practice deepens for the couples in the MBCP
course, mindfulness begins to seep into their relationship in unexpected
and often quite beneficial ways. As you and your partner practice, you too
may find old habits of relating begin to untangle as new, and often more
harmonious, options begin to emerge.

For years I have handed out a feedback form for each person to fill out
on the last night of class. It includes the following question: Have you noticed any changes in the way you relate to your partner since the course
began?

Here is a representative sample of the kinds of answers I receive.

"We are closer and more connected than before."

"I am more attentive, listen more, and am more helpful."

"Our communication has vastly improved—we can better articulate our
feelings."

"We are more compassionate with each other."

"Practice helps us reconnect, especially after stressful days."

"We forgive each other more easily."

"We now have a shared language and common mind-set for communicating."

Becoming more aware through mindfulness practice seems to support our natural desire for harmonious relationships, contentment, caring, and connection, allowing our basic goodness to emerge in our most intimate relationships.

It's the seventh session of the MBCP course, the class that takes place after our day of silent practice. As couples gather in the circle this evening, the trust, comfort, and familiarity are obvious.

Michelle is the first to speak. "I really couldn't wait to get to class tonight to share what happened with Josh and me this week. Remember that he missed the all-day session because he was on a business trip? Well, I was really looking forward to having him home again. I don't like being home alone, and now that the birth is getting closer, I really, really don't like it. And besides, I really miss him.

"As I was getting ready to go to the airport to pick him up, my cell phone rang. It was Josh, telling me that his plane had arrived a little early. And then he said, 'And I have some bad news. I just got a call from work. There's an emergency in the Seattle office, and they need me to fly up there first thing in the morning to see if I can straighten things out. I tried to get out of it, but they insisted. And I'm not sure I'll make it back in time for this week's class.'

"In that moment I felt myself getting really angry. My jaw clenched up, my heart started racing, and I could feel all this tension in my shoulders and in the back of my neck. I'm a person that really likes to be in control and I generally don't handle disappointment very well. Normally I would have just exploded—at Josh, at his boss, at the company he works for, at the fact that he might miss class again. I would have said all sorts of things I would have regretted later. And I probably would have started crying, right?" Michelle looks at Josh, and he nods.

"Even though I knew it wasn't his fault, and there was nothing he could do about the situation, that's what I would have done before taking this class. And the result would have been two miserable people. It would have turned into our standard fight about how he doesn't understand that I need him home more now, and how I don't understand his pressures at work. We've had that one so many times it's almost boring!

"But this time I did something different. I don't know why, or how, but the practice just kicked in. Instead of freaking out, I just came to the breath and said, 'Okay, I'm on my way to pick you up.' I still felt upset, but I was able to catch myself, right then in the moment."

Josh joins in. "Yeah, it was really amazing. I was dreading telling her, totally expecting her to be furious. I could hear in her voice over the phone that she was upset, but she didn't freak out. I couldn't believe it. When I clicked off our call I said to myself, 'Whoa, now *that* was different.'"

Michelle continues. "So on the way to the airport I just kept practicing, watching my mind spin out, letting the thoughts go, and coming back to the breath. I kept telling myself, 'It's okay. You're just going through a really big contraction right now. It'll pass. Notice how your body feels. Just keep paying attention to the breath.' And boy, it was some contraction. Definitely more than a minute—and definitely harder than ice cubes!" We all laugh, as Michelle continues.

"We live about fifteen minutes from the airport, and I kept practicing all the way there. Gradually I could feel myself calming down. And as I did, I realized that in that moment on the phone I had made a choice not to get all upset at Josh. And that I could just continue to choose how I was going to be when I picked him up at the airport. Then I started to think about how tired he must be after such a long trip, and I knew *he* wasn't happy about having to turn right around and go to Seattle in the morning and maybe missing class. By the time I got to the airport, I had totally calmed down."

Josh continues the story. "So there I was, waiting for Michelle to pick me up, and I kept thinking 'Well, she didn't freak out on the phone, but I'd better be prepared for the freak-out as soon as I get in the car,' so I started rehearsing what I was going to say. And then I realized I'm having a fight with her—and she isn't even there! So I just keep trying to come back to the breath. When she pulls up I open the car door, and she greets me with this 'Hi, honey' and a big hug. It was a miracle. Later she told me how she had used her mindfulness practice as she drove to the airport, and I told her how I had been using mine waiting for her. It felt so great to really communicate with each other instead of having a big blowup!"

◎

Life being what it is, the unexpected is always just around the corner, for ourselves and for the people we love. A partner gets laid off from work, a relative or close friend is diagnosed with a serious illness, a child breaks an arm at the playground, a baby takes a totally unexpected three-hour nap when you had planned to meet your friend and her baby for lunch, or a husband has to go on another business trip after being away most of the week.

Like Michelle, many of us go into reactive mode when we're presented with a situation we didn't expect and don't like. We look for someone or something to blame, or we lash out in anger or withdraw, feeling like a victim of circumstances beyond our control. Michelle's pattern was to turn her anger outward, but sometimes we turn it in on ourselves, falling into despondency or depression.

However, as we can see from Michelle's report, mindfulness practice presented her with a totally new option. Michelle had woven her inner mindfulness parachute, and it held her when she needed it. Her practice gave her the presence of mind to interrupt a long-standing and unhelpful pattern in her relationship with Josh. In that one moment of being present on the telephone, Michelle experienced freedom from her habitual reaction. As she observed her mind and body on her ride to the airport, she was able to expand her view and let go of her attachment to Josh being home for a while. In coming to terms with things as they are, Michelle is actually living the insight attributed to philosopher Viktor Frankl: "Between stimulus and response there is a space. In that space is our power to choose our response. In our response lies our growth and our freedom."

THE CONTRACTION OF I, ME, AND MINE: EXPANDING INTO AWARENESS

A more expansive view is in fact exactly where inner growth takes place and, as we see in Michelle's story, where mindfulness can help. When we are distressed, or when things don't go our way, our body and mind contract. Because Michelle had become more aware of her body through mindfulness practices like the Body Scan, she could describe precisely what parts of her body contracted when she received the upsetting news from Josh. She was able to be with the unpleasant, contracting sensations of *no* in her body and ride those moments with her breath, just as we learned to do with the ice. And it made a huge difference.

Looking deeply, we can see that the contraction Michelle experienced was related to disappointment over losing an imagined future and her lack of control over the situation. Looking even more deeply, we can see that what Michelle was contracting around was actually a sense of "I" or "me" that was losing something: the "I" wanted Josh to be at home with "me"; "my" reasons for wanting this were such and such; and "I" was definitely right to want it this way.

Now this is tricky stuff, but perhaps it could be useful to ask the question "Who exactly *is* this I that is doing all the contracting? And who is this me, and what is mine, really?" We can say that I am a mother, a father, a partner, a friend, a daughter, a son, a sister, a brother, a store clerk, a biologist, an office worker, a manager, a computer programmer, a teacher. These are socially defined roles, but are they *really* who we are? Well, on one level, yes of course, or so it seems. But on another level, perhaps not.

In daily life it can certainly feel like there is a person inside our head, the one who talks to us all the time, who seems to be in charge of this "I, me, and mine." But as we practice, slowly and over time, as we observe the inner workings of our own mind, its habits, its patterns, and in fact how completely inaccurate it may be at times, we may come to see that what we think of as "I" or "me" or "mine" is actually deeply connected to a story we have made up about who we *think* we are. The thinking mind, the one we can observe in meditation practice, can endlessly entertain or distress us with its stories about ourselves; all too often we come to believe that the stories are who we are.

However, as you can see from Michelle's story, being able to step out of the contraction of the emotions around I, me, and mine, even momentarily, also allowed her to step back from stories she had constructed about herself (like "I'm a person who really likes to be in control"). In coming to terms with things as they are, Michelle was able to soften around her sense of "I, me, and mine" just a bit and take a more expansive view, a view that included the reality of Josh in this situation. From this more mindful place, Michelle could see that Josh was probably tired and didn't want to get on a plane to Seattle the next morning either. From this expanded place within, Michelle could respond out of the goodness of her own true nature, from empathy and kindness. She wasn't repressing her disappointment or unhappiness about the situation; rather because she was using her mindfulness practice to work with her own reactivity, she could more skillfully navigate the life she and Josh were living right in the present moment.

By the time Michelle got to the airport, mindfulness had averted a reaction that might have caused a lot of unnecessary suffering for both of them. This is the gift that mindfulness practice can bring into our most intimate relationships, where it perhaps matters most of all.

Now it's important to be clear about this. There is nothing wrong with this "sense of self," and in much of life it serves us; in fact, it is critically important, sometimes even lifesaving, that we have a strong enough sense of who we are to protect ourselves or to speak up for what we need. This strong sense of "I" can help us move through some very rough times. But to think that this "I, me, and mine" is real, fixed, and unchanging because of a story we have constructed about "who I am" can severely limit us. The more tightly we cling to a fixed view of "who I am," the more we cut ourselves off from the process of *becoming*, which of course is what's happening in every moment.

This "I" often obscures a more expanded view, one that gives us a more accurate picture of reality, where we can see ourselves as whole yet also nested within the larger whole of the living universe. Albert Einstein described it this way: "A human being is a part of the whole, called by us 'the Universe,' a part limited in time and space. He experiences himself, his thoughts and feelings as something separated from the rest—a kind of optical delusion of consciousness. This delusion is a kind of prison for us, restricting us to our personal desires and to affection for a few persons nearest to us. Our task must be to free ourselves from this prison by widening our circle of compassion to embrace all living creatures and the whole of nature in its beauty."[1]

Through mindfulness practice we can sense this capacity for expansion, not only of the mind, but of the heart. And the latter is precisely what is required as you begin to care for your babies and children. It is your baby's developmental task to build a healthy sense of "I" and "me" and "mine" (a process that can present one of the more challenging aspects of parenting), while *our* developmental task is learning how to hold the larger view even when we *feel* exactly like our two-year-old, who is fiercely clutching "my toy," which belongs to another child, or is throwing a tantrum because she is not getting her way. As my wise husband, Kenji, sometimes says, "It doesn't matter whether you *feel* like the parent. The children *think* you're the parent, so you have to act like one."

Expanding the view from "I, me, and mine" to the "we" needed for family often begins with you and your partner in your dance of everyday intimacy. Who cooks what and how, who cleans what and how, who makes money, and who pays the bills—it all can be negotiated from the narrower perspective of "me" or the more compassionate, wider perspective that includes you *and* your partner. Once we have a baby, the task before each of us is to expand once again, to widen our sense of "we" into family, into seeing the whole, which includes empathy and compassion for our baby, our partner, *and* ourselves.

At a one-year reunion of an MBCP course, Ramona talked to me about life after her son, Mateo, was born. "I was completely blown away by how much my attention had to focus on what Mateo needs. Life is not all about *me* anymore. It's not about us, about Danny and me as a couple, anymore either. It's about the two of us growing into a partnership that takes care of each other and Mateo.

"This growing into 'mother me' really hurts sometimes," Ramona continued. "But just like labor, if I can embrace the change, it's much, much easier. I must use the practice at least ten times a day. How people survive this experience without a mindfulness practice is just beyond me."

OF FAMILIES, HABITS, AND PATTERNS

Michelle and Josh's story prompted Carla to share how mindfulness practice was affecting her relationship with Scott. "You know, since we began the class, I can see a change in Scott—and it's making life so much better for both of us." She turned to Scott and asked, "Can I tell them about our driving fights?" Scott nods a bit sheepishly.

"You see, Scott and I have had this ongoing fight about his driving. Basically, I can't stand the way he drives. First of all, he drives much too fast. And since I got pregnant I've been feeling more vulnerable, so his fast driving has been more difficult for me. And then he does the road rage thing, which just drives me nuts. He has tried to change but without much success. I've tried everything—yelling, refusing to ride in the car with him, or only being in the car with him if I drive. Something will work for a while, and then we're right back to fighting about it again.

"But since we started mindfulness practice, things have really changed. Last week we made an agreement that we would both make driving together one of our 'mindfulness in daily life' practices, like brushing our teeth. We agreed that Scott would drive mindfully—really paying attention to driving—and I wouldn't say anything but just pay attention to my breath and how uptight I was feeling. And it's working! He's driving much more slowly, and I've been much calmer. It's been so helpful!"

Now it was Scott's turn. "I kind of knew that I drove pretty fast, but it wasn't until Carla and I got together that it became such a big problem.

Driving as a mindfulness practice has taught me a lot. I realized that I actually don't even like driving that fast! If I drive in the slower lane, I get to see more things and feel more relaxed. I also realized that having my music blasting in the car was both distracting and jarring to my nerves. I'm starting to like silence. It's just more peaceful. And pretty soon our baby is going to be in the car too, so I'd better get it together."

Scott continues, sharing with us the history of his driving habits. "I learned the traffic anger thing from my dad. I remember how he and my mom used to have fights about his driving too, just like Carla and I were doing. I think as a kid I just thought, 'Oh, that's how you behave in traffic—cursing people and stuff.' But I realized I don't want to teach that to my kid, and I don't want him to see Carla and me fighting over it, either.

"The practice totally helps," Scott added. "The other day I was driving by myself, and this guy cut me off. That was the trigger. I saw all my angry thoughts raging up, and I felt the adrenaline and tightness in my body. It all happened so *fast*. But there was this split second before I reacted, just like Michelle was talking about, when I just decided to let it go, just to skip the whole drama. It's not that I didn't feel pissed off, 'cause I really did, but I knew it wasn't going to help the situation. The guy who cut me off didn't care; he was already halfway down the freeway. Getting all upset was just going to hurt *me*. And when Carla and the baby are in the car, it will just hurt them too. It's a small thing, but it's really important. Because if I can do lots of small things, then maybe it will add up to me being a different kind of father to my son than my dad was to me."

Indeed, little things do count, especially in family life. As Myla and Jon Kabat-Zinn write in their pioneering book *Everyday Blessings: The Inner Work of Mindful Parenting*, "Love is expressed in how we pass the bread, or how we say good morning. . . ."[2] It's not just that the little things count. It's that the little things are life!

Fear of parenting the way we were parented can be one of the biggest concerns we have during pregnancy—even bigger than giving birth. If you have this particular fear, mindfulness can be a key element to parenting differently. Indeed, mindfulness holds the very real potential for breaking intergenerational cycles of family dysfunction, both small and large.

Like it or not, we learn to parent from the way we were parented. If we were fortunate to grow up with parents who were, as the phrase goes, "good-enough parents,"[3] who saw and valued us for who we were and nurtured us to become all that we could be, we are indeed blessed. Many of us, however, begin our journey as parents with more difficult family histories.

Betsy is one such example. As she put it, "I grew up in a family with pretty severe abuse. There was a lot of yelling and hitting. I realize now, as an adult, that it wasn't about me; it was about whatever was going on for my parents. But I also realize that not having a mindfulness practice can mean so much negativity going out—toward your family, your loved ones. Mindfulness practice gives me the skills to do things differently. It's not easy, and sometimes I still feel like I'm channeling my mother when I behave in ways that I swore I never would. But that's not very often, and probably a whole lot less than I would be doing without my mindfulness practice. And when it does happen I have a way to forgive myself and start over again."

⟶ MINDFULNESS PRACTICE: A SPEAKING AND LISTENING INQUIRY ON OUR FAMILIES OF ORIGIN ⟵

We return to the form of the Speaking and Listening Inquiry that we used to explore fear and happiness in Chapter 6. The subjects you can explore about your childhood and your family are endless, so use this inquiry form freely, whenever you and your partner feel the need. It can help both of you understand a bit more clearly the patterns and habits each of you learned from the family you grew up in, and it can help clarify your intentions for the family you are in the process of creating. Giving words to what is otherwise implicit can help to initiate a conversation that you and your partner will be having for the rest of your lives and perhaps help each of you negotiate with more wisdom and clarity what is best for your children, yourselves, and your family as a whole.

While there is much talk about cross-cultural or "mixed" marriages or partnerships, in truth, *every* new family is cross-cultural because each of us grew up in a different family; it's just a matter of degree. The more different your upbringing was from your partner's, the more helpful it can be to bring unspoken assumptions, desires, and intentions to light so that you can find what is important to each of you as you move into this process of parenting together. The more awareness, intention, and shared vision you can bring to the kind of family you would like to create, the more likely it is that your children will enjoy a harmonious family life—and the more likely you will enjoy being parents together.

Begin by coming into silence and bringing attention to the breath. After three or so minutes of silent practice, begin the inquiry below.

Person 1: Please tell me one thing you *appreciate* about the way you were parented.

Person 2: (Answers.)

Person 1: Thank you. (Pause.) Please tell me one thing you *appreciate* about the way you were parented.

Person 2: (Answers.)

Person 1: Thank you. (Pause.) Please tell me one thing you *appreciate* about the way you were parented.

Person 2: (Answers.)

Person 1: Thank you.

Switching speaking and listening roles, continue with the series above, requesting and responding with your partner three times. When you have finished, close your eyes and come back to silence and the breath for three or four breaths, longer if you care to. Notice whatever thoughts, emotions, and body sensations are present. Then continue with the inquiry process.

Person 1: Please tell me one thing that was *difficult* for you in the way you were parented.

Person 2: (Answers.)

Person 1: Thank you. (Pause.) Please tell me one thing that was *difficult* for you in the way you were parented.

Person 2: (Answers.)

Person 1: Thank you. (Pause.) Please tell me one thing that was *difficult* for you in the way you were parented.

Person 2: (Answers.)

Person 1: Thank you.

Changing speaking and listening roles, continue together with the requesting and responding three times. When you have finished, close your eyes and come back to silence and the breath as before. Notice whatever thoughts, emotions, and body sensations are present. After some silence, continue once again with the inquiry process.

Person 1: Please tell me one way you would like to parent that is *similar* to the way you were parented.

Person 2: (Answers.)

Person 1: Thank you. (Pause.) Please tell me one way you would like to parent that is *similar* to the way you were parented.

Person 2: (Answers.)

Person 1: Thank you. (Pause.) Please tell me one way you would like to parent that is *similar* to the way you were parented.

Person 2: (Answers.)

Person 1: Thank you.

And switching speaking and listening roles, once again, continue with this request, asking for a response from your partner three times. When you have finished, close your eyes and come back to silence and the breath for three or four breaths. Notice whatever thoughts, emotions, and body sensations are present. After three minutes, continue with the inquiry process.

> Person 1: Please tell me one way you would like to parent that is *different* from the way you were parented.
> Person 2: (Answers.)
> Person 1: Thank you. (Pause.) Please tell me one way you would like to parent that is *different* from the way you were parented.
> Person 2: (Answers.)
> Person 1: Thank you. (Pause.) Please tell me one way you would like to parent that is *different* from the way you were parented.
> Person 2: (Answers.)
> Person 1: Thank you.

Changing speaking and listening roles, continue with the three request and response cycles as before. When you have finished, close your eyes and come back to silence and the breath for three or four breaths. Notice whatever thoughts, emotions, and body sensations are present. After three minutes, continue with the inquiry process.

> Person 1: Please tell me one way you might use mindfulness practice to help you create the kind of family you would like to live in, and the kind of family you would like your child to look back on and remember.
> Person 2: (Answers.)
> Person 1: Thank you. (Pause.) Please tell me one way you might use mindfulness practice to help you create the kind of family you would like to live in, and the kind of family you would like your child to look back on and remember.
> Person 2: (Answers.)
> Person 1: Thank you. (Pause.) Please tell me one way you might use mindfulness practice to help you create the kind of family you would like to live in, and the kind of family you would like your child to look back on and remember.
> Person 2: (Answers.)
> Person 1: Thank you.

Switching speaking and listening roles, once again, continue with this request and response cycle with your partner three times. When you have finished, close your eyes and come back to silence and the breath for three minutes, or maybe more. Notice whatever thoughts, emotions, and body sensations are present. After three minutes of silence, end this inquiry practice maybe with a hug or perhaps with some phrases of Loving-kindness, the practice you will learn in the next chapter.

The week after their class was given the Speaking and Listening Inquiry as their home assignment, Marie and Tony shared how much the practice was helping them. As Marie put it, "One of the ways the practice is helping us is that Tony is getting better at not interrupting me when I talk. It's something we've been struggling with for a long time."

Tony continues, "I got this insight during our day of meditation, when we did the Speaking and Listening practice. While Marie was talking, I kept thinking about all the ways I wanted to discuss what she was saying, like either talk her out of it or fix the things she was worried about. It was such a relief to let go of that and just to be present and listen. Having a form that didn't let me talk, that set up a situation where I was supposed to just listen, was really instructive. Now when we're having a conversation at the dinner table, I catch myself wanting to jump in and talk, but I just breathe and listen instead. Not all the time, but I'm definitely getting better." Marie smiles in agreement.

"And then, while we were doing the speaking and listening at home this week, I realized that part of the reason I interrupt Marie is because I grew up in a family with five kids. We were interrupting each other all the time! Being the youngest, I always had the feeling that if I didn't speak up, no one would even know I existed."

Marie says, "And I'm an only child, so I never had to share attention with anyone. I think that's why this is such an issue for us."

It's not hard to understand how Marie and Tony, given their family histories, might have a clash of communication styles. While this insight into the past is extremely helpful, the reactive pattern needs to be changed in the here and now. That's where mindfulness practice can help. After becoming more aware of your own deeply ingrained habits and patterns of behavior, mindfulness practice offers a way to actually change them, if you choose to. Is it easy? No. Is it possible? Most definitely.

Each of us has a family history, each of us has a story about what happened to us when we were young, and each of us has our own particular challenges when it comes to raising our children. Certainly some of us had more difficult childhoods than others, and our emotional triggers and automatic patterns can run deep. If these patterns hook into our partner's patterns in unhealthy ways, they can bring real unhappiness. The need to change is great, and sometimes the difficulties of making a change can feel almost insurmountable; trapped in an idea that these painful patterns are who we are, we can live them out over and over again.

Once we see that our ways of behaving come from habit, conditioning, and at the most basic level a desire to be seen or a fear of not being seen, mindful awareness can help free us from some of the inevitable friction that comes with any intimate relationship. Tony is not a bad person for interrupting Marie, nor is Marie a bad person for not wanting to be interrupted. The dynamic between Tony and Marie is just the all-too-human condition of two people from different families, with different habits, operating on automatic pilot. Even though such habits are deeply rooted, change is possible once we bring them into the light of awareness. With each of us taking responsibility for our own inner lives, we can learn and we can grow, separately and together. We can find the freedom to step out of old patterns of relationship and become the kind of person, partner, and parent we really want to be.

CHAPTER 14

It's All About Kindness

The true essence of humankind is kindness.
—the Dalai Lama

BY THIS POINT, the seventh session of the MBCP course, we have learned all the practices needed for whatever may come in the profound passage from pregnancy through childbirth and into parenting—save for one: Loving-kindness practice. This is the practice we will be learning now. The cultivation of kindness has been implicit in our mindfulness practice from the very beginning; Loving-kindness practice makes it explicit.

In the Buddhist tradition from which this practice comes, the idea of separating the mind from the heart is quite foreign; for example, when Asian meditation teachers talk about the mind, they often point to their chest. Perhaps because Eastern cultures have a long tradition of looking inward, they may know something about the mind and heart that we in the West are just coming to understand. In fact, mindfulness could just as well be translated as heartfulness.

The wisdom embedded in Loving-kindness practice stems from the basic understanding that all human beings on the planet want to be happy. Our forefathers recognized that the desire for happiness is so fundamental that they even listed it as one of the inalienable rights in the second paragraph of the Declaration of Independence. However, with all due respect to the Founding Fathers, it seems that happiness is not something we "get" from pursuing it—it's already inside us just waiting to manifest; as the title of meditation teacher Sylvia Boorstein's book puts it, *Happiness Is an Inside Job*. Loving-kindness practice helps us tap into and strengthen this already existing capacity.

When we practice Loving-kindness meditation, we silently repeat particular words and phrases that invoke a sense of friendliness and good-will, first for ourselves, then for particular beings, and ultimately for all beings everywhere. There are many versions of the phrases used in Loving-kindness practice, and the ones I offer in the MBCP course are as follows:

> May I be safe and protected.
> May I be healthy in body and mind.
> May I be happy.
> May I live with ease and in peace.

The phrases above are provided in the spirit of an offering or a suggestion. Loving-kindness practice is a very open, flexible meditation, and if there are other words or phrases that feel more genuine or natural for you, please use them. There are no "right" phrases in Loving-kindness practice.

Traditionally the phrases of Loving-kindness are first directed to ourselves. Then we shift the object of our well-wishing to a person or persons who have been teachers, guides, or mentors or to others who have helped or inspired us in some way. Next we direct them to a neutral person, perhaps someone we see in our daily life but with whom we have very little relationship, like a clerk at the grocery store or the teller at the bank. Then we direct Loving-kindness to a somewhat difficult person in our life, which is often rich territory for inner growth. Finally we expand our caring and compassionate wishes outward in all directions, to all beings everywhere who are suffering or in need, including all creatures on the planet—those of the land, sea, and air, those seen and unseen, born and unborn, near and far, everywhere—wishing them safety, health, happiness, ease, and peace.

Our Western culture instills in us very strong patterns of self-judgment, so in the beginning it can be challenging to direct the phrases of Loving-kindness to ourselves. For this and other reasons, in the MBCP course we use a variation of the traditional order of the beings we select to be the focus of our Loving-kindness practice. Rather than directing good wishes to ourselves first and then extending them outward to others, we begin our practice by offering these phrases first to our baby. After acknowledging the extraordinary vulnerability and preciousness of the new life growing within us or in our partner, we may tap into genuine feelings of caring and kindness that might not be as easily accessible at other times in our lives. It's almost as if now, during pregnancy, we have a superhighway into the true nature of Loving-kindness, if we choose to explore and expand it. Once we find a way in, we can extend Loving-kindness to ourselves and expand it outward to others.

As Matthew said in class the evening he first practiced Loving-kindness, "When you first told us about the traditional instructions, about starting with ourselves and then working our way out, I felt uncomfortable because for me it would have felt so unnatural if I sent Loving-kindness to myself first. I was so relieved when you said we would start with the baby—it just felt like such an obvious place to begin."

Loving-kindness was originally taught as an antidote to fear, and sending Loving-kindness to the baby does give us a way to directly address a basic fear that almost all expectant parents carry to some degree during pregnancy, the fear that "something will be wrong" with the baby. For some, this fear may be nothing more than a passing thought. For others, such as a couple who has a genetically inherited condition or may have experienced a previous pregnancy loss, worries about the baby may frequently occupy the mind.

Sometimes fears arise in pregnancy as a result of the very medical care we seek to ensure that all is well—a blood test that needs to be repeated, an ultrasound with suspicious shadows or a particular placental placement, amniocentesis results that take weeks to process. Fear can be present to a lesser or greater degree during pregnancy, and sometimes we wrap a sense of tentativeness around our pregnancy and our baby in the hopes of protecting ourselves from the many what-ifs the mind can generate in the face of the unknown. Loving-kindness practice can be an antidote to those fears.

✎ LOVING-KINDNESS MEDITATION ✎

When Loving-kindness practice is first introduced in the MBCP course, we learn the complete form, just as you will in the pages that follow. After we go through the form, if there is any part that particularly resonates for you, then return to it, and going deeper, dwell there. There's no need to complete the entire sequence of phrases in every session. One meditation teacher I know says that after she learned Loving-kindness practice she spent her entire first year of practice sending Loving-kindness only to herself. She confessed, "I needed it that badly."

After learning Loving-kindness practice, you may decide that on some days you will make it be your thirty-minute formal practice. On other days, experiment with bringing it into your practice by perhaps beginning or ending your meditation with three to five minutes of Loving-kindness. It's also a good idea to spend a few minutes each day sending Loving-kindness to your baby—perhaps when waking in the morning or as a practice before falling asleep. (It is said that one of the many benefits of Loving-kindness practice is that those who practice it "sleep well and have pleasant dreams.")

You can also make Loving-kindness practice part of your informal practice in daily life—perhaps when you pause during the day to practice being with the baby when you feel the baby move. I often practice Loving-kindness when I pass a homeless person on the street or when I'm standing in line at the supermarket—especially if I see a parent having a difficult time with their baby or child. Loving-kindness is also a great practice when traveling, especially in airports. I start practicing Loving-kindness as soon as I step into the security check line.

At the reunion for Jessica and Andrew's class, Jessica described how they had used Loving-kindness practice when she was in labor. "We heard this poor woman down the hall literally screaming in pain. We just looked at each other, and Andrew said, 'I wish she had taken the mindfulness class.' I said, 'Me too.' Then we both closed our eyes and sent Loving-kindness to her and her baby. Even though my contractions were two to three minutes apart, it was clear that she was in so much more pain than I was."

As you'll see, ultimately it doesn't matter to whom you direct the Loving-kindness phrases; you are cultivating a wholesome state of mind and heart within yourself, and that's what's most important. Go easy.

Begin the practice by settling into a position of comfort and ease. It's fine to practice either sitting or lying down, but as always, find a position where you can be comfortable yet won't fall asleep. Once settled, notice whatever body sensations, thoughts, and feelings are present, and let them be, just as they are, in this very moment. Now bring your attention to the sensations of breathing as you have been learning to do, perhaps at the belly. After focusing for some minutes on the rising and falling sensations of breathing, allow a felt sense of the baby within your belly, or an awareness of the baby within your partner's belly, to arise. If the baby is moving, focus on the actual sensations of the baby within your body. Whether the baby is quiet or moving, you might find it helpful to put your hand or hands on your belly, as you have been doing in the Being with Baby practice.

Silently direct the following phrases to your baby. Continue sending wishes for wellbeing to this new little person whom someday soon you will be able to see and hold in your arms. Observe any thoughts or emotions that may arise as you repeat the phrases below.

If an image of a baby arises in your mind's eye, that's fine. You may want to hold that image as you repeat the phrases below or the phrases you have chosen for yourself. If you lose track of the phrase you are repeating, not to worry. It's only a momentary distraction; just begin again.

May you be safe and protected.
May you be healthy in body and mind.
May you be happy.
May you live with ease and in peace.

As you practice you may access a deep sense of caring, protection, and kindness toward your baby. Savor those moments. Let feelings of warmth, love, caring—and perhaps gratitude—pervade your entire being. Recognize how much you wish for this being, your baby, to be safe and healthy, happy and at ease. Appreciate how vulnerable and precious this being is at this stage of life, and recognize that your baby will be subject to the same vicissitudes that life brings to all of us who are born: the joys and challenges of infancy and childhood; the experiences of growing up; the journey of finding love, connection, and meaningful work; and the trials of sickness, eventual aging, and death. Experience how much you wish for this being, your baby, to be as happy and as free of suffering as is possible in this life. Sending Loving-kindness to your baby from deep within your heart, softly and gently.

After perhaps three to five minutes, or longer if you care to, shift the direction of your love, kindness, and well-wishing to yourself. See if you can let yourself know deeply that just as you have wished for safety, good health, happiness, and ease for your baby, you wish these things for yourself as well. For at one point in your life you too were a baby growing within your mother's body, just as your baby is growing in your body (or your partner's body) in this moment. You were then—and still are—just as precious as your baby is now, and you need and deserve the same kindness and love.

May I be safe and protected.
May I be healthy in body and mind.
May I be happy.
May I live with ease and in peace.

Stay with these phrases, repeating them for another three to five minutes. Notice if there is any difference in feeling tone—even resistance—when you direct Loving-kindness to yourself. If you do notice any uneasiness, you may want to see yourself in your mind's eye as a baby or small child, and repeat the phrases of Loving-kindness and well-wishing.

You may also want to experiment with holding yourself and the baby in an expanded circle of kindness and unconditional care. See what it's like to place one hand over your heart and the other hand on your belly as you repeat the phrases to yourself and your baby for three to five minutes:

May you and I be safe and protected.
May you and I be healthy in body and mind.
May you and I be happy.
May you and I live with ease and in peace.

Now widen your circle of Loving-kindness, this time extending your well-wishing to those nearest and dearest to you—your partner, other children if you have any, your parents or others in your immediate or extended family of origin, and perhaps friends who are like family—all those to whom you feel connected in a deep way. Repeat the phrases of Loving-kindness for those near and dear for three to five minutes. And remember, you and your baby are included in this circle of Loving-kindness.

May we be safe and protected.
May we be healthy in body and mind.
May we be happy.
May we live with ease and in peace.

As you repeat the phrases, an image of the person or the people you are wishing well may arise in your mind's eye. Hold the image or images in your mind if you care to, but there's no need to force that to happen. Sometimes many people will arise in succession, or you may think of a group of people. This is a flexible practice, and there is no one right way. Whatever cultivates the heart for you is the direction to take.

You also don't need to actually feel caring and loving toward all these people, though you very well might. In fact, as you will see when we get to a difficult person, you may feel anything *but* loving and kind. View this as good information about your current inner state in relation to that particular person. What's important here is that you are planting seeds of Loving-kindness in your heart that will take root and grow in their own time. Everything is fine, just as it is.

Now shifting the direction of the phrases once again, this time toward someone who has really helped you in your life—a teacher, a guide, a mentor—or someone who has inspired you. Perhaps you can call to mind someone who helped you unconditionally or who really saw who you were and helped guide you in an important direction. Send this person your good wishes, perhaps noticing a sense of gratitude that this person came into your life.

> May you be safe and protected.
> May you be healthy in body and mind.
> May you be happy.
> May you live with ease and in peace.

Now see if you can call to mind someone in your life whom you consider a neutral person, someone you really don't know, with whom you have minimal contact. It could be the cashier who occasionally bags your groceries or the post office clerk you saw last week or the security guard in the office building you were in yesterday. You might be surprised by how difficult it is to find someone you feel neutral about. As you look deeply and become aware of this person's humanity, that he or she was also born to parents, had the many experiences of childhood, and has a world of relations, cares, and joys, hold this person in your mind's eye and repeat the phrases, as we have been learning to do, for three to five minutes.

> May you be safe and protected.
> May you be healthy in body and mind.
> May you be happy
> May you live with ease and in peace.

Extending well-wishing and friendliness to a neutral person, notice your experience.

Now shifting the focus of your Loving-kindness once again, calling to mind someone who may be somewhat difficult in your life. We all have people who can be challenging to interact with. This person may be a co-worker or your boss or a friend, a sibling, or a parent. You don't have to pick the most difficult person in your life. Just experiment, briefly perhaps and with curiosity, seeing what it might be like to send this difficult person wishes for his or her wellbeing. And notice what happens internally as you repeat the phrases below for three to five minutes.

May you be safe and protected.
May you be healthy in body and mind.
May you be happy.
May you live with ease and in peace.

Holding a contracted heart toward someone actually hurts you more than it does them. This person may not even have any idea that she or he is on your "difficult-people" list. See if you notice a wee bit of softening around the contraction of your own heart in relation to this person who poses a challenge in your life. Notice if that small easing increases your own sense of wellbeing.

And now widening your focus to include all expectant parents, who just like you will birth a baby. Begin with extending the phrases of Loving-kindness to the expectant parents in your community—perhaps those in a childbirth class or a prenatal yoga class—extending kindness and well-wishing to them and to their babies too.

May you be safe and protected.
May you be healthy in body and mind.
May you be happy.
May you live with ease and in peace.

Continuing to expand the openness of your heart, extending well-wishing beyond those in your immediate community to all expectant parents and their babies in the country and then to those in other countries, expectant parents all over the world who also carry hopes and concerns for their unborn child, just as you do.

Opening and expanding your heart, extending the feelings of well-wishing to all beings, those born and yet to be born, those of all colors, shapes, and sizes, those who are sick and those who are well, those who are in front of you, behind you, and extending in all directions—sending Loving-kindness to all people—to all those who may be suffering from sickness or scarce resources or war or violence of any sort—continuing to expand your wishes of friendliness and wellbeing to include all beings everywhere who have ever been babies, which of course includes all of us.

May you be safe and protected.
May you be healthy in body and mind.
May you be happy.
May you live with ease and in peace.

And if you care to, extending your well-wishing and friendliness even beyond human beings, wishing well to all the creatures of the earth, creatures of land, sea, and air, even extending Loving-kindness to microbes in the soil and inside your body. Radiating universal wishes of kindness into the whole universe in all directions, repeat the following for three to five minutes:

May all beings be safe and protected.
May all beings be healthy in body and mind.
May all beings be happy.
May all beings live with ease and in peace.

Now shifting from these most expansive phrases of friendliness and goodwill after three to five minutes, bring them back once again to yourself and your baby. Or just your baby. Or just yourself. Whatever you feel is needed. Whatever opens your heart.

May we be safe and protected.
May we be healthy in body and mind.
May we be happy.
May we live with ease and in peace.

WHAT IS KINDNESS?

It's interesting to reflect on what we mean by kindness. We could say that kindness is a very large tent, one that includes many qualities of basic human goodness. Like empathy, compassion, and gratitude, kindness is most available to us when we feel safe, protected, and at ease, when our very being resides in calm and connection.

As we practice meditation, mindful awareness strengthens and our nervous system calms down. By spending less time stressed out and self-judging and more time at ease within ourselves, we may find that kindness seems to arise quite spontaneously and with greater frequency. With practice, kindness may become our default mode.

LOVING-KINDNESS PRACTICE: AN ANTIDOTE TO FEAR

As with all the meditation practices we have been learning, Loving-kindness practice has its origins in the Buddhist tradition. The ancient texts, written more than five hundred years after the Buddha was alive, tell us that Loving-kindness practice was originally taught as an antidote to fear. Since so much of what we've been learning has to do with the many dimensions of fear, perhaps it makes sense to explore this aspect of this time-honored wisdom practice a little further.

Legend has it that after teaching mindfulness practice to a large gathering of monks, the Buddha sent them out into the forest to meditate for the duration of the rainy season, a period of about three months. When the monks came to the forest they discovered that it was filled with all sorts of sounds, which they attributed to tree spirits. Unable to meditate because of their fear that the tree spirits would harm them, the monks came rushing back to the Buddha to ask him what to do. In his wisdom, the Buddha sent them back into the forest with a practice that had the power to transform their fear. That practice was Loving-kindness. It is said that the tree spirits in the forest were so transformed by the monks' Loving-kindness that they happily took care of the monks while they practiced in the forest for the duration of the rainy season.

Of course we all have our own inner tree spirits, fearful thoughts and fantasies that we carry in our minds. In fact, if you did the Speaking and Listening Inquiry on fear in Chapter 6, you may have discovered a few tree spirits of your own, which could make you want to run just like the monks, to be somewhere other than where you are. Perhaps we can experiment with Loving-kindness practice and in so doing learn a way not necessarily to make our fearful tree spirits go away (that didn't work for the monks either) but to transform *our relationship* to them by befriending them. Perhaps it is possible, through practice, to come into a peaceful and harmonious relationship with the tree spirits in our mind.

LOVING-KINDNESS PRACTICE: AN ANTIDOTE TO OTHER DIFFICULT EMOTIONS

Even though Loving-kindness practice was originally taught as an antidote to fear, the practice can be used as an antidote to many other painful, contracted, negative mind states or emotions, such as anger, envy, jealousy, sadness, or disappointment. Because we are human, we all suffer at times from these difficult emotions. It's possible to see the pain of any contracted mind state as an opportunity to practice Loving-kindness toward ourselves, letting kindness serve as an antidote to whatever the painful state of mind might be. In Loving-kindness practice we can say to ourselves, "This is really difficult. I'm angry or scared or disappointed or in a lot of emotional pain, but this is just the way it is. It is hard, but I can be with it. It is just part of being human. I can hold myself with kindness and compassion right now, knowing that whatever it is will change. May I be safe and protected. May I be healthy in body and mind. May I be happy. May I live with ease and in peace."

I often use Loving-kindness in this way when I'm caught in a painful mind state and can remember to do it, or when I've clearly made a mistake—usually acting in a reactive way toward someone—and I'm relentlessly beating myself up about it. The ability to tap into Loving-kindness for ourselves is actually the root of our compassion for others. When we can be kind to ourselves in the face of our own reactivity, misperceptions, and mistakes, we are strengthening our capacity to tap into empathy and compassion for others when they react in similar ways. What we're really doing is learning to see ourselves and others with eyes of love. Again, this may not be easy, but it's well worth the effort.

RESISTANCE TO LOVING-KINDNESS PRACTICE

People commonly equate being loving or kind with a kind of accommodating or compliant niceness. Understandably, they resist a practice that may be about cultivating an acquiescent persona rather than being authentic or real. When it comes to Loving-kindness practice, this couldn't be further from the truth. This is a practice that asks us to hold *everything* that comes up within and outside ourselves—the good, the bad, and the ugly—while maintaining a fierce commitment to compassion and kindness for ourselves and others. Loving-kindness can be a very challenging practice, and it can also be deeply liberating.

On Not Feeling Loving or Kind

Feelings of Loving-kindness may or may not be present when you're practicing, even when you're sending Loving-kindness to the baby. Let's be honest: on any given day you could be wondering what in the world you've gotten yourself into by getting pregnant! Even having thoughts that maybe having a baby wasn't such a great idea after all. But as we've learned through practice, we are not our thoughts, nor are we our feelings. Thoughts and feelings come and go, and there is no need to judge or berate ourselves just because great waves of positive emotion don't arise exactly when we want them to. Like any farmer who plants seeds, we must be patient and have faith.

A core instruction of Loving-kindness practice is to go where it's easy, as you learned when we chose to begin by sending Loving-kindness to your baby. Some of us have been deeply wounded by the actions of others, and

it can take a long time to arrive at a place of openheartedness for those particular people. This is why I caution beginners *not* to pick the most difficult
person in their lives but rather to start with someone who is just somewhat
annoying. By not diving into the deepest end of the pool, you're choosing
the most loving and kind approach for yourself.

Bob reported on his first experience with Loving-kindness practice this
way: "It really surprised me how strongly I resisted feeling Loving-kindness
for this person who sometimes gives me a hassle at work. I was thinking
of this guy, and when I said to myself in the practice, 'May you be safe,' I
found myself saying, 'Yeah, I hope you're safe, but . . .' " Bob laughed. "I
mean, do I really wish something bad should happen to him? No, but like
you said, I can see that this meditation isn't so simple."

When Bob returned to class the next week he said, "You know, there's
something to this Loving-kindness practice. Remember that guy at work
I was telling you about last week? The one who I was having a hard time
with? Well, just for the heck of it, I decided to try sending him Loving-
kindness when I was at work. Every time I saw him, whether we were
interacting or not, I would send him a few phrases. To my amazement,
something shifted for me. I was suddenly able to see that all the stupid stuff
he did was just a way of covering up some major insecurities. And I started
feeling for the guy rather than just being annoyed. I even offered to help
him on a project, and he was very appreciative, in his own awkward way."

LOVING-KINDNESS PRACTICE AND SELF-JUDGING

The theme of kindness has come up before in relation to the harsh, judging mind that so many people discover during meditation practice. For
many of us, the judging mind is almost like a set point, the go-to tape that
runs automatically when we're not using our mindfulness practice to be
present. The judging mind can even make its appearance during the intensity of labor. Many times I've watched women meet the challenges of
labor with extraordinary strength and grace and still feel the need to apol-
ogize for every groan or utterance that wouldn't make it into Emily Post.

The silver lining is that such moments may push us in the direction
of authenticity and directness. As Myla Kabat-Zinn put it so beautifully
in *Everyday Blessings*, "Labor is an opportunity to take off the quiet, kind,
thoughtful, neat, taking-care-of-others, 'good girl' mantle so often adopted by women in our society, and allow ourselves the freedom to be
whoever and however we find ourselves, completely free to be inwardly

focused and fully engaged in the work at hand."[1] Part of the work of birthing mindfully is not only accepting the labor process but accepting *ourselves* as we pass through it, however we pass through it. As one class participant suggested in an email to the class just days after giving birth, "Give yourself more love and kindness than you ever thought you deserved."

LOVING-KINDNESS PRACTICE IN ACTION

Rachel and Eric took the MBCP course several years ago and found the mindfulness practice extremely helpful for their birth experience and for parenting their twenty-month-old son, Jessie. When they became pregnant a second time, they got in touch with me for an in-home before birth tune-up. As we settled onto their couch, our conversation turned to what was going on for Rachel in this pregnancy. "I seem to be having a lot of fears this time," she said.

"What kinds of fears?"

"Well, maybe *fear* is too strong a word. I'm just thinking about death a lot. I think it's because ever since we had Jessie, I keep thinking about my mother and my grandmother. My grandmother died during childbirth, and when I was a little girl my mother told me how much this affected her childhood. She was the oldest, and she ended up raising her three younger siblings beginning when she was only ten years old. I worry about what would happen to Jessie if I died in childbirth, and of course I worry about how Eric would manage. Ever since Jessie was born life just seems so precious and fragile. It feels like I have so much to lose now."

"Welcome to parenthood," I say, putting my hand gently over hers. "Seeing yourself in the context of time passing, and of life and death, is part of the territory. Not that other people don't grapple with these issues, but having children brings us into a closer relationship to mortality—ours and theirs."

"I know," Rachel responded. "We even started having conversations about life insurance and who we would want to raise Jessie and this baby if somehow something happened to both of us."

"My husband and I had exactly the same conversations, Rachel. Concern for the wellbeing of our children never goes away. My kids are grown now, so my worries about them have changed—instead of worrying that they will fall down the stairs I worry about them falling asleep behind the wheel. The specifics are different, but the desire to keep them safe and protected will always be with you."

Though Rachel and Eric had both learned Loving-kindness practice when they had taken the MBCP course, they said they hadn't really practiced it since then. I reminded Rachel that Loving-kindness practice was originally taught as an antidote to fear, and I asked if they would like to practice it now, while we were together. They were happy for the refresher. By the time we hugged good-bye, Rachel had decided to start doing Loving-kindness practice on a regular basis.

Three weeks later I received this email from Rachel:

Dear Nancy,

I wanted to drop you a quick email to let you know how incredibly valuable the Loving-kindness practice has been these past couple of weeks. A few days after we saw you I started having some spotting and cramping. I was only twenty-five weeks pregnant, and the doctors were worried that I might be having premature labor, so they admitted me to the hospital. I think Loving-kindness practice saved my life—or at least my sanity. Remember how we talked about my fears about death when you came to visit? Well, it was a good thing we did and that I had started the Loving-kindness practice, because fear really came up big-time once all this stuff started to happen! I was scared for the baby and for me too.

One night something happened that completely surprised me; it was actually quite beautiful, and it has really been helping me a lot. It happened after one of the nurses took me on a tour of the newborn intensive care nursery. The nurse said they do this when someone is hospitalized for premature labor because they think it's better for people to know what might happen, to make people less afraid.

Well, unfortunately, it had exactly the opposite effect on me. I saw all these tiny, tiny babies lying in their incubators all alone with all these tubes and wires in and on them, and the little stuffed animals their parents had put in with them, and it just broke my heart. It made me even *more* terrified of what might happen. So as soon as I got back to my hospital room I started my Loving-kindness practice. It was very easy—and very real—to send Loving-kindness to the baby and me, wishing that we'd both be safe and protected. And then I sent Loving-kindness to all the tiny and sick babies in the nursery, and their parents.

After that I just kept going, expanding the Loving-kindness practice to Eric and Jessie and to my mom, whose mother died when she was so young, and to my dead grandma, who I never knew. I wondered if she knew she was going to die and what that might have been like for her, knowing that she was going to die and leave behind her four children and her husband. When I hit this point in the practice I started crying. The tears just started rolling down my cheeks while I was lying there alone in my dark hospital room doing Loving-kindness practice.

After sending Loving-kindness to my mom and my grandma, I began sending it to all the women all over the world who might be in labor in that very moment, particularly to the ones who might be afraid—and to all their babies, wishing that they be safe and protected and healthy. And then I included all the patients and nurses and doctors in the hospital and all the people in the hospital kitchen fixing the food for all of us and the people who clean the hospital rooms—in my hospital and in hospitals all over the world. And I just kept on including people in my practice—all the people who couldn't get to a hospital or didn't have the money to go to a hospital, and then to all the parents whose children are sick, and all the children who are sick and maybe even dying, and to everyone in their extended families; I felt this love in my chest just keep getting bigger and bigger.

Then I decided to just keep going, to see what would happen. You know, I traveled a lot before Eric and I got together and I started seeing in my mind all these people from all over the world who had helped me in one way or another. I saw the taxi driver who helped me when my wallet was stolen in Mexico fifteen years ago and sent him Loving-kindness. I saw the woman I met seventeen years ago on the beach in Malaysia who took me into her home for a few nights when I was sick, and I sent her Loving-kindness. And then I did the same with their families.

And then I thought about the war in Afghanistan, and I started sending Loving-kindness to the people living there—and to the soldiers. I felt on a very deep level how each soldier, on both sides, had once been someone's baby and was still someone's child. It seemed so completely insane that they were trying to kill each other. By this time I wasn't afraid anymore—I was just terribly sad.

Now that I'm back home, the practice has continued to have an impact on me. I'm doing it every day, and it just seems like such a natural thing to do. I haven't had any experiences as intense as that one in the hospital, but it's continuing to affect my life, mostly I think by helping me settle down around that fear of death. Somehow being able to really feel that we all are going to die, and seeing that we are all here together for just such a short time, has made me less afraid of dying. I mean, it may sound crazy, but really, I'm not the only person in the world that will die. Or that has ever died. I certainly don't *want* to die, but something has shifted around the whole thing, and it makes each moment of being alive that much more precious. Being loving and kind to everyone is really the only thing that makes any sense, if you know what I mean.

I'm sorry this is such a long email—I didn't expect it to be—but I just wanted you to know how grateful I am for all your teaching. Thank you!

I hear Jessie in the next room waking up from his nap, so I've got to run.

Sending Loving-kindness to you,
Rachel

P.S. Eric sends his love too.

CHAPTER 15

Loss, Grief, and Healing Through Mindfulness Practice

Author's Note: This chapter is optional. Its primary benefit may be for those who have directly suffered the loss and grief of miscarriage, still-birth, infant death, or other heartbreaks related to birthing children into this world. Though relatively rare in modern industrialized societies, loss does happen. As we have seen, turning toward what is true, even when it is painful, is essential in mindfulness practice. Often this turning-toward can be an important part of the healing process. However, if you're feeling vulnerable at the moment or would prefer not to turn your attention in this direction for whatever reason, please skip this chapter and go on to the next.

> *Before you know what kindness really is*
> *you must lose things,*
> *feel the future dissolve in a moment*
> *like salt in a weakened broth.*
> —Naomi Shihab Nye

AS WE SAW in the chapter on Loving-kindness practice, Rachel found her practice very helpful at a time when she was experiencing tremendous fear—fear that her baby would be born too soon, would suffer, or would not survive at all. While in Rachel's case, as in most cases, everything went well, resulting in the birth of her healthy son, it is also true that events could have unfolded quite differently.

In this territory of bringing new life into this world, sometimes things happen that bring profound sorrow and the pain of loss. Fertilized eggs don't always continue to grow, and miscarriages happen. Sometimes they happen more than once to the same woman, and numerous complicated procedures and tests can follow before being blessed with a healthy pregnancy and a healthy baby. Sometimes babies are born much too soon, well before they are able to survive outside their mother's body. Sometimes babies are born with a congenital condition that entails the loss of an imagined future. And sometimes, quite unexpectedly and for reasons that likely will never be known, a seemingly healthy baby dies while still inside his or her mother's body. If you are coming into this pregnancy with a history of these or any other losses, you have already been chastened by your experience. You know all too well that there are no guarantees.

Mindfulness practice doesn't leave anyone or anything out—including those whose pregnancy ends through miscarriage, chosen termination, stillbirth, death from incidents occurring during the birth process, a baby with congenital anomalies incompatible with life, or anything else. In fact, if you have been through loss and the deep grief that follows, mindfulness practice may be exactly what you need to help you emotionally during pregnancy and to prepare for the birth ahead.

I'd like to tell you a little about Brooke and Todd's experience using mindfulness practice to prepare for the birth of their daughter, Sydney, almost two years after their son, Dylan, was stillborn at thirty-two weeks. As would be expected, their grieving process was intensely painful, especially for Brooke, who worked as a nurse in the fetal surgery unit at the UCSF Medical Center. While helping others manage their fears and losses, she was frequently reminded of her own. A year or so after Dylan's birth, Brooke and Todd had healed sufficiently to want to become pregnant again, and a few months later they conceived.

Knowing that they would both need some emotional tools to handle this next birth, Brooke and Todd signed up for the MBCP course. Feeling protective of the joyful anticipation of the other expectant parents, they worried about whether to share their experience with Dylan with the class. I supported them in sharing only what they cared to, including not sharing anything at all.

At our second MBCP class meeting they did in fact tell the class about their experience of losing Dylan. Brooke's complete honesty that evening allowed others to talk about their own pregnancy losses, including Ann, the mother-to-be who had had three miscarriages before this current pregnancy, and Kate, who had tried for several years to conceive the baby she was now carrying. Many expressed great appreciation that Brooke and Todd had created the space for, as one expectant father put it, "talking about the six-hundred-pound gorilla in the room."

Brooke wanted to fully experience this pregnancy as happily as she possibly could and to welcome her new daughter into the world with open arms rather than have her pregnancy and birth clouded by memories, grief, and fear. Both she and Todd were diligent about their mindfulness practice. And for Brooke, whenever a fearful thought or worry would come up, she would notice it, let it go, and come back to being aware of her baby's robust movements inside her. As she put it, "Mindfulness practice helped me to feel real happiness—and gratitude for being pregnant again."

When our class received the email announcement that Brooke and Todd's daughter, Sydney, had been safely born, we all rejoiced. At the reunion, Brooke described her experience. "Everything went quickly and smoothly. Focusing on the breath kept me anchored to the present, which was absolutely invaluable for getting me through the birth. I was able to keep my mind so focused that I only thought about Dylan's birth once, when I arrived in Labor and Delivery and wondered if they were going to put me in the same room where I had labored and birthed Dylan. They didn't, but to be perfectly honest, even if they had, I could have handled it. That was then, and this is now."

As a midwife, I know that one of the deepest lessons the birth process can teach us about life is that there are no guarantees, and sometimes our worst fears do come to pass. There is a well-known Buddhist legend that for thousands of years has brought comfort to those who have experienced the seemingly bottomless grief following the death of a baby, a child, or any loved one. In the story of Kisagotami and the Mustard Seeds, the universal lesson of impermanence is told through the grief of a mother whose beloved child dies. Although we can see in this story the cultural overlays of Indian society, the truth found in the tale is timeless and its wisdom universal.

KISAGOTAMI AND THE MUSTARD SEEDS

Once, long ago, there was a poor young girl named Kisagotami who lived in a small village in India. Thin and frail, she was often unable to do the hard work expected of girls of that time. Since she was also generally considered homely, the villagers were quite sure that poor Kisagotami would never find a husband.

One day a wealthy man traveling through town saw Kisagotami and was immediately taken by her inner beauty. To everyone's surprise, he asked her to marry him. Delighted by her good fortune, Kisagotami accepted.

Shortly after they were married, Kisagotami and her husband went to live with his family in another village, as was the custom of the time. However, because of her poverty, her low caste, her lack of physical beauty, and her inability to handle the hard work expected of a daughter-in-law, Kisagotami's husband's family treated her harshly. Understandably, Kisagotami was greatly distressed by this, especially because it created unhappiness for her beloved husband, who was upset by his family's treatment of his new wife.

All this changed dramatically when Kisagotami gave birth to an extraordinarily beautiful baby boy. Kisagotami fell deeply in love with her new son, her husband's family finally accepted her, and her husband's unhappiness disappeared. The baby became the light of her life, and Kisagotami reveled in caring for him. It was as if a great cloud had been lifted, and for the first time in her life Kisagotami lived in peace and contentment.

Then one day, when her son was about one and a half years old, he was bitten by a poisonous snake. Within hours he was dead, and the whole clan was plunged into mourning. Kisagotami was so overcome with grief, that her mind was unable to accept the reality of her loss. Obsessed with the delusion that her beloved son was merely ill, not dead, she wandered the village cradling her dead child in her arms, pleading at every house for medicine to make him well again. Frightened by her madness, the villagers closed their doors as she approached. "Go away. There is no medicine to bring back a dead child."

Finally, a wise and compassionate old man, a student of the Buddha, said to her kindly, "Dear Kisagotami, there is someone who might be able to give you the medicine you are seeking. Go see the Buddha. He is teaching in the next village."

Elated that she might finally find the help her son needed, Kisagotami started out on her journey. She walked through the forest all night, carrying her dead little boy, until finally, at midday, she arrived at the village where the Buddha was teaching. Pushing her way to the front of the large group that had gathered to hear the teachings, she laid her dead child at the Buddha's feet. A hush fell over the crowd. "Dear Buddha," Kisagotami pleaded, "I beg of you, please give me some medicine that will make my child well again."

The Buddha rose from his seat and approached her. Then, much to everyone's surprise, he looked gently into her eyes and said kindly, "I know of some medicine that will help you. But the medicine is not here. To get it you must first go into the village and collect a few grains of mustard seed from a house where no one—not a child, a parent, a grandparent, or any relative or friend—has been visited by death. Go now. I await your return."

Kisagotami was overjoyed. At last someone was going to heal her sick child. Still carrying her dead son in her arms, Kisagotami began going from house to house. When someone answered her knock, she would ask, "May I have a few mustard seeds from this house?" "But of course," the householder would reply, for mustard seeds were an inexpensive staple in every Indian household.

When she was given a few seeds, Kisagotami would ask the second question. "And can you please tell me if death has visited anyone in this household—a mother or a father, a son or a daughter, a grandparent, a relative or a friend?" And with that question, a torrent of stories of loss—of accidents, of sickness, old age, and death—poured forth. "Alas," the villagers replied, "the living are few, but the dead are many. It is good to share with you our deepest grief."

Finally, as night began to settle over the village, a weary and now hopeless Kisagotami climbed a hill and sat down by the side of the road with her child still in her arms. Looking out over the village at the houses whose candles would soon be extinguished by darkness, her heart broke open in compassion. Seeing clearly through the fog of her delusion, she exclaimed, "How blinded I have been by my own grief. I am no different from anyone. Death touches all beings and comes to us at any time."

That insight into impermanence, along with the ability to expand her grief into the larger space of compassion for all beings, freed Kisagotami's mind from her delusion and her suffering. She returned to the Buddha and sat before him. Neither spoke, but the Buddha could see by her softened face that her heart had learned what no words could have taught her. The Buddha rose, and together they carried the lifeless body of Kisagotami's child to the cremation grounds.

CHAPTER 16

Causes and Conditions
Navigating What Is

*Any experience, incident, or event exists only because of the existence
of other phenomena in an incredibly complex web of cause and effect
covering time past, time present, and time future.*
—*Samyukta Agama,* ancient Buddhist text

IF YOU'RE HAVING a normal, healthy pregnancy, your baby seems to be healthy, your intention is to give birth in a hospital, and your preference is to birth with minimal or no medical interventions, it's important for you to know that this is not the norm for a hospital birth in the United States. Childbirth in this country today (and in many other industrialized nations) has become intervention and technology intensive through the use of such things as electronic fetal monitoring (85 percent of births); induction of labor (40 percent of births); Pitocin (synthetic oxytocin) used to increase the strength and frequency of uterine contractions (70 percent of births); epidurals (rates as high as 80 percent in some hospitals); and a cesarean rate at an all-time high of *one in three* births in 2009, an increase of more than 46 percent since 1996. (The World Health Organization suggests that the cesarean rate should be about 15 percent.)[1]

Despite all these interventions, technologies, and the highest per capita spending on health care in the world, the United States is not doing well in the field of maternal-infant health—or for that matter, the health of the population in general. The preterm birthrate in this country continues to be very high; as does the number of low-birth-weight babies, who are more susceptible to health problems, particularly long-term ones; we have the highest maternal mortality rate among developed nations in the world (it increased from 8/1,000 live births in 1996 to 17/1,000 live births in 2008); and according to a 2010 World Health Organization study, babies born in the United States have a higher risk of dying during their first month of life than do babies in 40 other countries, including Cuba, Malaysia, Lithuania, and Poland.[2] This is pretty sobering stuff—and just one more symptom of an overall healthcare system that's severely broken—and that unfortunately is not going to be fixed before you give birth.

The causes and conditions for the medicalization of normal childbirth, and the attendant suffering it causes for normal, healthy mothers and infants *without improving their health outcomes,* are complex. The U.S. government has sponsored conferences and issued reports on the topic, organizations have been developed to address the situation, or at least parts of it, and professional and popular articles and books have been written about it, all in an effort to increase provider and public awareness of the situation. While awareness is increasing, real changes have been slow to arrive.[3]

For our purposes it's helpful to know that the factors that play into the medicalization of the childbirth process are multiple and complex. They include: the history of obstetrics and midwifery in the United States over the past century; the hospital as an institution and the protocols under which all its providers—doctors, midwives, nurses, and other allied health professionals—practice; the experience and culture of a particular medical and nursing staff in a particular hospital, whose perceptions of labor and delivery depend on where, when, and how they were trained, their skills, their experience, their individual temperaments, and their commitment to facilitating normal labor (not just deliveries); shared social and cultural beliefs and norms about what constitutes a healthy childbirth experience, suitable health risks, and health care in general; beliefs about the appropriate use of medical technology during childbirth; the very real and understandable fear of litigation on the part of healthcare providers who care for birthing women; and the general stress level of your particular healthcare providers (meaning their state of mind, their level of fatigue, and the degree to which they can be present) during the labor and delivery process itself.

As you can see, a tremendous number of external causes and conditions affect the dynamics of the labor process. In addition to these external factors, we must add what your unique body and mind bring to the mix, including the size and shape of your pelvis; the size and position of your baby; the strength (or lack thereof) of your contractions; how much you are able to move about during labor and the positions you can assume for birthing; the people you have chosen to be with you, all the mind-body ways you have learned to cope with the pain of labor; and the perceptions, intentions, attitudes, and commitments you are bringing to the birth process itself.

Because of the complexity of all these factors and more, if your intention is to birth with minimal to no interventions in a hospital setting, extra energy will be needed on your part to influence the causes and conditions of your birth experience.

Based on current research and my many years of clinical experience as a midwife, I have put together a list of evidence-based practices that you can do to facilitate the normal process of childbirth.[4] Some of these actions are recommended for you, and some are to be encouraged in partnership with your healthcare providers. The more of these steps you can take, and the more you can encourage them in others, the more you may be able to affect the causes and conditions of your labor and delivery experience, increasing the potential for birthing with minimal intervention.

Since all of these suggested actions and behaviors are interrelated, it's best to look at them as an integrated whole rather than become strongly attached to any single one of them. Consider these steps as options that, in consultation with your healthcare provider, you might work toward implementing, if you choose to or are able to. As one of the mothers from the MBCP course said after her birth, "You just get as many ducks in a row as you can and then let everything go, being as present as possible, fully participating in your labor and birth, however it unfolds, keeping an intention for safe passage for you and the baby. There's just a lot of random stuff that happens, and you can't control everything."

Remember, no single one of these behaviors—or even all of them combined—can guarantee that the use of medical technology or assistance will not be necessary or appropriate in the moment. In fact, given the constantly changing nature of the birth process, you may even choose in the moment to welcome and use that which can be offered. Sometimes that is a very wise thing to do.

If your intention is not to have a lot of medical intervention, it can be very comforting to know that the vast majority of the time the birth process goes well, with safe passage for mother and baby. Every woman and every partner does the best they can, and you will too, given who you are, the current health of your body, the particular baby you are birthing, the coping skills you have learned, your intentions and commitments, the choices available to you regarding a healthcare provider and place to birth, and the particular hand you are dealt when the time actually comes to labor and give birth.

Hospitals are incredibly complex institutions that employ hundreds or thousands of people, many of whom are highly skilled, extremely competent, and very caring. The orientation of a hospital is to care for those who are ill, offering treatment for acute diseases or conditions. Hospitals are organized much the way factories are, with employees who work shifts and need to get a certain amount of work done in a particular period of time. Whether they are run by a nonprofit corporation, a university, or a private company, hospitals are big business; in addition to providing a place for doctors and others to practice the art and science of medicine, they are run with an eye on the bottom line. In short, hospitals and the people who work in them operate on Industrial Time. They keep the factory humming by moving patients along, in and out of their surgical suites, treatment rooms, and hospital beds. Hospitals definitely promote Doing Mode over Being Mode.

This means that the hospital environment can pose a conundrum when it comes to a normal, healthy pregnant woman and a normal, healthy baby involved in a normal, healthy function of the female body—giving birth to a child. You and your baby, living in Horticultural Time, are navigating the birth process in an institutional environment oriented toward illness and disease that is operating on Industrial Time. At times the orientation of the hospital environment and those who work there and the nature of the birthing process itself can be a significant mismatch.

As we learned in Chapter 6, the unique ebb and flow of the labor process for any individual woman happens in the realm of Horticultural Time. Like the Japanese farmer who says he doesn't grow rice but creates the fertile conditions in his field so that the rice can grow itself, a healthy birthing woman with a seemingly healthy baby by and large needs a fertile environment in harmony with Horticultural Time to birth her baby.

Childbirth is but one more example of humans being more clever than we are wise with regard to the use of technology in relation to the natural world. Used skillfully, appropriately, and wisely, technology can be dazzling—and lifesaving—during childbirth. But technology used by humans who are operating on autopilot or who are under the illusion that there are only benefits and no risks to technology or who are caught in the mistaken perception that technology can fix everything without limits can cause real harm. It takes considerable wisdom, or applied common sense, to skillfully navigate the middle path between the Doing Mode of the hospital setting and the Being Mode in which this normal biological process of giving birth takes place. And it's one more way mindfulness practice can help you through your birthing experience.

USING BRANN

People who work in a hospital setting are often on autopilot just like we are. This may be the result of habit, certain belief systems, general stress, or the pressures inherent in Industrial Time. Those who will help you give birth may not even be aware that Being Mode exists. (You may not have been aware of it either before you began your mindfulness practice.) However, by learning and remembering to use the acronym BRANN, you can help yourself to make mindful and wise decisions *and* help your healthcare provider step out of autopilot and be more present as well.[5]

BRANN stands for the following: What are the *Benefits* of any suggested course of action? What are the *Risks?* What are the *Alternatives?* What about doing *Nothing?* And does it (whatever "it" is) need to be done *Now?* Unless it is a very rare emergency, there are *always* alternatives. There is no one right way for your healthcare provider either, and by engaging in respectful conversation, you can learn more about your provider's concerns and reasons for a recommended course of action, and you can maintain active engagement with the decisions that affect the course of your labor. In the best of circumstances you will enjoy a trusting partnership with your healthcare provider, and you will be a full participant in the causes and conditions of your labor and birth experience.

BRANN is also useful for navigating any medical advice, recommended treatments or procedures, and the healthcare system in general once your baby has been born. Unless you have given birth before or you have had significant health challenges in the past, pregnancy and childbirth may be your first real introduction to negotiating the complexities of a relationship with a healthcare provider and the healthcare system. Since you will be turning to a healthcare provider right away for guidance and health advice regarding your baby (such as vaccinations, medications, and other treatments), you are on the threshold of an important ongoing relationship. Not to mention that the choices you make regarding your baby's health will be pivotal in the attitudes she or he develops about how they will take care of their own body and health. At some point you might like to teach BRANN to them too.

During Pregnancy

If your preference is to have minimal technology or medical intervention during your labor and birth, one of the most important decisions you will make is who your healthcare provider will be. How your healthcare provider perceives the process of childbirth will determine their behavior and the advice they give you. (It's that old perception thing again.)

In general, the healthcare providers with the most expertise in facilitating the normal physiologic process of childbirth with minimal technological intervention are midwives, whose professional training and experience

focuses on normal birth. Midwives see themselves as working in partnership with the women and families they serve, balancing a woman's individual needs and desires with the best available evidence for clinical care.
In relation to childbirth, their approach tends toward being in harmony
with Horticultural Time, relying on patience, watchful waiting, and nonin-
tervention in normal processes whenever possible.

In hospitals, midwives work in collaboration with their physician colleagues as needed, employing appropriate, step-by-step use of interventions and technology if necessary. Having a healthcare provider whose
approach is in tune with your intentions can go a long way toward having
a birth with minimal interventions. Midwives who can attend deliveries in
a hospital are called Certified Nurse-Midwives (CNMs) or Certified Midwives (CMs). However, these midwives attend only about 7 percent of the
deliveries in U.S. hospitals today, so it is quite possible that this option will
not be available to you. If it isn't, follow the suggestions in this chapter, and
practice navigating what is.[6]

Early in your pregnancy I suggest you take one of the tours of the Labor
and Delivery unit offered to expectant parents at the hospital where you
intend to deliver. Find out about the hospital's rate for inducing labor as
well as its rate for administering epidurals and for performing cesarean sections. This will tell you a lot about the culture of that particular Labor and
Delivery unit, the culture in which your healthcare provider is practicing,
and the level of skill of the nursing staff with regard to facilitating normal
labor and birth. Ask lots of questions about what is possible and what is
not, particularly regarding protocols about being out of bed and moving
around during labor, the freedom to assume different positions for pushing,
eating or drinking during labor, and the routine use of fetal monitoring.
Discover if there is room for flexibility in the hospital rules. Sometimes
there is, and sometimes there isn't. If you are truly unhappy with what
you discover, use BRANN, consider the benefits and risks of your current
choice, explore your alternatives if there are any, and perhaps make a different choice about where you want to deliver. Or focus on what you can
do to optimize the conditions in your current choice, and practice coming
to terms with things as they are, including frustration, anger, sadness, disappointment, and fear.

If you are healthy, your pregnancy has been normal, and your baby
seems to be healthy, your alternatives may include a freestanding birthing
center or having your baby at home. Large population studies that compared
home birth to hospital birth have found that out-of-hospital birth is safe

for low-risk women. What's more, out-of-hospital births are associated with decreased rates of obstetrical interventions, reduced rates of maternal morbidities such as cesarean births, perineal trauma, or postpartum hemorrhage, and lower rates of newborn morbidities such as the need for resuscitation, admission to the Neonatal Intensive Care Unit, or need for oxygen therapy.[7] However, regardless of the setting you choose, the birth of your baby cannot be made completely risk free, and in your decision-making process you will need to weigh for yourself the risks and benefits of one setting or another.

Writing a Birth Plan to give to the hospital staff is frequently encouraged by childbirth educators, doulas, and other healthcare providers; you can easily find templates for them on the Internet. Reading about and considering writing a Birth Plan can be a way for you and your partner to educate yourselves about the culture and technology that surround birth in a hospital setting. However, the notion that you can have a plan for your birth experience doesn't fit with the reality that you cannot know how your childbirth will unfold. That said, a *Birth Preference Sheet* can be a way to communicate to those who will be caring for you during childbirth what your intentions and preferences are. After assessing the hospital culture you will be birthing in, if you think it wise to write a Birth Preference Sheet, use kind, flexible, respectful language, and keep it brief.

By and large, people who work in Labor and Delivery are there because they love their work and want you to feel safe and be happy with their care. Being aware of this can help you establish a relationship of trust with all the hospital staff members you encounter. Keeping this in mind can only improve the care you will receive.

Research clearly shows that women who have someone with them at all times during childbirth have shorter, less painful labors; use less medication; have fewer medical interventions or assisted deliveries such as forceps, a vacuum, or cesarean births; are more successful with breastfeeding; and are generally more satisfied with their birthing experience. Your partner may be able to take on this role, but truth be told, despite all the classes the two of you can take and all the books you can read, your partner is not likely to have much experience with hospitals, protocols, routines, and, most important, the skills necessary for guiding a woman through normal childbirth.

While a partner's presence is vital, it is not a substitute for a trained eye, particularly if your preference is to have a birth with minimal intervention in a hospital setting.[8] Historically, that trained eye was provided by a midwife who offered intimate, continuous care to a woman and her family throughout pregnancy, labor, birth, and the postpartum period. As there are comparatively few midwives in the United States today, the care of a pregnant woman, her partner, and her family through pregnancy, birthing, and the postpartum period is generally managed by an obstetrician, a highly trained specialist who has precious little experience or time available to facilitate a normal childbirth. A family practice physician may be an option for some, particularly if you live in a rural area, but the number of family physicians who practice obstetrics has been in serious decline over the past several decades.

A doula, a woman who is familiar with supporting a woman through the birth process, helps fill an unfortunate gap in care for the healthy pregnant woman seeking minimal medical intervention. Even if you have midwives caring for you in the hospital where you plan to deliver, the support of a doula can be invaluable.[9]

During pregnancy, consider hiring a doula. In addition to her trained eye, a doula will bring many other skills to support both you and your partner. If you plan to do a good bit of laboring at home, some doulas will come to your house to help you there. Birthing a baby, particularly a first baby, can sometimes take quite a while, and having someone involved in addition to your partner can be very helpful, especially at those times when your partner may need to take a nap, get something to eat, or just step out of the room for a bit. (In the MBCP course we sometimes refer to a doula as a "dude-la" because of her role in supporting the partner during the birth experience as well as you, the birthing woman.)

Some hospitals offer volunteer doula services; you might want to check into this. Also, doulas in training may have very low fees or may attend your labor without charge. A trusted family member or friend sometimes can take on some of the functions of a doula. If you decide to take the family member or friend approach, you might consider sharing this book with them so they can understand the mind-set you and your partner are taking in relation to your birth experience.

In Early Labor at Home

Set your intention to be as mindfully present for this experience as you can, whatever might unfold. If you have practiced mindfulness as outlined in this book, you have learned many skills, and now it's time to put what you have learned into practice. Give some thought to how you might like to spend your time in early labor. For daytime early labor, consider taking a walk outside, planting something special in your garden, baking cookies or a cake for your support people and hospital staff (chocolate is always appreciated), all done mindfully, of course. You might also spend some of this time in formal meditation practice, including yoga and Loving-kindness practice. Walking Meditation can be very helpful too. For nighttime early labor, sleep if you can, and practice the Body Scan if you can't. Time will pass, and day will come. You may even have a baby in your arms before sunrise. You just don't know.

Eat lightly to keep your strength up. Good suggestions include easily digestible foods such as hot cereal (oatmeal or cream of wheat), mashed or baked potatoes, bananas, white rice, and light soup.

Drink about one cup of liquid every hour. Juices, electrolyte replacement drinks, and water are all okay.

As your labor gets stronger, it's usually beneficial to be upright and moving about rather than being in bed. Of course if you're tired, lie down and take a rest. Then, when you feel rested, get up and move about some more. Use the breath and the pain practices to work with your contraction-expansions. Remember to let go of the wandering mind and come back to the breath, especially during the time between contraction-expansions. This is one of the most important contributions you can make to the normal physiologic process of childbirth.

When your labor seems to be getting stronger, keep doing whatever it is you are doing, including lying down to rest. Pay attention to your body. It will usually tell you what to do. Remember, there is no one right way.

Wait until you are in strong, active labor before going to the hospital. Then wait some more. How will you know? When your contraction-expansions are regular, frequent (every three to five minutes), when you can't talk or walk through them, and when you have the thought "This *really* hurts!" or "I'm not sure I can do this" or "It's time to go." If you have that last thought, then go, regardless of what anyone says. A doula can often help you sort this out if you decide to hire one. You may end up having much of your labor in the comfort of your own home. Or you may not have any early labor at all before the contraction-expansions become frequent and strong. You just don't know.

When you call the hospital to tell them you're coming in—or before that, if you talked to them when you were in early labor or went to the hospital to get checked—let them know about your intention to have minimal medical intervention, if that's what you want. Ask to have a nurse assigned to you who enjoys working with women who are approaching their labor and birth experience in this way. Helping a woman through childbirth without technology is labor-intensive (no pun intended), and some nurses have more experience and skill with it than others. Choosing midwifery care if possible and/or hiring a doula will ensure that these kinds of skills will be available to you, just in case there are no nurses with these skills on duty at the particular time you're in labor.

Your labor may go too quickly for any of the above recommendations to be implemented. If it does, let all of them go, pay attention to your body and mind in the present moment, and do what seems appropriate.

Early labor can sometimes take a while—even a long while, like a day or more. Sometimes it can be wise to go to the hospital to check that all is well with you and your baby. If you do go to the hospital, you might be offered some medication for rest or sleep. Sometimes this is a helpful option. Alternatively, you may be offered something to "speed things up." This too may or may not be a wise option; again, it all depends. Use BRANN. If you decide to take some medication for rest, see if you can take it at home, away from the tendency to "do," which can be so pervasive in the hospital environment. Or perhaps it makes sense to stay at the hospital and "do" something. Again, there is no one right way. Remain engaged, and remember: everyone is doing the very best they can, including and especially you.

In the Hospital

As soon as you get into your labor room, place a big sign over the clock that says NOW. Use that reminder to be in the moment for the duration of your hospital stay. Through your practice, you and your partner both know how much concentration it takes to be in the present moment and how to work with intense body sensations as they arise and pass. Maintaining a quiet, peaceful atmosphere can support your mindfulness practice as you labor, just as it does at home or in the classroom. Dim lights and drawn shades can be helpful. Your partner, your doula, or others who might be with you can help maintain an environment with minimal stimulation and distraction.

However, you may be a woman who is very vocal and energetic during labor. You may get to the hospital and be in such intense labor that you couldn't care less about peace and quiet in your labor room. If that turns out to be the case, stay in the moment, maintain your focus on your breath as best you can, and let go of any fantasy you may have had about your labor and birth. Anything you do to help yourself through the process is just what you do. Remember to practice non-judging, acceptance, and letting go.

Labor and Delivery nurses are sometimes the unsung heroines or heroes of the labor process. If you are assigned a nurse who has the skills to facilitate the normal labor process that you prefer, smile and thank her or him. Then thank her or him again. Gratitude is a healthy state of mind, and people respond positively when their efforts are recognized and appreciated. However, if you and the assigned nurse are not working in harmony, it is perfectly acceptable to ask, respectfully and kindly, for a different nurse. Use your mindfulness practice here. A doula also may be able to help facilitate a change if needed.

There will be a bed in your labor room. If you can get into it, you can also get out of it. Remember, research shows that your labor may be shorter and hurt less if you're upright. When you're upright, you're working with gravity, not against it. The uterus also works optimally when you are upright since it and the baby get more blood—which means more oxygen and oxytocin. Stand and move as much as you can during your labor. Walk, rock, lean, sway, do some yoga poses or stretching, rotate your hips, squat, or sit on a birthing ball. Then rest. Then do it all over again. Getting on all fours can help get the baby into an optimal position for birthing, and it can *really* be helpful if you are having back pain or back labor. Child's Pose (which you practiced in the yoga sequence) can also be very comfortable during labor and is particularly helpful if you are having back labor.

It is well documented that receiving fluids through an IV during labor does not improve birth outcomes for a healthy pregnant woman. Being attached to an IV and its pole is also cumbersome when you are up and moving around, which you will probably be doing a lot. Your healthcare providers may not be aware of these research findings, and it may make them nervous if you don't have an IV. A heparin lock (a thin, flexible catheter that is inserted into your arm to administer medication if it becomes necessary) may be a nice compromise. Discuss this with your healthcare provider before labor. Depending on how your labor unfolds, you may not use the heparin lock at all. Or you may. In any case, keep drinking that one cup of clear fluid every hour during labor. Little sips are fine.

There may be protocols at the hospital where you are delivering that don't permit eating during labor. The data clearly shows that eating and drinking in labor is okay. Most women in active labor aren't interested in eating, so this may be a moot point, especially if you were eating and drinking at home before going to the hospital. But if you're hungry during labor in the hospital, easily digestible food is fine. If you're worried about this, discuss it in advance with your healthcare provider.

You might want to bring your own food and energy bars with you to the hospital. Even if you aren't hungry, others on your birth team might be.

Also, you might be really hungry very soon after the baby is born, and food cooked in your own kitchen is usually tastier than hospital food.

An electronic fetal monitor (EFM) is a machine that monitors your uterine contractions and the baby's heart rate during labor. You are connected to this machine by two cords attached to two belts strapped around your belly (one belt for your contractions and one for the baby's heart rate). As mentioned earlier, continuous electric fetal monitoring is routine in most U.S. hospitals today (85 percent), but it is not necessary during labor for a baby whose mother has had a healthy prenatal course. In fact, multiple studies show that continuous EFM is associated with more frequent use of forceps, vacuums, and cesarean births. Being attached to an EFM machine often leads to spending more time in bed (did I mention that being up and moving around during labor are important?). It's also a lot more comfortable to be free from belts strapped around your belly when you are in labor.

The alternative for checking your baby's heart rate during labor is intermittent auscultation (IA). This means that a nurse or a midwife will listen to your baby's heart rate with a handheld Doppler device before, during, and after a contraction—usually about every half hour during active labor and more frequently when you're pushing your baby out. According to the American College of Obstetricians and Gynecologists (ACOG) and the American College of Nurse-Midwives (ACNM), this is a totally acceptable way to check on the baby's wellbeing.[10]

For those taking care of you, practicing IA may take them out of their habitual or automatic routine and therefore out of their comfort zone. Again, discuss all of this with your healthcare provider before labor. Find out about the hospital protocols during your tour of Labor and Delivery. See if there is room for negotiation. There may or may not be. You might be able to negotiate something during the birthing process itself, especially if the baby appears well. It all depends. Remember, no one of these actions or behaviors is a make-or-break situation. Stay upright if you can, be in the moment, use BRANN, and do what makes sense at the time.

A situation can arise during labor where it's prudent to monitor your baby using EFM. Even if this is the case, remember how important it can be to continue to move around and stay active during labor. You needn't stay in bed just because you're connected to a machine. In fact, it may be even more important for you to be upright if there is concern about your baby. Remember the increased blood flow, oxygen, oxytocin, and help from gravity that you and your baby get when you're upright.

In some hospitals, healthcare providers who are on automatic pilot may routinely break your bag of water by briefly inserting a small instrument into your vagina to make a tiny hole in the amniotic sac. This is called artificial rupture of membranes (AROM). The procedure is very simple and not painful. The reason for this routine behavior is the mistaken belief that AROM speeds up labor. The research shows that AROM does not shorten labor, nor does it decrease the number of cesarean births. Left alone, the amniotic sac usually breaks late in the first stage of labor, during transition, or when your cervical dilation is between seven and ten centimeters.

There are some situations during childbirth when AROM may be totally appropriate and quite helpful, allowing the baby's head to descend further into your pelvis and put pressure on your cervix from the inside. You may be involved in one of those situations. Remember BRANN. If the reason given for breaking your bag of water is "to speed up your labor," you may want to decline the offer. If another reason is given, you may want to consider it. You can't know now. You and your partner will listen, learn, and decide in partnership with your healthcare provider what is best for you and your baby in the moments when you're in labor.

Warm water during active labor can be very helpful in facilitating the normal physiologic process of childbirth. Warm water can aid relaxation and decrease the need for pain medication. Evidence shows that it is safe to be in water during labor. Water is often very helpful when labor is most intense. If you have the thought, "I'm not sure I can do this," remember, it's just a thought. If you speak that thought aloud, others around you may take that as a signal that you need an additional way to cope with the intensity of the sensations of labor. This is an excellent time to get into warm water.

A shower can be as effective as a tub during labor. After being in the shower or tub, you may find you have renewed energy, determination, and courage. Or you may want to ask for some pain medication through that heparin lock. Or you may surprise yourself and decide that you want to use an epidural after all, even though you were pretty sure you didn't want one before labor. It's usually a good idea to have someone do a vaginal exam before you go ahead and have an epidural, as you may be very close to complete dilation and almost ready to push your baby out, which feels very different from the way you are feeling in that moment. A lull in the contractions may not be far away. Since we just don't know, you can decide in the moment. You will find your own way.

Read one book about common birth technology, interventions and drugs, and the situations when they might be recommended. Remember,

85 to 90 percent of births are normal. You don't have to become an expert on everything that can go wrong. That's the job of your healthcare providers; that's why they went through many years of professional training and why you hired them. However, if you need to have a BRANN conversation, it can be helpful if you know a little bit about the territory of medications and interventions. For a well-reasoned, balanced, and evidence-based approach regarding technology, interventions, and drugs as well as non-pharmacological alternatives, I recommend *Our Bodies, Ourselves: Pregnancy and Birth* by the Boston Women's Health Collective. Other books and online resources with helpful information are listed in Appendix B.

In the Second Stage of Labor

After complete dilation, there may be a slowing of labor contraction-expansions before you feel the urge to push. The contraction-expansions won't stop: they just may become farther apart. This is normal. It is your body's way of giving you and your baby a rest before taking on the next phase of birthing, the pushing phase. This lull can last as long as two hours for women having their first baby and up to an hour for women having a subsequent baby. Enjoy the rest, using your practice to stay in the present moment. Your baby is probably enjoying the rest too.

Research clearly shows that honoring this lull is associated with a reduced need for forceps, less trauma to a woman's perineum, less maternal fatigue, and fewer worrisome variations in the fetal heart rate. However, sometimes well-meaning healthcare providers who may not know about this lull may tell you, "You're completely dilated. It's okay to push now," or "Go ahead and push now." If you feel the urge to push, by all means do so. If you don't yet feel the urge to bear down you can say, "Thank you, but I'll wait until my body tells me to push. It's nice to have a little break." Then do a Body Scan. Take a little nap between contraction-expansions. There's more work ahead.

Learning to push can take a while; by paying attention to your body and following its lead, you will learn how. If you have practiced mindful pooping, you may get the hang of pushing sooner than if you didn't do that particular mindfulness practice. During this stage, try lots of positions, including pushing on a birthing stool or on the toilet. Research shows that bearing down in an upright position is associated with a shorter time needed to push a baby out. Guidance from an experienced provider—a doula, a midwife, a nurse, or a physician—while you're bearing down may be quite helpful.

Watch out for the judging mind before, during, and after labor, and if it appears, practice letting go. Practice Loving-kindness toward all who are participating in the birth of your baby, especially you. Your body, mind, and heart are doing something quite remarkable however the labor and birth are unfolding. You're about to begin your lifelong journey of parenting. Being fully present for beginnings is important. (Being fully present for middles and endings is important too.)

USING BRANN FOR PAIN MANAGEMENT: AN EXAMPLE OF NAVIGATING WHAT IS

Birthing in a hospital means that you'll have many options for pain management in addition to your mindfulness practice, should circumstances arise where it is appropriate or advisable to use them. Your reading and BRANN should give you enough background in procedures and medications to be able to have a conversation with your nurse, midwife, physician, or anesthesiologist between contractions during labor, if you wish to do so.

An epidural is just one of many options for pain management. It's also the most high-tech option and requires a lot of technology to be used safely and well. Because an epidural is the most common way to manage labor pain in hospitals today, sometimes other, simpler options (such as a short-acting narcotic) are overlooked. (It's autopilot once again.) Such alternative options for pain management could be appropriate in your particular circumstance and are worth exploring.

If you do receive an epidural, an anesthesiologist or nurse anesthetist will give you an injection of Novocain to numb an area over your spine where a long needle will be inserted into the epidural space that surrounds your spinal cord. Once that's done, a small thin plastic tube or catheter is threaded through the needle and the needle is removed, leaving the catheter in place in your back. A pump will be attached to the catheter so you can receive the anesthesia, which temporarily blocks pain messages from your spinal cord to your brain. Because of this, the endorphins your brain normally makes in response to the labor pain from your contraction-expansions will be significantly reduced.

If you have an epidural, in addition to being hooked up to the pump, you'll need to be attached to an IV to get fluids into your veins, to an electronic fetal monitor machine with its two belts around your belly to monitor the baby's heart rate and your contraction-expansions, and to a blood pressure cuff that will stay on your arm to monitor your blood pressure every fifteen minutes or so. In addition, because you'll no longer be able to feel the urge to pee, you'll need to have a thin plastic catheter periodically inserted into your bladder to empty it. Sometimes, if there are concerns about the baby, a very tiny screw with a wire will be attached to the baby's scalp. The wire will come out of your vagina, be taped to your thigh, and then attach to a fetal monitor machine. You may also have a thin plastic catheter threaded into your uterus to monitor the strength of your contractions. That's between five and seven tubes and wires, plus all the equipment they are attached to, on or in your body during your labor. Epidurals are fabulous when they are needed, and they usually work well. Sometimes they even prevent a cesarean birth. But they are not so simple and not without risks.

Here is an example of how you might use BRANN in relation to the decision to use or not use an epidural.

What Are the Benefits?

- An epidural, when it works well, takes away your ability to feel the pain of uterine contractions within about fifteen to twenty minutes. Usually you will not have any pain sensations from just below your breasts all the way down to your toes. There is no way to know if the epidural will work well for you until you have one. Generally they do.
- Not feeling the pain of labor means that you can take a rest from the labor process and gather your strength. This can be especially helpful if your labor is taking a long time. You can sleep, sometimes for several hours, when you have an epidural.
- If your labor is not progressing, meaning that dilation of your cervix is not continuing, the relaxation provided by an epidural may help you to completely dilate so that you can move into the next stage of labor, pushing and birthing your baby.
- If you need a cesarean delivery, you can be awake during the surgery and can see your baby as soon as she or he is born.

What Are the Risks?

- Even with all the care taken, there's a small chance of infection at the site where the needle is inserted into your spine. A serious infection could cause paralysis or even death; the risk of this happening is tiny.
- In rare cases, the needle used to insert the plastic catheter could hit a nerve and cause nerve damage or paralysis.
- If the catheter in your back is placed too high up, or if anesthesia accidentally gets into your spinal fluid, you may lose the sensations of breathing

and have to be put onto a ventilator to keep you breathing regularly. This too is very rare.

- The epidural increases your chances of getting a fever during labor. Usually this "epidural fever" if it occurs is in response to the epidural, but occasionally a fever occurs that means you or your baby has an infection. Because your healthcare provider can't tell if your fever is from the epidural or from an infection, if you do get a fever the baby may have to be tested and observed for infection. This could entail anything from having one blood test and being checked by the nurses more often during the first twenty-four hours to a potentially several-day admission to the Neonatal Intensive Care Unit (NICU) for an IV and multiple blood tests. This of course means that the baby will experience physical and emotional pain from being stuck with needles and from being separated from you. Depending upon how aggressive a particular doctor or the culture of the hospital is, the baby might have a spinal tap to check for infection in the spinal fluid.

- Sometimes an epidural can considerably slow down or stop your labor. Then you will need the hormone Pitocin through your IV to start the contraction-expansions again or to make them strong enough to dilate your cervix.

- Your legs will be numb, and you won't be able to stand or walk anymore during labor. With an epidural it can be challenging to change positions in bed too. (There are variations in the way anesthesiologists give epidurals that can keep you from losing all sensation in your legs, but you can't count on this. Ask about it on your hospital tour.)

- If your baby is not in the most optimal position for birthing, the total relaxation of the pelvic muscles provided by the epidural may mean that the baby will not rotate her or his head into an optimal position for birthing. This means that the baby can get stuck in certain positions and you can't help it get unstuck by moving around. This can increase your chances of needing a vacuum or forceps to help you birth your baby.

- Since you have limited sensation in the lower part of your body, pushing your baby out may take longer. Sometimes the epidural can be turned down so that you can feel more sensation and move about a little for pushing, but usually you'll have to stay hooked up to all the machines and won't be able to get out of bed.

- There is a 1 to 2 percent chance that you will get a spinal headache after birth with an epidural. A spinal headache is a severe headache that starts one to two days after the epidural. If you are at home, you may have to return to the hospital to have a procedure called a blood patch; this usually stops the headache almost immediately.

- No one knows exactly why, but babies of mothers who have had an epidural seem to have a harder time breastfeeding in the first few days after birth.
- Some women feel quite distressed by the unfamiliar loss of feeling in the lower part of their body during the epidural. By contrast, some women are absolutely delighted to have most or all of the sensations of labor taken away.

Even though the list of risks for epidurals is quite long, when an epidural is needed, it can be a true blessing.

What Are the Alternatives?

Assuming you have done all the non-pharmacological things that help a normal labor along (mindfulness practice, being upright, warm water, continuous labor support, and so forth), there are still other options, such as short-acting narcotics, just to get you through a brief intense period. Nitrous oxide, a gas you can inhale (used a lot in dentistry), may be one of those options. Ask your healthcare provider about its availability at the hospital where you plan to deliver.

What Would Happen If You Did Nothing Now?

Sometimes you just need a little more time to do what you're already doing and things will change all on their own. Or you need to do everything you've been doing *again* to get through a rough patch. (Most women have a rough patch at some point during their labor.) You might choose to do *Nothing Now.* Wait a little longer—say an hour or so—and then reevaluate the situation. Sometimes you have reached the limit of your endurance, and an epidural is the wisest and most compassionate course to take. Nothing in life is risk free, even getting out of bed in the morning. If you really need help (and only you, in consultation with your healthcare providers at that time, will know), fully accept the technology with gratitude, and work with the doctors and nurses to do what they are well-trained to do. Use your practice to work with the judging mind and any negative emotions— fears, sorrow, disappointment, frustration, anger, or blame—that may arise. Hold those emotions with kindness and self-compassion.

CARE OF YOUR BABY DURING DELIVERY

Remember that everything changes, including the practices physicians and midwives use during childbirth. For example, in the 1950s and 1960s it was fairly routine for a woman in labor to receive an enema, have her pubic hair shaved, labor on her back, be strictly confined to bed, and be given an episiotomy. Currently two delivery practices are in flux: the timing of cutting the umbilical cord after birth and the use of the bulb syringe to suction your baby's nose and mouth during and immediately after delivery.

Evidence continues to accumulate that waiting until the cord stops pulsing after a baby is born (sometimes called "delayed cord clamping") is protective against iron deficiency anemia in infants for as long as four months after birth.[11] In addition, vigorous suctioning of your baby's nose and mouth to "clear the airway" right after your baby's head and body are born is also coming to be seen as an unnecessary practice—and perhaps even a harmful one. Vigorous suctioning, which is done with a bulb syringe, can hurt the sensitive tissues inside your baby's mouth and throat, causing it to swell and thereby making it difficult or painful for your baby to suck, swallow, or nurse after birth.[12] Your healthcare provider, the physician or nurse (midwives usually wait until the cord stops pulsing and rarely do vigorous suctioning) attending your delivery may have been assisting women during childbirth for many years and therefore may have deeply ingrained habits and attachments about "the right way to deliver babies." As you yourself are coming to see, it is not easy to change habits. Have a conversation with your healthcare provider about the kind of care you do or do not want your baby to experience during and immediately after delivery, and remember, this is *your* baby, for you to keep safe and protected from the very beginning.[13]

CARE OF YOUR BABY AFTER DELIVERY

One of the most challenging situations to navigate in a hospital setting can be what happens to your baby—where your baby goes and how she or he is cared for—immediately after birth. The routine in most hospitals today is to let you hold your baby for a few minutes after birth before taking her or him away to a crib or a table with very bright warming lights for an initial examination. There your baby is vigorously dried, weighed, measured, and banded on the wrist or ankle with a little plastic identification bracelet. Antibiotic ointment is quickly put into your baby's eyes and vitamin K injected into your baby's thigh. Then your baby is diapered, dressed, tightly wrapped in blankets like a little burrito, and given back to you.

You may be able to see everything that is happening with the baby from across the room—or you may not. You may also be birthing the placenta during this time. The baby may cry during these procedures, which is the baby's way of communicating distress.

This standard process is your baby's first experience of life outside your body. There is a kinder, gentler, and more mindful option, one that not only honors and respects the preciousness of these first moments of your baby's life in this air-breathing world and your life as newly born parents, but is actually healthier and more in tune with the millions-of-years-old instincts and physiological programming deep within you and your baby.

If there is no cause for concern about your baby—meaning that your baby has a healthy color, is vigorous, and is breathing well within a few minutes after delivery—you can have your warm, wonderfully wet and slippery baby placed directly onto your chest or abdomen, skin-to-skin. Your baby's back can be gently dried as your baby rests on your warm body, all the while hearing the familiar sounds of your voice, and your partner's, as you see, touch, listen to, and smell your baby for the very first time. You can slide your baby so that you and your baby can look into each other's eyes. You can marvel at the baby's face and examine his or her little hands, fingers, feet, and toes. You can wonder at the miracle that is your new son or daughter. This is a way you and your baby could first experience each other in the world outside your womb.

Multiple research studies have found that babies who are kept skin-to-skin with their mothers after they are born cry less in the first hour after birth, initiate breastfeeding more easily, have improved early sleep patterns, and stay warmer than babies who receive routine hospital care. The research also shows that mothers are less distressed and seem more attached to their babies if they have skin-to-skin contact immediately after birth.

Once again, before you give birth it's a good idea to educate yourself about the routine hospital procedures and care the staff expects to give your baby immediately after birth. You can find out about this on your hospital tour or from your healthcare provider. Use BRANN, and think about what you want for your baby. It's perfectly acceptable to ask to delay all the hospital's routine procedures—the eye ointment, the injections, the dressing, and any bathing of the baby—for several hours after birth. This will probably be inconvenient for the nurse caring for you since it will disrupt her usual Industrial Time work routine and it would be kind of you to acknowledge this. However, none of the hospital procedures for the new-born are urgent. You and your baby are still living predominantly in Horticultural Time and have some very important work to do—breastfeeding for the very first time. Hospital routines and procedures can wait.

BREASTFEEDING

Most perinatal healthcare providers and organizations that promote optimal maternal-child health, including the World Health Organization, encourage new mothers to breastfeed their baby within the first hour after birth if at all possible. For a healthy newborn and a healthy mother, there are precious few reasons this should not be possible. After birth, particularly an unmedicated one, your baby will usually settle into a quiet, alert state, which is optimal for her or his first breastfeeding experience. Colostrum, the pre-breast-milk fluid in your breasts that is filled with extraordinarily important protective antibodies, is also very important for encouraging your baby's digestive system to begin functioning, helping to eliminate meconium, the thick, tarry, green-black first contents of your baby's intestines. Skin-to-skin contact and the sense of smell helps your baby recognize you, find and latch onto the nipple, and learn to breastfeed right from the beginning. This is another reason for your baby not to be taken away to be dried, washed, and dressed. Remember, though, while it's optimal for your baby to stay with you skin-to-skin immediately after birth, babies need to eat, and they'll learn to breastfeed even if they don't go straight onto your belly or are separated from you for a time after birth.

The role of oxytocin, the hormone that was so fundamental to the birth process, continues to be essential in breastfeeding. Stimulated by your baby's sucking, oxytocin helps your uterus contract immediately after birth, thereby decreasing the amount of blood you lose after delivery. Oxytocin is also fundamental to the beautifully complex dance that helps you, your partner, and your baby become attached to each other. It's not called "the love hormone" for nothing. Breastfeeding helps you maintain an open, receptive state, similar to what you may have experienced in meditation practice. Through breastfeeding the intimate relationship between your body and the baby's body can continue in a new way, a way that can be deeply nourishing to the two of you in the days, weeks, months, and years to come. (Oxytocin levels increase in men during the postpartum period too.) Bottom line: maintain skin-to-skin contact and breastfeed your baby within the first hour after birth, if at all possible. You'll read more about breastfeeding in Chapter 18.

While breastfeeding right after birth is optimal, and we certainly do want to aim for optimal, we don't always get it in this life. The reality is that some babies need help right after birth. Your baby may be able to get that help in the room where you delivered, but sometimes the healthcare providers taking care of your baby observe things that cause them to recommend your baby be taken to the nursery for observation or treatment. That means that you and your baby are separated right after birth. If this is the case, your partner can go with your baby to the nursery; even though you can't be with them right now, knowing that your baby and partner are together may bring you some comfort. If you can, go to your baby in the nursery as soon as possible, or have your baby returned to you as soon as possible. In a busy hospital environment, this can take some persistence. If so, be persistent. Again, a doula or midwife may be able to help you negotiate this.

Your baby is born from a sterile environment, your womb. As she or he passes through your birth canal, your baby begins to be colonized by your microorganisms. This process continues after birth and is one way your baby becomes part of the microecology of your family. It's healthier for your baby to be colonized by the microorganisms that live on your skin and in your body and those of your partner than those that live in the hospital nursery. Remember, even if well-meaning hospital staff offer to take your baby to the nursery "so you can get some rest," you can politely decline. You may not be able to do so, but if you can, keep your baby close while you're in the hospital.

One of the keys to breastfeeding success, besides nursing in the first hour after birth and keeping your baby with you, is not giving your baby anything to drink other than breast milk unless medically indicated. According to a 2011 U.S. Centers for Disease Control and Prevention (CDC) report, nearly 80 percent of U.S. hospitals give healthy breastfeeding infants formula even when there is no medical reason to do so. Again, keep your baby with you—and *on* you, if possible. If you and your baby must be separated, have your partner go with the baby and post a big sign on the baby's crib that says BREAST MILK ONLY, PLEASE.

Hospitals, especially large ones, can be busy, noisy places. Postpartum nurses check in on you frequently. Nurses caring for the baby do the same. The midwife or doctor who assisted you at delivery will stop by to examine you. The pediatrician will come to examine the baby, and you may have a visit from a lactation consultant if the hospital has one. The person who administers the routine newborn hearing test needs to get that completed before you go home, and the person whose job it is to make sure the birth certificate is signed and sent to the state may also come to visit. Then there is the lab technician who comes to draw your blood, the people who deliver your food and clean your room, and the family and friends who want to come to congratulate you and to meet your new baby.

Needless to say, all this coming and going is not conducive to rest or sleep for either you or your baby; neither is it conducive to learning to breastfeed or to your recovery in general, especially if you've had a long, challenging labor. Taking in information when you're exhausted isn't easy, and during the postpartum period your body and mind are in tremendous flux. It's perfectly acceptable to post a sign on the door that says Mother and Baby Sleeping. Please Do Not Disturb. That said, a visit from the in-hospital lactation consultant, if there is one, can be invaluable.

You might consider staying in the hospital only a minimal amount of time, especially if you have good help at home. Some doulas make home visits and are skilled at helping you with early breastfeeding. You may also have private lactation consultants in your community who will come to your home during the first few days after birth. Some hospitals have a home visiting program, where a nurse will come to your house three to five days after delivery. Some cities and counties have home visiting programs for new mothers; ask during your hospital tour or hospital stay whether such a program is available to you. If it is, take advantage of it.

Paying attention, getting to know this new person in your life, learning to breastfeed, and resting and recovering are your main labors now. You may want to get yourself home where you can be quietly nurtured and peacefully be with your baby and partner (and possibly other children) as you begin this new phase of your life.

USING YOUR PARACHUTE: A BIRTH STORY

Just as I was completing the writing of this chapter, the email below arrived from Sarah and Steve, who had taken the most recent MBCP course. It's such a wonderful example of how they used their mindfulness practice for the birth of their son, Gus, that I'm including it here.

Dear Mindful Birthing classmates,

Sarah and I are delighted to announce the arrival of Gus! He showed up like a champ on Sunday just after 7:00 P.M., weighing in at 7 lbs 10 oz. Everyone's doing great!

Sarah's water broke without her realizing it on Thursday evening. By Friday she thought, "Gee, that's a lot of pee." Her OB was firm about admitting her to the hospital, so right off the bat our birth "preference" for laboring at home was out the window.

We spent Friday to Sunday at the hospital trying various methods of inducement, mostly to no avail. Our best move may have been to insist on totally unhooking Sarah from IVs and monitors on Saturday night and to use that opportunity to eat a real meal and to get some uninterrupted sleep. By Sunday, Sarah's cervix was fully effaced and a bit dilated. With a second round of Pitocin, Sarah labored from 3:00 P.M. until about 7:00 P.M., and then WHAM, she was pushing—and out came Gus!

The mindfulness techniques were an enormous help, in a variety of ways. For one thing, we brought our class CDs right into the room and did a few guided meditations during the long wait between being admitted and going into labor. During labor, we worked our way from mindful stroking to applying pressure to Loving-kindness and up to Sounding. (Sounding just "happens." WOW!) Sarah found that being with her breath between contractions—and using Loving-kindness practice to remind her of what this was all about—were especially helpful. She labored in Child's Pose, on all fours, on the birthing ball, leaning on me, leaning on the bed, and finally on a birthing ball in the shower. Hot water was absolutely key.

We experienced two other lessons that are worth mentioning. First, we used BRANN over and over again to slow down discussions of intervention. Absolutely everyone at the hospital was warm and helpful and well intentioned, but we found that interventions were generally presented as foregone conclusions. Without the formula, we would have found it difficult to assert ourselves in these conversations. Second, our doula was a tremendous resource in every possible way. We both found it incredibly reassuring to have a steady presence through an otherwise revolving cast of characters.

Gus is a pretty great guy. We can't wait for you all to meet him!

With love,
Sarah and Steve and Gus

A SUMMARY
MINDFULNESS AND SKILLFUL ACTION

DURING PREGNANCY

- Learn and regularly practice mindfulness—both formal meditation practice and informal practice—for decreasing stress and worry, strengthening your calm-and-connection system, and preparing for the transformational pain of childbirth ahead.
- Choose a healthcare provider who you trust is in harmony with your preferences for your labor, birth, and the care of your baby. This person should support you in general and in such specific desires as late cord clamping, skin-to-skin contact, and minimal to no suctioning of the baby at or immediately after birth. Trust is also important when choosing a healthcare provider for your baby.
- Choose a birthing environment that engenders a sense of safety.
- Early in your pregnancy take a tour of the birthplace you've selected so you can assess the culture of the institution and the support (or lack thereof) for normal physiologic childbirth. If you are unhappy with what you discover, research your options, choose another place to birth, or come to terms with things as they are.
- Consider hiring a doula.
- Read one book to inform yourself about common medical technologies and interventions used during childbirth. If you notice that your reading begins to induce fear, use your mindfulness practice to work with it. Also ask yourself: What is the evidence that supports what I'm reading? If the information is evidence-based, pay attention. If it is not, be a bit more cautious about the information given. These guidelines apply to watching birth videos and assessing information on the Internet as well.
- Read one book about breastfeeding, and apply the guidelines above.
- Read other books about pregnancy and childbirth because you are curious, not because you feel you have to master huge amounts of information. You are not taking a final exam; you are having a baby.
- Ask your healthcare provider when she or he wants to be notified that you are in labor.
- Go to a breastfeeding support group or a La Leche League meeting during the second half of your pregnancy.

(continued)

- Be sure you have the name and number of a lactation consultant or a breast-feeding support group in your community *before* giving birth.
- Eat well, take your prenatal vitamins, get plenty of sleep, exercise regularly, and practice mindfulness, formally and informally.
- Slow down, be present, pay attention, and be happy—or as happy as you can be.

DURING LABOR AT HOME

- When the sensations of labor begin to call your attention, use your mindfulness skills for being with them, *remembering to bring your awareness to the moments of ease and peace between the sensations.* Sounding is okay.
- Alternate between periods of being upright and active and periods of rest.
- If it's nighttime, sleep if you can; practice the Body Scan if you can't.
- Notify someone that you are in labor according to your healthcare provider's advance instructions.
- Call your doula if you hired one.
- When you contact the hospital, ask to be assigned a nurse who has the skills to facilitate a labor with minimal interventions, if this is your preference.
- If you are hungry, eat lightly.
- Drink one cup of liquid every hour, even if you are not thirsty.
- Do all of the above mindfully.
- Remember the half-smile practice. Be happy. You and your baby will meet each other soon.

DURING LABOR IN THE HOSPITAL

- Continue to use your mindfulness skills for being with the powerful moment-to-moment sensations of labor and with the moments between those powerful sensations. Remember, sounding is okay.
- If you made a Birth Preference Sheet, give it to your Labor and Delivery nurse.
- As soon as you get into your labor room, put a big sign over the clock that says NOW. Do your best to follow your own instructions.
- Negotiate the use of intermittent fetal monitoring (IA) and a heparin lock.
- Stay out of bed as much as possible.
- Lie down and take a rest when you need to.
- To support your inward focus and minimize stimulation of the thinking mind, keep your labor environment quiet, and keep conversation to a minimum.

- Experiment with warm water for relaxation, especially when the sensations of labor get very intense.
- Remember Loving-kindness practice for yourself and your baby. You might also consider including in your Loving-kindness practice your partner, your nurse, your doula, the midwife or doctor helping you, the woman in labor in the room next to yours, and the three hundred thousand other women on the planet giving birth to their babies on this very same day (or night).
- Wait to begin pushing until your body tells you to begin. Try lots of different positions for pushing, especially if your baby is slow in being born.
- Use BRANN for all suggested interventions.
- Be as fully present for your experience as you can, one breath at a time.
- Practice non-attachment to hopes and fears.
- Sadness and disappointment are possible emotions in relation to your childbirth experience. Practice non-judging and Loving-kindness, especially if thoughts of "failure" or self-judgment arise.
- Remember that the powerful sensations you are experiencing are a sign that you are part of the life-transforming process that is bringing your baby into your arms. It will not last forever. Guaranteed.

AFTER GIVING BIRTH

- If at all possible, put your baby skin-to-skin immediately after giving birth.
- Keep your baby skin-to-skin with you for a good long time—at least during the first hour or two.
- If at all possible, breastfeed your baby within one-half to one hour after birth.
- Again, if at all possible, delay all hospital procedures for your baby, such as injections, eye ointment, and bathing, for at least one to two hours after birth.
- If you have a cesarean birth, skin-to-skin contact is still important. Put your baby on your body as soon as possible for as long as possible. Nurse your baby as soon as you are able.
- While in the hospital, keep your baby with you at all times unless conditions necessitate otherwise.
- If your baby must go to the nursery and you intend to breastfeed, put a sign on his or her crib that says, Breast Milk Only, Please. The please is important.
- A visit from a lactation consultant while you're in the hospital can be very helpful.
- If there is too much coming and going in your postpartum room, post a sign

(continued)

outside your door that says, "Mother and baby are sleeping. Please do not disturb." This is perfectly acceptable.

- Consider going home sooner rather than later if you have good help at home.
- Eat. Sleep. Nurse (if you have chosen to). Pay attention. Be present and allow yourself time to begin the process of falling in love with your baby. Partners can be encouraged do the same (except for nursing).
- Live within the oxytocin calm-and-connection system as much as possible, now and for the rest of your life. Your friend the breath will always be around to help with that.

CHAPTER 17

Your Baby, Your Mindfulness Teacher

"There is no such thing as a baby"—meaning that
if you set out to describe a baby, you will find you
are describing a baby and someone.
—Donald Winnicott

COUPLES ARE GATHERED, chatting, laughing, and munching on snacks. Even though we have two more class meetings, there's already a sense that these weekly gatherings, which have become such a regular part of their lives, will soon be no more. By this point everyone has learned all the formal mindfulness practices and understands well the importance of mindfulness for decreasing stress in their lives and for supporting the normal physiology of labor. They know how to work with and even welcome the challenging sensations of childbirth and any fear or other emotions that might arise. They have learned on an experiential level that change is a constant; that there are no guarantees about the future—in childbirth or anything else; that there is a difference between reacting and responding; and that with mindfulness practice we have a choice about how we will relate to the birthing process and to anything else in our lives.

Tonight we are moving on, both in the class and here in this book. It's time to talk about life after birth. For whatever is to happen, the moments of birth will come and go for these couples—and for you as well. And then you will be living the next moments of the rest of your life. Jack Kornfield, a wise meditation teacher, titled one of his books *After the Ecstasy, the Laundry;* in our case, we could be thinking "after the birth, the laundry."

And so we turn our attention to how you might use your mindfulness practice for living with greater ease in the new life you've been birthed into. Perhaps by now, it will come as no surprise that the mindfulness instructions for after birth are actually no different than they were before birth: to practice being as awake and present as you can be, learning, growing, and changing one moment at a time.

"So what have you heard about life after you have a baby?" I ask the assembled group.

Maya raises her hand. "I've heard it's exhausting. That you never get any sleep."

"Well," I reply, "it's true that your sleep will be interrupted, fatigue is common, and being tired is certainly an unpleasant state. And I've had expectant parents worry a lot about not getting enough sleep, only to find, to their surprise, they are managing much better than they expected. Caring for a newborn is pretty labor intensive, and each baby has his or her own sleep rhythm, just as you do, so you'll just have to see how it goes. This parenting business is so much about who this particular baby person is, and what they need.

"A general rule of thumb," I continue, "is for you, the new mom, to sleep when the baby sleeps. This can be a challenge if you're not accustomed to napping, and the Body Scan or some Awareness of Breathing can help with that. When the baby sleeps, you may find yourself trying to get back into Doing Mode instead of napping yourself. The healthier and perhaps wiser course in the first couple of weeks is to realize that you and certainly your baby are living primarily in Horticultural Time. This is where healing from the birth takes place, and where you and your partner grow into new parents. Taking care of yourself, including napping, is more important than any of the doing tasks you may be feeling urgent about.

"Sometimes I hear women say, 'Nobody told me how much time it would take to recover and get my body back after the birth.' So let's get that out of the way. It took your body almost a year to grow your baby and then give birth and sometimes it can take a while to physically recover from the process—like four to six weeks, maybe even longer. It all depends on your age, your general state of health, how challenging your birth experience was, how easy or stressful initiating breastfeeding is, whether you or your baby have any unexpected health challenges after birth, how much care and support you and your partner have in the adjustment time after your baby is born, and your baby's temperament and general state of health. Just like giving birth, that's a lot of unknowns about the future, and you'll just have to take it moment by moment.

"So, what else have you heard?" I ask.

"I've heard it can be really lonely sometimes," Heather says. "My friend told me that after her husband went back to work she'd sometimes be alone at home all day. Some days she never even got out of her pajamas or took a shower! And then, at the end of the day she would look back and think, 'Where did the day go? I didn't get a thing done.'"

"It sounds like your friend could benefit from learning about non-judging and Being Mode. Maybe there are some lessons that can be drawn from our day of silence that might help us adjust to this new life. Maybe there's a way of just being with your baby, of letting go of Doing Mode and just allowing the day to unfold for you and your baby, moment by moment. It might be useful to know that after birth you are living in the season called Baby Time. And like all seasons, this one will pass too, and perhaps all too quickly.

"In Baby Time," I continue, "you will still experience contractions—like when the baby cries and you can't seem to comfort her or him or when you are really tired from a challenging night and can't rest the next day. But even in the midst of a difficult day, by remembering your mindfulness practice, you will likely be able to find some wonderfully peaceful, calm moments, moments of love and connection with your new baby, perhaps during a feeding or while you're resting with the baby next to you. If you framed a day of taking care of your baby as a day of mindfulness practice in everyday life, maybe the experience would take on a very different quality. After all, is keeping your baby alive, loved, and well cared for *really* doing nothing?" I ask.

"Well, when you put it that way, I guess not."

"We have this very strange notion in our culture that caring for babies and children isn't important work, despite everything we know about how critical these early years are for laying down the foundations of mental and physical health and wellbeing. These attuned moments of interaction between you and your baby and between your baby and intimate others are forming her or his neurological pathways, pathways that develop their capacity to form strong social bonds, tell them that people can be trusted and that the world is basically a safe—and pretty interesting—place. It's part of setting a tone for their entire lives. That doesn't sound like 'getting nothing done' to me.

"What else have you heard?"

Sam speaks up. "We have friends who say that they can't believe how much fun they are having since their daughter was born. They told us that they can't wait for her to wake up in the morning, that they never knew they could love somebody so much!"

"When conditions are right we certainly do fall head over heels in love with our babies. And babies play their part by smiling at us and just being so amazingly cute! Like my husband, Kenji, says, 'Being cute is their profession,' and they're really, really good at it. They have to be. Their survival depends on us falling in love with them. One way you can help this process along is by taking the time to just be present, paying attention to who your baby is and what she or he is trying to communicate, especially in the early weeks, months, and years after being born."

WHO IS THIS BABY PERSON, AND WHAT DOES SHE OR HE NEED?

Over the course of the last thirty years or so, all sorts of experts—pediatricians, psychologists, neuroscientists, child development researchers, and even anthropologists—have been looking at what might be the optimal need for raising healthy and happy human creatures. Though so much more is known now about babies and what they need, most new parents still know precious little about how normal babies develop over time. As dedicated as new parents are to taking care of their babies well, the vast majority of us are still pretty baffled by this astonishingly cute yet hard-to-decipher creature who has been catapulted into our lives.

Jeremy described this moment of realization in an email to his MBCP class shortly after his son, Tobias, was born. "We feel incredibly blessed that the birth was so straightforward and that Toby and Laura are both healthy and well! I remember this intense moment when we were fumbling to put Toby into his car seat for the first time. The nurse was helping us, and all of a sudden it hit me that they were sending us home with this baby, *our* baby, *all alone.* They assumed we could take care of him, but I knew we didn't have a clue! I mean, we'd read a bunch of books and everything, and we'd had some time in the hospital when people taught us some stuff, but really, we were about to be totally on our own. We were both really excited and really scared at the same time.

"And then I remembered Nancy saying, 'You are giving birth to your mindfulness teacher,' and I realized that all we had to do was pay attention to him and Toby would show us what he needed. Thank goodness for that. We've trusted that, and it's pretty much what we've been doing since we got home—practicing paying attention to our mindfulness teacher. And we're happy to report that everything has been going pretty smoothly! There's a lot of being with the breath, especially when he cries, and a lot of living in don't-know mind because every day is different. We've just been figuring it out moment by moment, and now we can pretty much tell what he needs most of the time. And if we take care of that, he is pretty content. Mindfulness practice rocks!"

Dr. Kevin Nugent, director of the famed Brazelton Institute at Children's Hospital in Boston, puts it this way in the introduction to his wonderful book, *Your Baby Is Speaking to You*, which I highly recommend to every new parent: "Parents and other caregivers lament, often with some hard-won humor, that babies do not come with an owner's manual. But in fact your infant does come with caregiving guidelines embedded in his behavior, which can tell you what he needs to survive and thrive. These guidelines do have to be decoded, however. And because each infant is different, with a distinctive disposition and sensibilities, each one's guidelines are unique. As you learn to decode your baby's behavior, he will offer you precious information about his preferences, needs, and expectations—about who he is!"[1]

Though you won't be able to decode your baby all the time—no parent can—your mindfulness practice will help you see and actually enjoy all the fascinating, moment-to-moment nuances of your baby's behavior and will truly help you decode, attune to, and sensitively care for this very small new person in your life.

Part of your challenge in taking care of your new baby is learning how to be in relationship to this small person's constantly arising and passing states and to respond appropriately to his or her needs. When you lapse into autopilot and just go through the motions of changing a diaper, you may miss the messages your daughter or son, who is right before your eyes, is giving you. However, with your mindfulness practice, you can drop into the moment, perhaps more frequently, being aware of your baby and yourself during *this* diaper change, *this* moment of nursing, *this* moment of rocking and cuddling, and *this* moment of exhaustion or frustration or confusion.

Sensitive caring for a newborn requires a crash course in nonverbal communication, and you can use your mindfulness practice to pay attention to the baby's sounds, cries, facial expressions, and body language as well as your own body sensations, thoughts, and emotions in this fascinating and sometimes stressful new job of yours—parenting. Remembering impermanence, the ineluctable truth that all things change, can help you keep your perspective through the difficult times and to fully live the moments of joy in parenting. When you are exhausted or frustrated you might remind yourself that these precious days, even if they have moments of challenge, will quickly pass. Infancy is brief. Childhood is brief. Life is brief. Don't miss it.

Jeff, one of the fathers who took the MBCP course, put it this way: "Babies are a real test of your mindfulness practice, especially of observing without judging. If Kira is tired and fussy, she's just tired and fussy. She's not trying to push my buttons. That's just the way babies are sometimes. My job is to use my mindfulness practice to keep from taking it personally, to notice my reactivity, my habits, my patterns of resistance to whatever is, and act like the parent anyway. I'll take her for a walk, rock her, check to see if she needs a diaper change or is hungry. Sometimes I'll even take her for a ride in the car if that's what she needs," he says laughing. "It's acceptance of things as they are. The more I fight what is happening, the more stressed things become—for her and for me!"

NEWBORN STATES OF BEING

Just as we cycle through states of being throughout our day—states of wakefulness and sleepiness, of hunger and ease, of more or less energy, of interest and boredom—your newborn baby cycles through states of being too. The patterns of these cycles are very different from those of an adult, and it can be helpful to know about them. The basic states are: deep sleep, active sleep, quiet alert, active alert, fussing, and crying.[2]

Each state has its unique characteristics, and as your baby lives through them you read her or his cues as best you can, making adjustments in your response, moment to moment in this constantly changing dance of caring. There is nothing rigid about the order of these states, and sometimes your baby may skip one or even two—for example, going from active alert to deep sleep with barely a fuss. Like knowing the stages of labor, knowing something about what you might expect from your newborn baby without becoming attached or thinking that this is the way it should be may help you navigate living in Baby Time.

Deep Sleep

A newborn baby sleeps anywhere from sixteen to twenty hours a day but rarely for more than four to four and a half hours at a stretch at least to begin with; sleeping in cycles of two to three hours is the usual pattern for a breastfed baby. There are two kinds of sleep states: deep sleep and light sleep. Deep sleep is restorative and is associated with lower oxygen consumption and the release of growth hormones. Your baby has the capacity to screen out sound, which means that in this state of deep sleep, she or he will be very hard to rouse.

You will often see this state of deep sleep right after you feed your baby. In breast milk the prolactin and oxytocin are a kind of soporific, but this state is induced simply by feeding and digesting, so it will also happen if your baby is bottle fed. I usually refer to the state right after feeding as "drunken bliss." To find out if your baby is in this state, pick up his arm just a tiny bit and let it go. If it falls limply, without eliciting even a twitch, he's in it: drunken bliss.

Active Sleep

Active sleep is the REM, or rapid eye movement, part of the sleep cycle. You will know your baby is in active sleep in all sorts of ways: your baby's eyes move underneath her eyelids; she stretches and tightly squeezes her eyes; or she moves her mouth and tongue as if she is nursing. I call this the "dreaming of Mommy" state, even though we don't know for sure if babies actually dream. About half the time your baby is asleep she is in this part of the sleep cycle. Many who study sleep in babies believe that active sleep is associated with brain stimulation and with processing and storing information.

At some point in this active sleep phase the baby will wake up. This can be a gradual process, moving through drowsiness to wakefulness, or if wakefulness is prompted by the internal sensations of hunger, your baby can wake up fussing or crying in distress. Her or his body knows it needs to eat to stay alive, and for a baby, the decidedly unpleasant sensations of hunger are all-consuming and stressful. The highest concentration of the parasympathetic nerves in our body are around the mouth, and feeding your baby will bring her back from the agitation of the sympathetic nervous system's stress reaction into the balance of oxytocin's calm-and-connection system once again. When feeding happens right after sleep, the baby is usually wide awake and fully concentrated on the task at hand.

Quiet Alert

The quiet alert state is an absolutely magical time of calm and connection, when your baby is relaxed, present, and at ease. This state often appears after a baby has been fed and is well rested, warm, dry, and free from any internal discomfort. The quiet alert state is your baby's time for taking in the world—for learning and especially for interacting with you and the other important people in his or her life. It is in this quiet alert state where you will probably see your baby's first simple smile, the smile that appears sometime between the first and third or fourth week of life. This smile is different from the fleeting smile you see in REM sleep or the full-on social smile, which comes between one and two months of age, but it is a smile of pleasure nonetheless. It is your baby's earliest recognition of *you*.

For some newborns this quiet alert state may last for only about five minutes; for others it may last as long as twenty. However long this state of being is, it's a delicious time to be present with your baby, gazing into his eyes, quietly talking or singing to him, and just enjoying these special moments together. If you are nursing, the prolactin and oxytocin released by your brain can heighten your enjoyment of these moments of peaceful interaction and connection. If you plan on practicing infant massage, which can be a wonderful mindfulness practice for you and your baby, this would be the optimal time for it.

Active Alert

Sooner or later your baby will transition out of quiet alert and into an active alert state. I like to think of active alert as "baby yoga time." Your baby has a lot of work to do in order to strengthen all the muscles in her body. She has to strengthen her neck muscles so she can better hold up and move her head (which is one-third of her total body mass), her back muscles so she can roll over and eventually sit up, her arm and hand muscles so she can reach for and hold objects, and her leg muscles so she can eventually roll over, crawl, stand, and walk. And she gets all this done in about a year to a year and a half. That's a lot of work in such a short time! The amazing thing is that her body just does it. Just as no one had to teach your body to give birth, you don't need to teach your baby to roll, sit, crawl, stand, or walk. However, your affectionate attention and appreciation of this process can definitely increase the joy of your baby and of your parenting experience.

In active alert you'll see all sorts of vigorous movements—like arm waving, kicking, and bouncing up and down with her feet while being held up on your lap. Your baby will also practice making sounds and calling to you. Then, as time passes, she starts to get tired. Or hungry again. Or both. Now stop for a moment and think how *you* feel when you have worked really hard and are both tired and hungry; this is the standard recipe for an everyday, garden-variety, cranky, fussy baby.

Fussing

Whatever the cause—hunger, fatigue, or other sensations of discomfort—your baby has moved into this next state of being, fussing. As we've seen, he may be tired from his workout in active alert or hungry again or both. Or maybe he's in an uncomfortable position and needs to be picked up or needs a diaper change. Or maybe he's lonely and just needs some cuddling. Or perhaps the environment has been overly stimulating and his nervous system is a bit stressed, or maybe he's bored and needs a change to something interesting for a short while.

Whatever is going on, your job in these moments is to try to decipher what will bring peace and ease back to this small, dependent person. Since awakening roughly an hour or so ago, your baby has engaged in a lot of activity. He has eaten, perhaps been burped, undoubtedly has had a diaper or full outfit change or even a massage or a bath, which may have included a shampoo. Perhaps he has spent some time in a sling or been outside in the fresh air. He may have exercised his body quite vigorously, and had a variety of stimuli from the external world come into his senses, and quite frankly, he's done. Enough awake time. The transition he needs now, probably from active alert or fussing or crying is to sleep. This is where your intuition, your creativity, and your capacity to be mindful of your baby's cues really come in handy.

Crying

Of all the challenges of parenting, especially new parenting, your baby's crying is probably the most distressing. As the birth process taught us, transitioning can be hard. Some babies transition from one state to another more easily than others, and transitioning to sleep can be, for some babies and their parents, one of the more challenging series of moments of the day or night. Here is another time when your mindfulness practice can be a lifesaver.

A baby is hardwired to cry when in distress, and we as adults are hardwired to feel distress when we hear the sounds of a baby crying, particularly if it is our own. From a mindfulness perspective, crying is the result of something in your baby's internal or external environment that creates a state of imbalance. Your baby's crying is a way of alerting all within earshot that the experience of distress is present.

We may be hardwired to hear a baby's cries, but how—or even whether—we respond to those cries is largely culturally determined. In Western industrial societies it is common to view a baby's cries through the reactive lens of judgment. A baby who is easily soothed or has an easygoing temperament is described as a "good" baby while a baby who has a more sensitive nervous system, who may need more care and attention to find calm and ease, is described as a "difficult" baby. For the parent whose baby is not easily soothed, all sorts of unpleasant feelings—anxiety, frustration, fatigue, anger, bewilderment, and helplessness—can be triggered. Negative thoughts can also be part of the package: "I'm a bad parent; my baby doesn't love me; what have I gotten myself into?"

When crying goes on for a long time, the stress can send a parent over the edge. It has been documented that the behavior known as shaken baby syndrome, where a baby is shaken so vigorously that she or he suffers brain damage, is almost always preceded by a long bout of crying. Without the inner skills to regulate his or her own reactivity, the beleaguered parent can do lasting harm.

Perhaps more than at any other point in your newborn's life, and yours, it is here, when your baby is crying, that the qualities cultivated in your mindfulness practice—especially patience and kindness—can be essential. Our ability to self-regulate and be with whatever unpleasant emotional state *we* may be experiencing, riding the wave of emotional contraction with patience and kindness for ourselves and our baby, can make all the difference in the world.

I think of Mark, who took the MBCP course many years ago with his wife, Geneen. A lively, humorous, and loving partner, Mark was very much engaged with mindfulness practice and very excited to become a father. When Geneen and Mark returned to the class reunion, with their infant daughter, Stacia, they were obviously very much in love with her. As we do at the reunion, we took turns around the circle naming what was joyful and what was challenging. When it was Mark's turn to speak he said, "I knew babies cried, but I didn't know that it would be so difficult for me to hear. Sometimes when I can't get Stacia to stop crying I feel so helpless that I get really angry. One time I was swept up in an incredible rage. Thank goodness in that moment I remembered the breath. I followed it for a moment, then I said to Geneen, 'I think you'd better take her.' Even now it upsets me just to think about what might have happened. For the first time in my life I can really understand child abuse. All I can say is, 'Thank God I had my mindfulness practice!'"

There was a pause, as if everyone was taking a collective breath in the wake of Mark's deeply honest admission. Hearing this story, I thought, "It's so hard sometimes to be a parent. And it's really hard sometimes being a baby." Parenting is such a constant practice of compassion—for ourselves as parents, doing the best we can given who we are, and for our babies, who are doing the best they can given who they are. This being human, at any stage of life, can be a pretty intense business.

'ROUND AND 'ROUND AND 'ROUND IN THE CIRCLE GAME

In the MBCP class I describe these early infant states of being to expectant parents using the circle you see in Diagram E. Then I take the marker pen

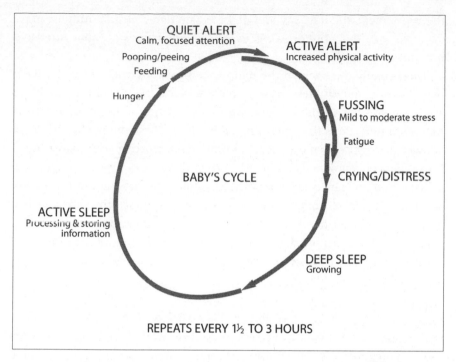

QUIET ALERT
Calm, focused attention

Pooping/peeing

Feeding

Hunger

ACTIVE ALERT
Increased physical activity

FUSSING
Mild to moderate stress

Fatigue

BABY'S CYCLE

CRYING/DISTRESS

ACTIVE SLEEP
Processing & storing information

DEEP SLEEP
Growing

REPEATS EVERY 1½ TO 3 HOURS

Diagram E: Infant States of Being

and make another circle slightly overlapping the first. Then another one, then another, over and over again . . . eight, nine, ten, eleven, twelve circles. Assuming the typical sleep-wake cycle for a breastfed baby, you, your baby, and your partner will live through eight to twelve of these sleep-wake cycles in a twenty-four-hour period. That's one day and night of your life and your baby's life, moment by moment: feeding, burping, changing a diaper, playing, interacting, talking, singing, being present, rocking, soothing, swaddling, walking a crying baby in your arms or in a sling, soothing, feeding, burping, changing a diaper, helping your baby transition back to sleep; feeling moments of joy, love, exhaustion, frustration, awe, boredom, confusion, fear, amazement, calm, connection, irritation, ease, and wonder. And sometime, somehow, within one or another of the cycles you try to take a shower, eat a meal, drink water, take a nap, take a sitz bath to help heal your perineum if you need to, try to go out for a walk around the block, actually go out for a walk around the block, make a phone call to the pediatrician, or think about taking a glance at your email or smartphone but never actually do. And so it goes, again, and again and again around the cycle, night and day, day and night as you live your mindfulness practice, taking care of your growing, ever-changing baby, one labor-intensive mindful moment at a time.

This is really the heart of the matter, and in many ways why you have been learning mindfulness skills in the first place. For it is in the quality of attention and the attuned caretaking that you bring to these moment-to-moment interactions that parenting takes place. These moments with your baby begin to lay down the actual neural architecture in your baby's brain for resilience, happiness, and health. When this oh-so-dependent creature called a human baby is fairly consistently enfolded into the calm and connection of his or her mother and other caregivers, your baby slowly grows and develops his or her own inner resources to grow and thrive. Through repeated interactions of affectionate attention, your mindful parenting can nurture your baby to grow and develop the inner foundations for a happy and healthy mind and body.

THE BIRTH OF THREE BABIES

In the moments that your baby comes into this world, three babies are born: two baby parents and a baby son or daughter. If you are birthing a second or third child, or beyond, you are still giving birth to a new life as a larger family with a unique child to care for. Just as newborns need to be nurtured, sensitively cared for, and protected, your baby family does too. As you think ahead, beyond the birth itself, the question for you and your partner becomes, Who will you turn to for this nurturing, protective care? With whom will you feel most comfortable in this tender, vulnerable time after the baby is born, when you are all in recovery from the intense physical and emotional experience of giving birth, not to mention the very steep learning curve needed for breastfeeding and taking care of a newly born infant?

While we usually think of pregnancy and birth in terms of expansion and growth, it can also be helpful to know that this period is also an end, the dissolution of an old order that is completed by giving birth. In this early time after birth (sometimes called the fourth trimester), you and your partner are gradually putting the pieces of your life back together in a new order. The person you thought you were is in the process of profoundly transforming. Someone else besides a baby has been born.

You both need time and space to get to know this new little person and to feel your way into becoming this baby's parent. Not having had the direct physical experience of being pregnant and giving birth, a partner may especially need time in order to feel connected. I always encourage partners to stay at home as long as possible after their baby arrives to have time and space for attending to this reconstruction and reconstitution phase after birth. Two weeks off from work is good; a month or longer is even better.

Since it is optimal for the two of you to just be on Baby Time together with your new infant, having people around to help can be quite wonderful. Because our society puts so much emphasis on being independent rather than on accepting the truth of our interdependency, asking for and accepting help postbirth can be a mindfulness practice in and of itself—both a challenging and a heart-opening experience. If there was ever a time to ask for and accept help from family and friends, this is it.

What you need is actually quite simple: nutritious food, help keeping your home reasonably clean, and someone to do simple tasks, like running a few loads of laundry or picking up a few things from the grocery store. If parents or parents-in-law are coming to help, you are fortunate indeed, depending on your relationship, of course. This is a time to make your needs and expectations clear—that it is your wish that they focus mostly on cooking, cleaning, and caring for the two of you so you and your partner can focus your attention on learning how to take care of your new baby.

It can also be helpful to assess the comfort level, knowledge, and attitude parents or in-laws have about breastfeeding. In this intimate time of learning new skills, it is not helpful or confidence building to have a visiting mother or mother-in-law who didn't nurse her own babies hovering skeptically about, wondering aloud if you are producing enough milk or feeding the baby too often.

Being fed well is primary, and baby showers are an excellent opportunity to organize friends who will bring food after your baby is born. In my neighborhood, when someone is close to delivery, we send around an email with a meal sign-up list, ensuring that food is delivered several times a week for at least the first month after a baby is born. Each neighbor takes the food they have prepared to the new parents' home between five and six o'clock in the evening, leaving it in an ice cooler on the front porch or doorstep.

The key to postpartum support is to clearly assess who you can call on for care and what you think would be best for your newly birthed family given who you are, who is offering to help, and how you feel in their presence. If you feel tense and worried that you will be judged or that old family patterns might make their unhappy appearance, perhaps receiving care from friends or from a postpartum doula is a wiser initial choice, opting for a visit from family after you have established some confidence in taking care of your baby. On the other hand, the birth of a baby can provide an extraordinary opportunity for growth and healing, especially if this is a first grandchild. A new baby can bring a radical shift in family dynamics as everyone enters a new phase of life and takes on new roles.

One of our class members, Leslie, was ambivalent about her mother coming to visit right after her baby was born. Though her relationship with her mother was okay at the moment, it had been strained in the past, and Leslie didn't want to risk any problems. "I don't think I want my mother around right after I have the baby," she told the class. "She didn't nurse any of us kids, and she tends to have very strong opinions about things. So Dave and I have arranged for her to visit about six weeks after the birth, when we have a better sense of what we're doing."

At least that was the plan. But Leslie's mother had other ideas, and much to everyone's surprise, she showed up right after the baby was born. As it turned out, Leslie had had a long and difficult labor, and in the beginning, breastfeeding was challenging. At the reunion Leslie reported, "I couldn't believe it when my mother showed up. Dave and I had planned on taking care of the baby by ourselves, but truthfully, we were pretty overwhelmed. And it turned out that my mom was great, taking care of us and helping with the baby. She cooked, and she supported me in the middle of the night when I was having trouble nursing and Dave had to sleep so he could go to work the next day. And she was just so sweet with Miriam. It was a very special time for me and my mother, and I feel something really important shifted in our relationship. It's not all about her and me anymore. We share Miriam now, and as a result we feel much closer to each other. You just never know, do you?"

POSTPARTUM DEPRESSION: THE JUDGING MIND RUNS WILD

Sometimes giving birth causes us to get so out of balance that we can spin into a downward emotional spiral. Commonly known as postpartum depression, this state can provide the judging mind with a field day. Depression during the postpartum period is essentially the same as any major depressive episode; it just happens after giving birth. (Sometimes depression starts during pregnancy.) It's a terribly debilitating condition that affects a mother's ability to feel happy, to care, and to connect with her baby—or anyone else. Some 10 to 15 percent of women are subject to depression during the first year postpartum, and it can have serious long-term consequences for the healthy emotional development of a baby and for a mother's feelings about herself.

Although researchers have identified a number of risk factors for depression during the postpartum period, accurately predicting depression for one particular woman rather than another is difficult. We do know that women who have a history of depression, have a difficult or traumatic birth experience, lack social support, or have a high degree of stress during pregnancy and after giving birth are more at risk for developing depression in the postpartum period. Though it looks somewhat different in men, depression after a baby is born also affects a surprising number of new fathers.[3]

Fortunately, depression postpartum is very treatable, so if you're feeling sad and listless much of the time or no longer find pleasure from things you used to find enjoyable (when you have the time to do them!) or are feeling disconnected from your baby and these feelings persist for two weeks or more, it's important to seek professional help. It's also good to know that mindfulness practice can play a helpful role in this situation. In another adaptation of the Mindfulness-Based Stress Reduction course, Drs. Zindel Segal, John Teasdale, and Mark Williams have developed a highly successful eight-week Mindfulness-Based Cognitive Therapy (MBCT) program, which teaches mindfulness skills to prevent depressive relapse for people who have had a series of depressive episodes in their life. This MBCT course is now the treatment of choice for prevention of relapse in depression in the British National Healthcare System and has proven to be as effective as the drugs used to treat depression.[4]

Yet another program, currently being developed and studied by Sona Dimidjian, PhD, at the University of Colorado and Sherryl Goodman, PhD, at Emory University, expands and adapts the MBCT course (including some of the practices used in the MBCP program) into an innovative prevention program specifically geared to women at risk for postpartum depression. Their approach is already showing promising preliminary results. Training in mindfulness skills may in the not-too-distant future become an important preventive measure for perinatal depression and offer an alternative to drugs and traditional one-on-one psychological therapies for depression in the perinatal period.[5] By learning mindfulness practice now, you may actually be doing something both preventive and protective of your mental health and wellbeing in the postpartum period and beyond.

CHAPTER 18

Breastfeeding
A Dance of Connection

I maintain . . . that we are born and grow up with a
fondness for each other, and that we have genes for that. . . .
Societies are noisy affairs, drowning out the sound of ourselves
and our connection. Hard-of-hearing, we go to war.
—Lewis Thomas

THE FIRST TIME I saw a woman breastfeeding her baby was in Patzicia, Guatemala, in the summer of 1962. Patzicia was a small market village several hours north of Guatemala City; I was living there with eleven other Americans, learning the ways of the local people while increasing my fluency in Spanish. Our work that summer was gender specific: the young men of our group would go off every morning to work with the local men making bricks to build a school while the women stayed in the village, buying food in the market, learning to cook local dishes, and making friends as best we could with the women and children. I was nineteen years old, and I didn't know that milk came from a woman's breasts.

That morning I took the big straw basket from a hook behind the door and walked the few blocks to market. Farmers from surrounding towns had arrived by bus very early, and by the time I got there the central plaza was filled with vendors, their wares spread before them on woven mats. I approached a woman sitting behind mounds of fruits and vegetables. Her black hair was parted in the middle and arranged in complicated braids, and like the other women of the village she wore a traditional, elaborately embroidered blouse called a *quipiel*. Tied diagonally across her chest was a brilliantly striped green, blue, and fuchsia serape, which bulged in a way that made it clear a baby was nestled inside.

After we negotiated the price of some oranges, the mother bent forward to count them out. In that moment the baby became visible. Holding onto her mother's breast much the way an American baby would hold a bottle, the baby swiveled her head to get a better look at what was transpiring while continuing to keep the breast's pliable nipple in her mouth. Her bright black eyes locked on mine, and I smiled in both surprise and delight. The baby, who was about seven months old, continued to suck and gaze at me intensely while her mother, oblivious to our interaction, placed the oranges in my market basket.

It all seemed so totally natural, but it was a remarkable sight for this American girl who had grown up in the suburbs of Los Angeles after World War II, where the modern thing to do was to feed babies with a bottle of formula on a rigid four-hour schedule. Years later I was to hear of a study on the frequency of nursing babies in Guatemala, which was something like sixty-four times a day! The authors were trying to make the point that like many mammals, human babies might be considered continuous nursers when they have unlimited access to the breast.

Fast-forward about fifty years to the eighth meeting of our MBCP class—the session on breastfeeding. By this point in the course I know that all of the women in the room intend to breastfeed. I also know that this basic mammalian way of feeding our young sometimes poses real challenges.

"Breastfeeding is a huge subject," I begin, "one that's impossible to cover in one class, so what we're going to do tonight is focus on the physiology of breastfeeding from a mind-body perspective and how your mindfulness practice can help optimize the normal physiology of breastfeeding, just as we did with labor and birth. I'll also share a couple of things to keep in mind so that hopefully your breastfeeding relationship gets off to an easy start. Sound like a plan?"

Everyone beams, so I continue. "So what do you already know about breastfeeding? What have you read or heard about it?"

"Well, I've heard that breastfed babies are healthier," Marissa says. "They don't get hospitalized or sick as much, and they don't get as many allergies as babies who don't breastfeed. I've also heard that they have higher IQs."

"All that is true," I reply. "And you can add to that list a reduced risk for diabetes, asthma, SIDS, obesity, and lots of other things. The American Academy of Pediatrics (AAP) recommends exclusive breastfeeding for the first six months of your baby's life and then continuing to breastfeed for a year or longer.[1] Breast milk is a very healthy first food for a baby."

"I've heard that breastfeeding is really good for mothers too," Louise says. "That it helps your uterus go back to size after pregnancy, and it helps you lose weight after the birth."

"Yeah," Patricia joins in. "My friend says it's the only thing you can do to burn calories while sitting down." Laughter follows.

"And mothers who breastfeed have a reduced risk of breast cancer, rheumatoid arthritis, heart disease, diabetes, and postpartum depression," I add.

"I've heard that breastfeeding is a lot cheaper," Jason offers. "And that breast milk is always the right temperature. I think the whole thing is pretty amazing."

"I'm happy to hear your attitude, Jason, because the research is quite clear that women whose partners are supportive of breastfeeding are much more successful at it than women whose partners aren't."

"I've also heard that it helps you bond with your baby. That it's good for your emotional relationship," Anna says.

"Again, that's true too. Remember back to our calm-and-connection system, where oxytocin plays such a vital role? Well, oxytocin steps front and center again when it comes to breastfeeding. It's what helps stimulate your milk supply and causes your milk letdown—and of course it contributes to feelings of love, calm, and connection between you and your baby.

"But we do have to be careful here," I continue. "While it's pretty clear that breastfeeding is the healthiest choice you can make, it's also important to know that you and your baby can fall in love and you can be a wonderful, caring mom even if breastfeeding doesn't work out. Touch, skin-to-skin contact, and mindful awareness can do wonders. Being connected, attuned, and nurturing is ultimately what matters, and that can still happen without breastfeeding.

"Looking at this life-sustaining process from a mind-body perspective we can learn a lot. The logical place to begin is with your home and your baby's home—your body—and in this particular case, we can focus on the organs we call the mammary glands, or breasts. Just as we learned how our uterus and brain worked together during childbirth—and learned how we could support the normal physiology of childbirth by using our mindfulness practice—we can do the same for breastfeeding. Our breasts and our brain are as intimately interconnected in the process of breastfeeding as our uterus and brain are during labor."

At this point, much to the amusement of the tech-savvy folks in the classroom, I pull out a cart with an overhead projector and set it facing the blank wall. "I'm sure I'll figure out how to get these things onto a PowerPoint someday," I say lightheartedly as I set a couple of transparencies on the cart,

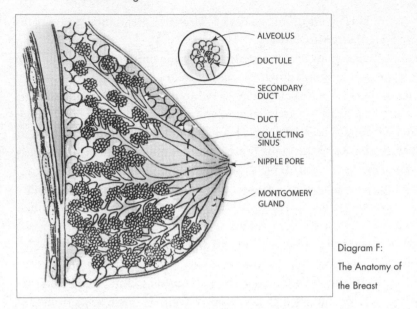

ALVEOLUS

DUCTULE

SECONDARY
DUCT

DUCT

COLLECTING
SINUS

NIPPLE PORE

MONTGOMERY
GLAND

Diagram F:

The Anatomy of

the Breast

"but obviously that day hasn't arrived yet. As old-fashioned as they are, overhead projectors and transparencies still work just fine. Just like breasts."

THE ANATOMY AND PHYSIOLOGY
OF BREASTFEEDING

If you look at Diagram F, you'll see the anatomy of the breast. You can see the ribs, the muscles between the ribs, the muscles of the chest wall, and then the breast attached to those muscles. All female mammals are born with the capacity to nurse their young, and so are you; the structures for nursing grew in your breasts when you were still inside *your* mother's womb. If you are having a daughter, the structures that will allow her to nurse her children (and your grandchildren) one day, should she decide to have them, are growing right now too.

During puberty, the structures inside your breasts grew under the influence of estrogen and progesterone, but it isn't until now, when you have really high levels of those hormones (they're the ones that keep you pregnant), that the breastfeeding structures fully mature. That's why your breasts have gotten bigger since you became pregnant, and by the time you give birth, your breasts will be ready to produce milk. In fact, your breasts are ready to produce milk by the twentieth week of your pregnancy. It's one of the more remarkable things about breastfeeding that if you were to give birth at, say, the thirty-fourth week of your pregnancy, you would produce breast milk that is perfectly suited in its nutrient composition to feed your thirty-four-week newly born baby.

It may be helpful to know that the size of your breasts has absolutely nothing to do with your ability to produce breast milk. Your breast size, as you can see in Diagram F, is determined by the number of fat lobules in your breasts, which is genetically determined; it's the other structures in your breasts that produce milk. If you give birth, which you will, your breasts will produce milk. Period. Of course your baby needs to stimulate your breasts by sucking to get the process fully established, and needs to continue to suck frequently so that your breasts continue to produce milk, but we'll get to that in a moment.

After breast milk is produced, it flows like a stream through small tributaries called ductules, finding its way to larger ducts that lead toward the collecting sinuses behind your areola, the darker area around your nipple. Erectile tissue in the nub of your nipple firms up so your baby can grasp it with his or her mouth. Then a complicated movement of your baby's tongue stimulates the milk to "letdown," which means that the milk is squeezed from the milk-producing alveoli, goes down the ducts, and is ejected into the baby's mouth like a little shower from the ten to twelve nipple pores at the tip of your nipple. This is called the letdown reflex, and it happens multiple times during one nursing session.

Now let's look at the areola and nipple a little more closely. As you've probably noticed, there are little bumps scattered on the surface of your areola. These bumps, called Montgomery glands, are amazing little structures that secrete lubricant to keep the nipples soft and pliable. That's what allowed the baby in Guatemala to keep the nipple in her mouth even when she turned her head abruptly to look at me while she was nursing. This lubricant also has antibacterial properties, which help prevent bacteria from passing through the nipple pores and entering the breast ducts, reducing the chances of a breast infection, or mastitis. Still, it's really important to remember to practice good hygiene while breastfeeding, making sure to wash your hands after you use the toilet or after changing the baby's diaper.

If you know your baby is hungry or it's time for a feeding, try not to wait too long to put the baby to your breast; otherwise the hunger sensations your baby is feeling may make him or her so frantic that he or she will cry instead of suck. Crying is actually a late sign of hunger—the earlier signs are fussing noises, sucking on her or his fists, and "rooting," or bobbing her head looking around for the breast.

Within three weeks after you give birth, your extraordinary body will be producing about a quart of milk every twenty-four hours, which means that you need to continue to eat really well after the baby is born. You actually need about five hundred more calories a day to nurse a baby than you did to grow one.

As discussed in the previous chapter, hanging out in the calm-and-connection system of rest, recovery, growth, and healing as much as you can in the few weeks after your baby is born is a really good plan. Minimize phone use. Don't bother with email. Forget the food shopping and house-cleaning. Keep stress levels down. Have supportive help available. Nurse your baby frequently, enjoy lots of skin-to-skin contact, and chances are good that you will produce lots of oxytocin—and lots of breast milk. A good mantra to live by in the early postpartum period? Eat. Sleep. Nurse. Love.

MINDFULNESS AND BREASTFEEDING

Now let's look a little more closely at breastfeeding from a mind-body perspective. Diagram G can help us understand this connection a bit better.

There are two basic aspects to breastfeeding: milk production and milk release (or the letdown reflex). For both of them, we need to go back to our old friends from childbirth, the hypothalamus and the pituitary. Basically, the hypothalamus needs to get a message to produce the hormones prolactin and oxytocin—prolactin for breast milk production and oxytocin for breast milk ejection—and to send those hormones to the pituitary gland (the oxytocin goes to the posterior pituitary and the prolactin goes to the anterior pituitary) so it can release them into the bloodstream. Fair enough. But how does the hypothalamus get that message? Believe it or not, from the baby. Here's how it works.

In one of the most basic examples of physical and emotional interconnection, when your baby sucks on your nipple, the fourth intercostal nerve, the main nerve that innervates your nipple, sends a message to your hypothalamus to make oxytocin. Oxytocin stimulates prolactin, which gets the whole production process going and keeps it going. It's also critical for ejecting the milk. So this is the all-important take-home message about breastfeeding: *your baby's sucking makes your milk.* The more the baby sucks on your nipple, the more the fourth intercostal nerve gets stimulated, the more messages get to the hypothalamus to make oxytocin, and the more prolactin you will make. The more prolactin you make, the more milk you will have. You and your baby are interdependent in a system that's elegant in its simplicity *so long as you don't restrict the baby's sucking.*

Think about it. A mother cat doesn't feed her kittens on schedule or keep track of how many times a day her kitten nurses. Neither does a polar

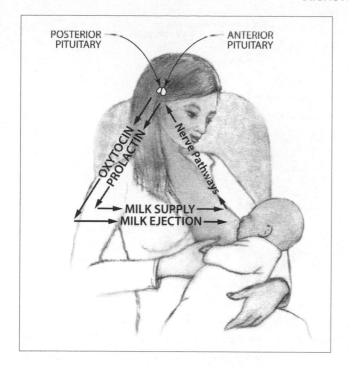

POSTERIOR
PITUITARY

ANTERIOR
PITUITARY

OXYTOCIN
PROLACTIN

Nerve Pathways

← MILK SUPPLY →
← MILK EJECTION →

Diagram G:
The Physiology
of Breastfeeding

bear or a chipmunk or, for that matter, the mother in Patzicia so many years ago. If you put your baby to your breast often and let the baby suck for a good length of time—this can be as long as twenty to thirty minutes in the beginning, when you are getting your milk supply established—you will make lots of milk. Usually. Except if you are one of those very few women who don't produce enough milk, for all sorts of reasons.

Just as in childbirth, many, many factors are at play here, including your particular physiology, the kind of birth experience you had (including whether you used medications or not), your baby's weight at birth, how much milk she or he will be needing in the beginning, the structure of your baby's mouth and tongue, and your overall stress level, which of course means your state of mind. We simply don't know what interrelated causes and conditions will be present after the two of you have gone through your particular birthing experiences.

So that's the production side. The second aspect of breastfeeding, getting the milk out of your breasts and into your baby's mouth, also involves the brain. Diagram H is a picture of a little grapelike structure, an *alveolus*. Lined with special milk-secreting cells called *secretory alveolar epithelium*, the alveoli are where your milk is actually produced once the cells have been stimulated by prolactin.

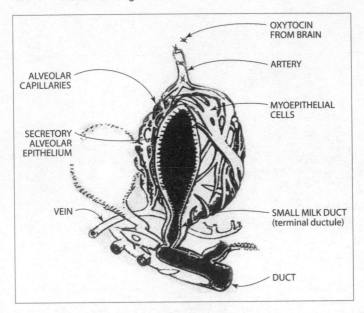

OXYTOCIN
FROM BRAIN

ARTERY

MYOEPITHELIAL
CELLS

ALVEOLAR
CAPILLARIES

SECRETORY
ALVEOLAR
EPITHELIUM

VEIN

SMALL MILK DUCT
(terminal ductule)

DUCT

Diagram H:

A Milk-Producing

Alveolus

In the diagram you can see a basket weave of cells around each of the alveoli called *myoepithelial cells*. Now this is the part I totally love. Do you know where else myoepithelial cells are located? Your uterus! And what are myoepithelial cells sensitive to—both in your uterus and around the alveoli in your breasts? Of course: oxytocin.

If you look closely at Diagram H, you can see that there is another network around each of the alveoli. These are alveolar capillaries, which bring blood with prolactin and oxytocin from the pituitary to the cells that make the milk *and* to the myoepithelial cells around the alveoli so that they can contract to eject the milk. After your milk supply is established, you may actually feel tightening or tingling sensations throughout your breasts about ten to fifteen seconds after your baby starts sucking. That's all those little alveoli contracting.

With the contraction, the milk is squeezed out of the secretory alveolar epithelium, down into the small milk ducts, then into the larger ducts leading to the collecting sinus behind the areola, and when the baby moves its tongue and gums on the nipple, voilà! Out comes the milk into your baby's mouth! Expansions and contractions—sound familiar? Now it's the expansion of your breasts filling with milk and the contraction needed for you to feed your baby.

And where does mindfulness fit into this? In Diagram I you'll see that an important part of breastfeeding is being calm and at ease. If

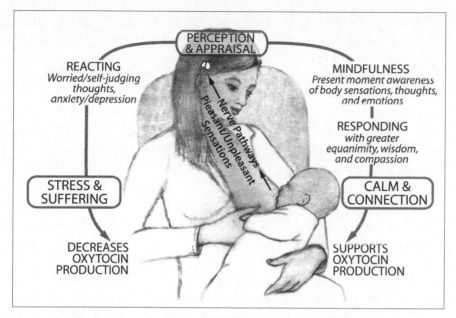

REACTING
Worried/self-judging thoughts, anxiety/depression

PERCEPTION & APPRAISAL

MINDFULNESS
Present moment awareness of body sensations, thoughts, and emotions

Nerve Pathways Pleasant/Unpleasant Sensations

RESPONDING
with greater equanimity, wisdom, and compassion

STRESS & SUFFERING

CALM & CONNECTION

DECREASES OXYTOCIN PRODUCTION

SUPPORTS OXYTOCIN PRODUCTION

Diagram I: Mindfulness and the Normal Physiology of Breastfeeding

during breastfeeding, especially during your initial learning period, you are stressed, if your mind is filled with worried thoughts about the future or unhappy thoughts about the past, if you are anxious about nursing or in pain (more about that in a moment), the fight-or-flight system goes to work. Just as it does in childbirth, the production of oxytocin decreases and alters blood flow. Only this time, it's away from the breasts and into the large muscles in preparation to fight or flee. Once again those distressing thoughts work against the normal physiology, in this case, the physiology of breastfeeding. The result is less milk produced and less milk ejected.

However, if we make breastfeeding a mindfulness practice, this may not be so. If we remember to stay anchored in the present moment, if we decide to pay attention to our new mindfulness teacher, our baby, we can decrease stress and discover moments of deep pleasure during breast-feeding, just as we did with the birth process. In the quiet moments of oxytocin-enhanced calm and connection during nursing, we may experience some of the most pleasurable emotions we humans are capable of: joy, awe, gratitude, bliss, contentment, ease, peace, connectedness, openheartedness—and love.

Katrina, who took the MBCP class with her husband, Thomas, before the birth of their second baby, Elise, described how nursing became a mindfulness practice for her. "I was so much more in tune with Elise than I ever was with Nick. We didn't take a mindfulness class before Nick was born, and I was just so distracted that I didn't pay any attention to his cues. I would be nursing him, and suddenly look down and say, 'Oh, look at that, he's asleep.' But with Elise, it's so different. Nursing is my time to just be with her. Lots of times I'll just take her into the bedroom, close the door, lie down with her, tell her how much I love her, maybe do a quick little meditation—Body Scan or some Awareness of Breathing—and settle in to just being with her while she is nursing. It's such a peaceful, special time; it's nourishing for both of us."

PAIN AND OTHER BREASTFEEDING CHALLENGES

As always with mindfulness, it's important to tell it like it is, and the process of breastfeeding is no exception. Not every bodily sensation associated with breastfeeding is pleasurable; nor is every emotion associated with breastfeeding positive. Sometimes the sensations of breastfeeding, particularly at the beginning, can be downright painful, and since breastfeeding is a human experience, other emotions can arise as well.

If pain is your experience in the beginning phase of breastfeeding, or if you have difficulties of any sort, your mindfulness practice can help sustain you through what can feel like an emotional roller coaster. There is nothing quite like being completely committed to nursing your baby (for all the reasons we discussed earlier) and not having it go well. Whether it's pain during nursing, pain of sore nipples, a bout of mastitis, too little milk or too much, a baby who seems discontent at the breast or is not sucking well or not gaining weight—all these situations and others can easily trigger a cascade of thoughts and emotions that cause us to suffer. The mind can spin incredibly harsh tales of self-judgment here, creating fears about the future and severely undermining our confidence as a mother. The specifics of the potential problems with breastfeeding are as endless as the potential problems with childbirth, but all of them can be ameliorated to some degree with mindfulness practice.

So if after giving birth you do run into breastfeeding challenges, there are two tracks to take: a problem-focused coping strategy and an emotion-focused coping strategy. With the problem-focused coping strategy, you get help and get it quickly. For this you can turn to an abundance of information, highly trained lactation consultants, wonderful La Leche League leaders, and breastfeeding support groups. But for the moment-to-moment distress, it's the emotion-focused coping strategy of mindfulness practice that can see you through. Just as with childbirth, you have woven your inner parachute, and this is the time to use it. Breathe with the physical or emotional pain, observe the thoughts and emotions that are creating suffering, and come back to the moment. The moment may be difficult, perhaps even very difficult, but you know it will change. Giving birth has already taught you that. Just take it one breath at a time, one suck at a time, one nursing at a time.

And please be gentle with yourself. You are learning. You are doing the best you can. And so is your baby. Remember your Loving-kindness practice. Send Loving-kindness to yourself and your baby, over and over and over again. The situation, as unbelievably challenging as it may be, is what it is. As Pema Chödrön says, "Welcome the present moment as if you had invited it. It is all we ever have, so we might as well work with it rather than struggling against it. We might as well make it our friend and teacher rather than our enemy."

WHO IS BREASTFEEDING WHOM?

Five decades have passed since that morning I bought oranges in Guatemala, and in that time a lot of very intelligent, dedicated, and caring people—research scientists, physicians, nurses, midwives, lactation consultants, the La Leche League community, to name but a few—have been paying attention to the breastfeeding process, encouraging and supporting mothers to do it for the present and future health of themselves and their babies.

However, for those of us who assist a new mother and baby in their breastfeeding relationship, there's a bit of a mystery here: Why is it that something as essential to life as feeding one's baby can sometimes be so difficult and painful? Mechanically the reasons often focus on "the latch," the actual connection point between the mother's breast and the baby's mouth. It's difficult not to see this as a metaphor for a society where human connection can seem so puzzling.

However, a striking evolution is taking place in the thinking of some who work with nursing mothers and babies. They are moving away from the notion that breastfeeding is a skill that experts must "teach" to a new mother (so she "finds the proper latch," or holds her baby in a particular position), for this approach implies that there is a right way or a wrong way to breastfeed.

In this new view, which is based on the research and thirty-five-year clinical experience of British midwife Suzanne Colson, PhD, *breastfeeding is seen as a unique relationship between a mother and baby.* Named Biological Nurturing,[2] this way of seeing breastfeeding is holistic—an approach based on the understanding that there are inborn, intuitive behaviors in both mothers and newborns that are stimulated and enhanced by a combination of conditions: skin-to-skin contact immediately after birth and for the first several days; nursing postures of relaxation and ease for both mother and baby, postures that are in harmony with gravity and each other's body shape and preferences; and allowing the baby to use its inborn reflexes to "find" the nipple as the mother instinctually assists her baby as needed. Biological Nurturing "suggests that maternal-infant positional interactions release some 20 neonatal reflexes as well as what appear to be emerging patterns of maternal instincts."[3]

Seeing a mother and her baby as the experts co-creating their own way of nursing while using healthcare providers for assistance and information if need be, Biological Nurturing offers a mind-body approach to breastfeeding that holds great promise for alleviating some of the most common difficulties in breastfeeding today. If you find yourself having challenges with breastfeeding, it may be worth exploring this approach.

Betsy experienced continual pain while nursing her son, Milo. After consulting one expert after another without results, Betsy finally came to realize that she had forgotten to consult the two people most expert in the situation: herself and her baby. "Finally, after one more person gave me one more theory and suggestion that didn't work, I gave up. I decided to stop running around from one expert to the next, trying to find someone out there to fix things. I just took Milo home, closed the door, and trusted that together we could figure things out—or not. I even told myself that if I didn't end up nursing him it would not be the worst disaster in the world. I think I *really* let go—of everything.

"And what happened was really interesting. After two or three days of really paying attention to him when I put him on the breast, watching him, breathing with the pain, and trying a bunch of different things—I'd definitely learned a lot of useful stuff from all the folks who had tried to help me—something finally seemed to just click and the nipple pain stopped! Actually, the hardest part was not the nipple pain, it was all the awful stories I had been telling myself—that I was a failure as a mother, that I would miss this wonderful experience with him, that he would be scarred for life, or that his immune system would be messed up forever. In the end it really came down to my mindfulness practice—paying attention—and trusting myself, and him."

CHAPTER 19

Endings and Beginnings
A Last Class

What we call the beginning is often the end.
And to make an end is to make a beginning.
The end is where we start from.
T. S. Eliot

AS YOU CAN SEE, there are not many more pages to read in this book. We're coming to the end, and I hope that something of what you have read has resonated with you and that you are perhaps motivated to begin (or return to) a regular mindfulness meditation practice. Though the seeds of practice may have been planted during your reading, the only way these skills will take root and grow deep is through your experience with the practice itself. In the spirit of T. S. Eliot, coming to the end of this book can also be a beginning—a beginning of making the practice your own now, of keeping it alive in your life through your birthing experience and hopefully beyond.

The formal MBCP classes you've been reading about are also coming to an end. In this, our last class, it is not unusual for expectant parents to express surprise, tinged with sadness, that our nine weeks together are ending. Bonds have been formed through this learning journey, and a sense of caring and good humor now permeates our time together. We have laughed as we heard how Katrina's dog Pepper seems to be becoming more attentive and affectionate, as if she knows that her days as an "only child" are numbered. We have felt sorrow with Cindy and Joe when they shared the news that Cindy's beloved grandmother had been admitted to hospice care and may not be alive to meet her great-grandchild. We have been happy for Lydia when she told us how mindfulness practice helped her with a breakthrough in her relationship with her in-laws, and we've felt Shauna and Todd's disappointment when they told us that their obstetrician was unable to turn their breech baby last week and that it is likely Shauna will have a cesarean birth instead of the one with minimal drugs and technology that they had hoped for. Whatever the circumstances are now in the lives of these expectant couples, they have shared a deep, collective learning experience, cradled by the intention to be more present and awake in their lives. In short, we feel connected.

This evening I have set up the chairs a bit differently. Moving my own chair to the side, I've placed four chairs in the usual teacher's spot, since two couples and their babies from a previous MBCP class will be joining us. These new parents with their babies will be our mindfulness teachers tonight.

We settle in for a period of sitting before our guests arrive. This evening we practice without any meditation instructions from me, for by now everyone has learned how to practice on their own. There is hardly a rustle of clothing, or the squeak of a chair, and this deep stillness is a testament to the intention, commitment, and effort of each expectant parent during our weeks together. I find my heart opening with gratitude and joy.

I have left the door ajar, and toward the end of our sitting we begin to hear unmistakable baby sounds that signal the arrival of our teachers. I ring the bells to close our practice, and everyone opens their eyes. Judy and Marc, with their newborn son, Luke, and Amanda, David, and baby Stella are gathered at the edge of the circle. I beckon them to come take the teachers' seats. Stella is fussing a bit, and David unwraps her from the sling he has been wearing as Amanda reaches into the front of her shirt to unhook her nursing bra. David passes her to Amanda saying, "Sorry, little girl, I just don't have the right equipment."

"I hope nobody minds if I nurse while we talk," Amanda says in an off-hand way.

"Not if you don't," I reply.

"I don't mind. One of the things that's gone completely out the window since I've had Stella is modesty. I mean, after giving birth, who can care about modesty anymore?" Amanda laughs, and we join in.

I introduce our teachers to the class and invite them to tell us about their birth experiences and their mindfulness practice. But before they do I say a few words to the class.

"As we hear about the births of these babies, I'd like to encourage you to listen to Judy and Marc and Amanda and David mindfully, meaning being aware of your thoughts and emotions as best you can while you listen. Remember, these birth stories are their unique experiences, and yours will be different: not better, not worse, just different. So watch what your mind says as you listen. Do you hear yourself thinking, 'I hope that happens to me'? Or 'I hope that *doesn't* happen to me'? Or 'I would *never* do that'? Hope and fear, grasping and aversion, judging and comparing: the ingredients for suffering are ready to appear, in any moment. As you listen, do your best to pay attention to how Judy and Marc and Amanda and David used their mindfulness practice and what they—and you—can learn from that."

I turn toward our four teachers in expectation and invitation. Amanda says, "Judy, since I'm still nursing Stella, why don't you start?" And so Judy begins.

"Well, first I suppose I should tell you that Luke is my third baby, so I had some past experience to guide me. And maybe I should also tell you that I'm an obstetrician, so I had a lot of work to do from that angle—to stay in beginner's mind and not let everything I 'know' bring up all sorts of fears that could get in my way.

"So in the week leading up to the birth, I started to get pretty anxious, as I have in the past, thinking that the worst things possible were going to happen to Luke or to me. I even got to the point of firmly reminding Marc that I was an organ donor, stuff like that." Judy laughs. "So the practice was super helpful during that period, just to watch all the fear arising and patting it on the head.

"In reality, the birth turned out to be a pretty quick and easy affair. I was swimming laps at 3:00 P.M., and four hours later I was holding Luke! I started having contractions after my swim and called Marc to come home. I wanted to head over to the hospital sooner rather than later—the hospital is about an hour's drive from our house—even though I knew there was a chance I might get sent home. With my other two births I did a lot of serious labor in the car, and I just wasn't up for it this time.

"Marc's mom lives about a mile away, so she came over pretty quickly and took our daughters—Clare is four, and Vivian is two—to her house. Marc and I got in the car at about 5:30 P.M. I had been so busy getting the girls ready and saying good-bye to them that I didn't really start using the mindfulness practices for pain until we were in the car. First I counted the breaths through the contractions—one on the inhalation, two on the exhalation. That was really helpful because I knew that by the time I reached twenty the contraction would be over—it was about ten full breaths per contraction. Between each contraction I did a Body Scan—and I remember being completely amazed that I could feel so comfortable during that time. Finally, as things got more intense, I moved directly into the pain, noting the actual sensations of pain, specifically, burning in my lower pelvis. It's interesting because I never liked practicing that technique with the ice in class; it always seemed to make the sensations feel more intense, but this time it helped me to just acknowledge that burning was all I was feeling, and not lots of other, different—and scarier—sensations.

"When we got to the hospital, the midwife—she was just so wonderful—checked me, and I was eight centimeters. I was so surprised—and relieved! They put me on the fetal monitor for about twenty minutes—Luke was doing just fine—and just as they were unhooking me from the monitor I started to feel the urge to push. The timing was perfect because they do water births at this hospital, and I wanted to get in the tub as soon as I could. They filled the tub really quickly, and I got in just in time for the delivery. It was a godsend!

"With my other two births the transition from being mindful of contractions in the first part of labor to actively pushing took some intention and coordination. I know I tend to hold back because of the fear of the pain, but this time I remembered mindful pooping right away, and it really helped me direct my pushing. Because I was in the tub, I was kneeling so I was able to guide Luke's head out of me with my hand. That was really amazing, delivering my own baby's head—I could push and know exactly how much to push from both the inside and the outside so I wouldn't tear. It was really a great way to feel present in those last, very intense burning moments as the head was crowning.

"Luke came out really quickly. I'm lucky because I grow little babies, and little babies definitely come out easier. He was seven pounds three ounces, which is big for me; both the girls were about six and a half pounds. I sat in the warm tub with him for a long time, just amazed at him and the miracle of birth. And I do have to say, everything is so much easier the third time around—the birth, the nursing. You do learn how to do this, you know.

"And Marc was just incredible too, right by my side the entire time, a rock, the best birth partner I could ever have." Judy turns to Marc and gives him a big, affectionate smile.

"Well, I don't know about that," Marc says, reddening slightly. "She was pretty incredible herself. I used the practice too, to just be there and do whatever Judy needed me to do, which honestly wasn't much, besides taking pictures—she was pretty insistent that I do that because our last daughter came so fast we didn't have time to take pictures. It's pretty amazing how in the moments of birth everything else just seems to fall away."

"Thank you for telling us about your experiences. And how about you two?" I say, turning to Amanda and David. "How was it for you?"

"Well, my experience was pretty different from Judy's," Amanda begins. "I remember reading about her birth experience on our group email list and thinking it's great to hear that it gets easier because we definitely want another baby. My labor was very different from what I had imagined it would be, yet we're completely okay with it. I had about thirty-six hours of on-and-off labor at home with very little sleep. The mindfulness practice was so important during that time to keep me centered and grounded and just working with the pain. David was really with me, and the doula was great. I loved having these two people there just for me. It was a very new experience, feeling so taken care of.

"When the contractions finally became strong and regular we went to the hospital, and when they checked me I was only three centimeters dilated. That was a big emotional setback—I was really disappointed that after all that time I wasn't further along. But I kept reminding myself to just take it one breath at a time, which really helped. I tried counting my breaths, like Judy, but it didn't work for me as well as just feeling the breath in my belly. I also visualized that wave-contraction diagram that you did on the whiteboard that night in class when you told us about the pleasure between the waves of contractions. I think that helped me stay in the moments between and to experience the time of real peace in the process.

"When the contractions got really strong I started saying 'transformational pain, transformational pain' to myself over and over. I remember being struck by the whole notion of transformational pain when you talked about it in class, and the words just came to me when I was in labor. I knew the pain was taking me to my new life as a mom.

"After about six more hours of labor, in and out of the shower, standing, rocking, leaning over a chair, doing Child's Pose on the bed, lots of sounding, the doula and David massaging me, I was still only about four centimeters dilated. At that point the doctor came in. She was great. She sat on the bed, and we talked about my options. She thought I needed some Pitocin to help me along.

"I remembered to use BRANN in that conversation," David interjects. "And it really helped us figure out what we wanted to do."

Amanda takes up the story again. "I was so exhausted. I knew I had reached my limit and needed something, so I opted for the epidural. What I had learned in class had given me the strength to persevere for a really long time and then to make a clear decision when I needed to. There was some trouble after the epidural went in—my blood pressure dropped, and the baby's heart rate didn't look so good during contractions. And then my contractions stopped, and they were afraid to give me the Pitocin, which was probably just as well because I got a few hours of sleep, and I really needed it. After a while the contractions picked up on their own, and about five hours later I started to feel like I really had to push. David was so funny when I told him how it felt—he goes, 'Hooray for mindful pooping!'

"I pushed for about an hour and a half, and I really used the practice for pushing into the sensations. I could actually move around more than I thought I would be able to with the epidural. For the birth itself I used that side-lying position from the yoga sequence. The birth was just amazing—and Stella got to come right onto my belly! She was a lot bigger than anyone thought she would be—nine pounds two ounces."

"It sounds like you made good use of your practice," I say.

"Absolutely," Amanda replies. "Even though things didn't go the way we would have preferred, I feel that under the circumstances I did really well. Another thing that helped me were the emails from our class, when everybody shared their birth experiences. There were so many different experiences in the group, yet it was absolutely clear that everyone rose to their particular challenge, used their practice, stayed involved, and did what they needed to do to get their baby born. The non-judging support of the group has been so positive."

"How about you, David? Did you use the practice during the labor?"

"Absolutely. It helped me be very present the entire time, which was a very powerful thing for me. I think I was able to stay pretty calm." He looks toward Amanda, who nods her head affirmatively. "In general I didn't get caught up in worries about what might happen when it seemed to be taking so long—and it was especially useful in that flurry when they were concerned about the baby after they started the epidural. And I do wonder if the practice has something to do with the deep and amazing love that I felt for Stella right away, which just keeps getting stronger."

"Maybe," I smile. "Remember way back how some people's hearts opened when they paid attention to their raisin? It's pretty amazing what focused attention can do. And how have the two of you been using the practice since Stella was born?"

Amanda answers. "Stella calls on us to be in the moment all the time. She is definitely our mindfulness teacher. We are not so caught up in our own petty problems like we used to be. We need to be there for her.

"She also teaches us a lot about letting go. She's always changing, so we have to do the same. If we get too attached to how we think things should be or want things to be too different than how they are, we just get stressed. Mostly, if we stay flexible and pay attention, we can usually figure out what she needs. Not always but usually. She's a pretty easy baby.

"I connected a lot with her during pregnancy—when I would stop and take those mindful moments with her throughout the day, all her little kicks and rolls—I was just so excited to see this little person who had been inside me all that time. Now I get to watch all those little kicks and rolls outside my body and learn even more about who she is. It's pretty unbelievable."

"I've been practicing most when Stella cries," David says. "Her crying is really hard for me. A lot of times I'll put her in the sling and just do some Walking Meditation with her. I think the slow movement and her feeling my breath and that I am calm is soothing to her."

"And how about you?" I turn to Judy and Marc. "How have you been using your practice since Luke was born?"

"I think I can say for both of us that the practice has been invaluable. I don't have as much time to focus just on Luke as I did with the girls when they were babies because they need so much of our attention now. I'm so glad I have the practice for those precious times when it is just Luke and me—like in the middle of the night. You know, juggling the needs of three kids can feel pretty crazy sometimes." Judy and Marc both laugh as Judy says this. "But we try to just take it one child at a time, one moment at a time."

I see that it's getting late, and I'm mindful that these parents need to go home. The night is still ahead, and who knows how much or how little sleep they will get. After some last questions from the expectant parents, I thank our guests for coming and invite them to stay for a snack if they care to. As we break a small crowd gathers around them, eager to ask a few more questions and get a closer look at a real newborn. The visit has definitely made what is to come seem very real.

During the break I assemble the objects we will need for the small closing ceremony that has evolved over the years as a way of ending our time together. After placing a large round mirror in the center of the circle, a mirror that represents the reflective quality of mindfulness that we have been cultivating together, I put a pile of smooth black stones in its center. The stones represent being grounded in the present moment and our ability to smooth our own rough edges through practice. I also set out small tea candles, which represent the insight that can come when we strengthen our capacity to look within.

Tonight each person will speak about what they have learned during our nine weeks together and then will exchange their small candle for one of the stones in the center of the mirror. The stone is theirs to keep, a re-minder of mindfulness practice and of our time together. It's their diploma.

Gathering everyone together for this last time before giving birth, I be-gin. "None of us know how things will unfold in the weeks ahead," I say, "but I do know that we will be holding each other in our thoughts and our hearts. We are coming full circle, and I'd like to invite each of you to join in a guided reflection at the well we visited eight weeks ago."

I notice how easily these expectant parents settle and drop into silence now. After guiding them to imagine a well once again, I say, "Now, picking up a stone, let it become the question 'What have I learned? What will I remember from our time together that I will take with me as I live the mo-ments, days and weeks ahead?' Let the first splash of an answer come, and just wait. Once again, see if an answer comes from a deeper place as the stone drops and settles."

As my own stone falls I too wait for an answer. Although I have done this reflection many times before, I learn something new from every class, and I'm always curious to see what will come up. Tonight the answer that arises is "The power and the gift of sharing the present moment with others."

Before too long I ring the bells, and everyone opens their eyes.

"Now I invite each of you to share what arose during the reflection."

Our sharing ceremony lasts about forty-five minutes. Many speak of the joys of slowing down and of being more fully present in their lives. Some describe how the practice feels like coming home to themselves. Others speak of discovering a new inner peace and the need to reevaluate daily life in order to bring more of that calm into it. Kelly says, "I'm so grateful for the practice. Before this I never knew what it meant to live without anxi-ety. I feel normal for the first time in my life."

Catherine says, "I learned that I don't need to learn how to have a baby. I know how even if I don't know." Many people thank the group for the open, sharing community they have become, and several partners say they had no idea that they themselves would learn so much. Others express how much they appreciate the common language and perspective they now share with their partners. Jack observes, "I thought our relationship was pretty good—we've been together for seven years—but the practice took us to a whole other level."

Will is the last to speak. He says simply, "My initial thought when I began the class was that this would be a birth class that I might get something else out of. What it's ended up being for me is a life-perspective-altering class that's going to help with our birth. Leaving the class now, it's a complete reversal. It's not about the birth anymore. It's going to help us with the birth, but it's not about the birth. It's about our lives."

The room falls silent once again. There doesn't seem to be anything more to say. Yet the hour is getting late, and I know that we'll need time for lingering good-byes. So I say, "I want to thank each of you for all your hard work over the past weeks. It's been a joy to be with you as you've come to know yourselves, each other, and this way of being that is possible through the cultivation of mindfulness practice. As we become less reactive, we learn how to be in wiser relationship with ourselves and each other. Ultimately the practice of mindfulness is about kindness, compassion— especially self-compassion—wisdom, and peace. Because of your practice over the past nine weeks, the world is a little more peaceful because you are a little more peaceful. My deepest wish is that each of you gives birth in good health and with ease and that you and your babies are safe, protected, healthy, and happy. I hope that you will continue to practice between now and the time you give birth—and for the rest of your lives. May your practice serve you well."

And for you, dear reader, I have exactly the same wish. So I invite you to take a moment right here, right now, and reflect on what you've read, much the way the expectant couples did in their class. Ask yourself: What have I learned from this book? What have I learned from practicing mindfulness, however much or little as I have practiced? What might I take with me into my life? What might I commit to in the moments, days, and weeks ahead that will contribute to my being more awake and alive for myself, my partner, my baby, my family, and all whom I encounter in my daily life?

And after some time in silent reflection, perhaps two or three minutes, open your eyes. And share your reflections with your partner, if the two of you have been learning and practicing together.

And then you might read this poem aloud to each other; it's a poem I often read to close the MBCP course, and I use it here to send you on your way, in peace.

For the Children

The rising hills, the slopes
of statistics
lie before us.
The steep climb
of everything, going up,
up, as we all
go down.

In the next century
or the one beyond that,
they say,
are valleys, pastures,
we can meet there in peace
if we make it.

To climb these coming crests
one word to you, to
you and your children:

stay together
learn the flowers
go light

—Gary Snyder, *Turtle Island*

CHAPTER 20

Life After Birth
A Reunion

*A new moon teaches gradualness
and deliberation and how one gives birth
to oneself slowly. Patience with small details
makes perfect a large work, like the universe.*

*What nine months of attention does for an embryo
forty early mornings will do
for your gradually growing wholeness.*
—Rumi

IT'S THREE MONTHS later when the day arrives for the reunion. Our gathering today is set for 1:00 P.M., though experience has taught me that it is a rare trio that arrives on time. These new families are living on Baby Time now, and there is no telling what adventures will precede their attempts to get here. Gone are the days when one grabbed a purse or a wallet and rushed out the door. Leaving the house now requires planning, coordination, multiple decisions, and exquisitely choreographed teamwork.

One by one, each new family arrives. What joy it is to see them again, safely on the other side of childbirth! I'm always struck by how dramatic the physical changes are post-pregnancy. For those who gave birth many weeks ago, the maternity clothes are gone along with some of the extra pounds. Some women have cut their hair short in a style more convenient for a hardworking new mom who barely has time for a quick shower and blow-dry. But mostly I'm struck by a certain something in the eyes, something I can only call maturity—an inner sense of knowing that wasn't there before. A transformative challenge has been encountered, fully met and transcended.

When the time seems right, I ring the bells in the familiar signal to take our seats. "How wonderful it is to see you all again, and to see all these beautiful new babies! Life is certainly different from the last time we sat in this room together, isn't it?" Wry laughter follows this statement of the obvious. "There was no way out but through, and now you are on the other side," I continue. "Congratulations."

"What I'd like to do," I say, "is begin like we always have, with practice." Some people seem genuinely surprised at the notion of practicing with the babies present. I continue, "Much has changed, but the present moment is still right here, right now. And we can still drop down into Being Mode by stopping, noticing our body sensations, our thoughts, our feelings and coming to the breath—holding them all in present-moment awareness.

"Some of you will be doing Being with Baby Practice, just being present with your baby, taking care of him or her when he or she needs something. The rest of us will just sit."

Except for the sounds of the babies—a grunt or a small cry, a burp or a hiccup—stillness settles in the room. The babies do seem content in this quiet space, and I can't help but wonder if they learned the power of meditation practice before they were born. And with that thought comes a memory. Roughly twenty years ago I attended a gathering of several hundred people in the Berkeley High School auditorium with a well-known meditation teacher, S. N. Goenka. After his talk there was a question-and-answer period. A man in the far back raised his hand, and when called on, he stood and asked, "At what age should you teach children to meditate?" Without missing a beat Goenka smiled and said simply, "In the womb."

After a short while I ring the bells. "Gently moving your fingers and toes, stretching a bit, and when you are ready, opening your eyes," I say, bringing the meditation to a close.

Suddenly Jerry, whose baby is five weeks old, says, "Wow! That was great. We've been so busy these past few weeks that I'd forgotten how good it feels just to sit. Thanks for the reminder."

"You're welcome. I'm sure you're mostly doing lots of informal mindfulness practice these days, but it can be helpful to be reminded that there is truly something beneficial about formal practice too—even a really short one.

"What I'd like for us to do now is to have a bit of a check-in about life as you are living it now. Let's each start by introducing our baby, when and where he or she was born, and then share the following about your new life: something that is joyous; something that is challenging; something you appreciate about your partner; something you appreciate about yourself; and how you are using your mindfulness practice, including in your relationship to each other, if you are, in this new life."

THE JOYS

Far and away the most frequently mentioned joy for both parents is seeing their baby smile. Carin says, "It just breaks my heart open," and Nathan adds, "There's nothing like the moment when I come home after a long day at work and she smiles at me." Others mention cooing and interacting, saying, "It's like a payoff for those first weeks before she got herself fully here." And Jamie observes, "I just love our time together, the three of us in bed in the morning—how we're this little family now."

Some mothers say that their joy is that a long-standing fear of motherhood has been resolved. "I wasn't sure I was going to like being a mom, but I really do. I just like being with him." Many report how satisfying an experience breastfeeding is, though it sometimes comes with a qualifier like, "But it was a real struggle in the beginning. I sure used my practice for that."

Fathers and partners often mention how having a baby has brought a new perspective to their lives, and of course there's lots of humor that comes from the beginner's mind in this new life. "I can't believe how much poop a baby can make!" Nathan says. "The first time Tamara really cut loose it blew me away!" Ted chimes in with "I didn't expect I'd be living in the house with a topless woman. She never puts a shirt on anymore." Elena says, "I never knew how many things I could do with one hand—go to the bathroom, pull down panties, wipe, pull up panties, wash hands. Talk about mindfulness practice in daily life!"

THE CHALLENGES

And then, because this is life, and because caring for a new infant can be just plain hard work, there are challenges. The most commonly mentioned challenge is lack of sleep and the process of discovering how to help their baby go to sleep. Fatigue can definitely be one of the more unpleasant sensations for new parents, and it's important to take it seriously, for constant sleep deprivation affects our sense of wellbeing and can contribute to suppressing the immune system as well as to depression. Leah says, "The Body Scan has been a lifesaver. I've never been much of a napper, but it really helps me to fall asleep when I need to."

Of course other challenges of parenting come up, like when the baby cries and can't be comforted, and the challenge of staying mindful of their own feelings of distress, so as not to exacerbate the situation. "Once we're satisfied that the basic checklist has been taken care of—diaper dry, baby fed and burped, not too hot or too cold, no fever or other sign of illness—then all that's left is for Jim and me to be present," Ellie says. "With affectionate attention, as best you can," I chime in. "Yep, that's the practice. We know that this crying session, even if it lasts an hour or more, isn't permanent. Sometimes we do a lot of breathing. But it always passes, thank goodness."

Lucy tells a particularly touching story. "One day I was right outside the supermarket holding Katie, and she was just crying and crying. I had tried everything, and I just couldn't get her to stop. I was beside myself, completely caught up in the judging and worrying mind, blaming myself for being a complete failure as a mother, worrying that something was seriously wrong with her—I was so upset I couldn't even think! By this time I was crying myself—so I called Tom. He said, "How about putting her in the sling and going for a walk?" I had tried everything else, so I just did it. There I was, walking down the street crying with a crying baby strapped to me, and this guy pulls up to the curb in his car, rolls down the window, and looks right at me and says in this very sweet way, 'Just take a breath. It's going to be okay.' It was amazing! Right then and there I decided that the next time I see a parent in the supermarket with a crying baby I'm going to do the same thing—to say that I know it's hard and that it's going to be okay."

Stacey, who had very specific plans for returning to work, tells us how she is completely reevaluating her life. "I can't believe I'm even considering being a stay-at-home mom—at least for much longer than I ever imagined I would." As with giving birth, life after our baby is born can be very different from what we imagined it would be, and non-attachment, beginner's mind, and letting go may give us the flexibility to find our way.

Michael says his greatest challenge also has to do with work. "Truth be told, I would much rather be home with Trish and Aiden than having to go to work." Andrew chimes in with his work challenges. "Me too. Before Sophia was born I was traveling a lot for my job, but now it's really hard to be away. I talked to my boss, and we are figuring out how to change that." Then Daniel says, "Sometimes I have to leave really early in the morning before Jackson wakes up, and I come home after he's asleep. I was feeling all this sadness around that, and then I realized this is what it was like when I was growing up: my father was never home. I'm not sure what we're going to do about it, but at the very least it makes me want to be really present for the moments I do have to be with him."

APPRECIATION FOR OUR PARTNER

Tears often begin to flow when new parents are given an opportunity to express appreciation for their partners. It is not often we hear ourselves deeply appreciated by our partner in a public setting, and it always feels like a privilege to be present during these heartfelt moments. Among the most common appreciations expressed by partners is awe at the enormous strength they observed during the birth process. Sam says, "I knew Julie was strong, but I didn't know how strong until the birth." Others frequently express appreciation for their partner's "amazing capacity for patience" in caring for the baby. "Kari has so much more patience than I do," Jonathan says.

Julie speaks up. "I knew Sam would be a great dad, and it's true. I so appreciate how sensitive he is with language. Like if James is crying, I might start saying, 'It's okay. You're all right.' But really, that's not true. In that moment he's totally and completely unhappy. When I say that to him I'm really just trying to calm myself. So we are trying to practice being present with James and breathing with our own upset when he's unhappy, and naming what he might be feeling. The question we ask ourselves is, 'Can we let him have his unhappy moments and still let him know we are here for him?'"

APPRECIATION FOR ONESELF

As joyous and heart opening as parenting can be, it takes a tremendous amount of time, energy, attention, sensitivity, and plain hard work to raise a happy, healthy child. As Jon and Myla Kabat-Zinn say in their book *Everyday Blessings: The Inner Work of Mindful Parenting*, "Parenting is one of the most challenging, demanding, and stressful jobs on the planet. It is also one of the most important, for how it is done influences in great measure the heart and soul and consciousness of the next generation. . . ."[1]

Sometimes a little encouragement is needed for new parents to hold themselves in the light of appreciation, but when gently encouraged, they do. New mothers particularly appreciate the capacity of their bodies to grow and birth a baby, grateful that their babies are healthy and that the whole experience of giving birth and becoming a mother has brought them into a new and deeper understanding of the fragility and preciousness of life itself. Other new parents name and appreciate, sometimes with surprise, their capacity for patience, perseverance, and joy—all of which have been nurtured by their mindfulness practice and their growing connection and attachment to their new baby.

MINDFULNESS PRACTICE WITH EACH
OTHER IN THIS NEW LIFE

When the time comes for these new parents to share how they are using their mindfulness practice in their relationship with each other, couples describe how invaluable it has been. Robert and Jessica say that they've been using their practice to address some of the issues that come up in their relationship. "I have to really give Robert space to find his own way with Jared," Jessica reports. "I can get pretty bossy and think I know what's best for Jared because I spend so much more time with him. That only makes Robert feel unsure of himself, and it's not good for their relationship or ours. So I'm trying to make my practice coming back to the breath instead of reactively telling Robert what to do. It's not easy for me, especially when Jared is crying, but usually if I can just stay put and breathe, within about five breaths Robert usually figures out what to do in his own way. It's like breathing through a contraction!" Everyone laughs.

Amy speaks up. "I'm finding that practice helps the two of us find ways to support each other. Sometimes we can feel overwhelmed, trying to keep up with everything. Usually when one of us is feeling that way it's because we're just exhausted, so we try to remember to come back to Loving-kindness, for ourselves and for each other. And we try to spell each other. Last week Jerry took Violet for a whole morning so I could go to a yoga class. It's amazing how being away from her for such a short time can rejuvenate me. Even a ten- or fifteen-minute walk can make such a big difference."

Trish takes a turn at speaking. "We've been using the practice to deal with the stress of me having to go back to work. I really didn't want to, but financially we needed me to. We have this great day care, but last week Aiden got his first cold and we started feeling totally guilty that he's in day care. But we just reminded each other to just breathe and be here now. It's just a runny nose, for heaven's sakes, not the end of the world."

Stacey continues, "When I'm home it feels like the day is broken up into all these little increments of time. If I think, 'I'm always getting interrupted,' I can start to feel annoyed or resentful, but if I just stay in the flow of the moment, everything is so much easier. Last week I was home with Marcus while he was taking his morning nap. I was having a cup of tea and just sitting looking out the window at this tree I love. And I started to think, 'This isn't going to last very long. I'm going to be interrupted at any moment.' And then I realized that I was worrying about the future instead of just enjoying my cup of tea right now. So I stopped and just enjoyed it. I actually sat there for a good ten minutes! Well, maybe seven would be more accurate. But it was lovely."

The afternoon is passing quickly, and it's already time to share that most basic of human activities—eating. We take a break for a snack.

CHILDBIRTH: A PROCESS TO LEARN FROM

I ring the bells calling everyone back into the circle. There is one more essential activity for us today—to reflect on the lessons of our birth experience.

"Though so much of what we learned together has to do with being in the present, reflecting on the past can help us toward greater understanding of who we are and what it means to be human. This may be a good time to remind ourselves that when we recall the past, we are selecting only certain moments and that many moments, of necessity, are left out. Stories can be extraordinarily powerful, for better and for worse, but they reside in memory. They are not the reality of now, and it is in the now that we are living. Mindfulness practice is about stepping out of the story that our minds have constructed and reflecting on the past not as story making but *as an experience to learn from*; deeply reflecting on the past is a way to glean wisdom from experience.

"So in that spirit, let's do a short guided reflection." I wait a few moments until babies and mothers settle into breastfeeding or the last moments of a diaper change are completed. As we rest here in our chairs or on cushions on the floor, quiet punctuated by baby sounds prevails. "Now, into this stillness and quiet, I invite you to drop a question. And the question is, 'What did I learn about myself through my experience of giving birth or of helping my partner give birth?' Or even let the question be, 'What did I learn about life itself? Am I grateful for anything about my birth experience? Is there more to learn from the experience?'"

After a short time I ring the bells.

"Would anyone like to share what came up for them? Let's see if we can look at your experience within the spaciousness of Loving-kindness and the wisdom that comes from reflection. The direction here is to be sparse on details and abundant with wisdom."

IT'S NOT WHAT HAPPENED
BUT YOUR RELATIONSHIP TO IT

Trish takes a breath and begins. "Well, I think the biggest thing I learned is how strong I actually am. Even though my anxiety about giving birth went down a lot with practice, I still had this lingering feeling that other women could do this but not me. There were certainly some moments of doubt, like when I got to the hospital and suddenly my contractions slowed way down. But I stuck with it, used the practice, and all in all it was pretty straightforward. Mostly I think I gained a new sense of trust in myself. If I can have a baby, I can do anything!"

Michael says, "You know, I have to say almost the exact same thing. I knew Trish was strong, but I really underestimated how strong she actually is. I was just so in awe of her and what the female body can do. To think that that's the way we all got here! It was just amazing. I walked around for a couple of days afterward just looking at her and everything differently."

Julie takes her turn. "I think the main thing I learned from the experience is how much I love Sam. He was right there with me every step of the way. And my mom was there too, which was really special. We even asked her to cut the cord. She was so honored."

Stacey speaks up again. "There are a couple of things that I tell my friends about childbirth now: first of all, get a mindfulness practice so you can absolutely be present and involved in the process and everything and anything that happens. And that what you really want is safe passage for yourself and your baby—and to be treated with kindness and respect by the people taking care of you. And we got all of that. I certainly didn't get the birth experience I thought I wanted, but I definitely got a whole lot . . . a healthy baby, a healthy me, and maybe a little wisdom too. I feel grateful and at peace with the way everything turned out."

COMMUNITY: IT'S ONLY NATURAL

All too quickly the reunion comes to an end. Already there is talk about another get-together in a month's time. Julie says to me, "It is such a relief to sit in a room with a group of people and be honest about what's really going on. I especially love it that we are here together with our partners."

We gather for group photos that include the babies. Hugs of good-bye are not far away. Coming too are the bittersweet moments for me, moments that most every midwife feels who accompanies a woman and her partner along the intimate journey through pregnancy and birth; my work is done, and it's time for letting go. I'm heartened by knowing that these new parents have learned skills that they will be able to draw on for the rest of their lives.

Looking at this group of newly birthed parents and their babies through the camera lens, I take a breath in, saying silently to myself, "May the contractions of your lives be few and manageable." As I push the camera button down I breathe out, saying silently, "May you and your babies be safe, healthy, and happy. May you live with ease and in peace."

CHAPTER 21

Birthing a Mindfulness Practice

A half-hour a day of meditation is essential, except
when you are very busy. Then a full hour is necessary.
—Saint Francis de Sales

WHAT FOLLOWS HERE are basic guidelines for establishing a mindfulness meditation practice, along with a week-by-week guide to the nine-week MBCP program as it has evolved over the past fourteen years. I have included it in case you wish to develop your mindfulness practice in the same structured way the expectant parents do in the MBCP course. With a deep bow of gratitude to Jon Kabat-Zinn, who originated this way of teaching mindfulness in a secular context, I highly recommend that you follow the sequence of practices in the order given here. There is deep wisdom and even a certain genius embedded in the course structure itself. Each week builds on and informs what you learned before, and learning in this way will help you begin and deepen your mindfulness practice as you go along.

This book includes all the information you need to start and maintain a formal mindfulness practice as well as guide you in a way to bring more awareness and presence into your daily life. As mentioned in the Introduction, if you think audio guided meditations would be helpful as an aid to your learning, you can order the same guides the expectant parents use in the MBCP course from the MBCP website listed in Appendix B.

If you would like to take the nine-week MBCP course with an instructor and one isn't available in your area (check the MBCP website listed in Appendix B for locations), consider taking a Mindfulness-Based Stress Reduction (MBSR) course if one is available in your area. Then use the information and practices in this book to help you apply what you are learning there to your pregnancy and future birthing experience. Or, as I mentioned in the Introduction, you might consider organizing an MBCP course yourself with a few other expectant parents. You could meet week by week, working your way through the outline of practices given here, supporting each other and sharing your experiences with mindfulness practice throughout pregnancy and early parenthood. Online courses may be available in the future, so check the MBCP website for developments.

MAKING A COMMITMENT

To shift from reading about mindfulness to actually making a commitment to a formal mindfulness practice is no small matter. It takes real determination to begin this inner work, followed by a certain discipline and patience to sustain it. The tug of old habits, patterns, and stories we tell ourselves can be quite strong, and a certain intention and energy are necessary to overcome obstacles as you find your way.

The key to this kind of learning is consistent, regular, daily practice, whether you feel like it or not. As you know, those who sign up for the MBCP course are committed to formally practicing meditation thirty minutes a day, six days a week. If you want to take up this way of preparing for childbirth and parenting, it would be ideal for you, or you and your partner, to make that kind of commitment too. In addition to daily formal practice, there are also informal practices to use throughout your day. Ultimately, you may come to see this as a somewhat arbitrary distinction, for mindfulness practice is not about either formal or informal meditation practice but about a way of being in *every* moment of your life.

That said, even five minutes a day of formal practice on a consistent basis can make a very real difference. It can keep you in touch with your intention to be more awake and present in your life, and it can help you drop into a mode of calm abiding with things as they are that is always available whenever we can remember to access it. Of course, the more you practice, the more robust your capacity to be mindful will be and the more readily you will be able to drop into that way of being during your childbirth experience.

WHEN IN PREGNANCY SHOULD I BEGIN TO PRACTICE?

From a childbirth education point of view, the MBCP program is designed to fit into the time period when most women and their partners sign up for a childbirth class—typically during the second half of their pregnancy. However, it's never too early to begin reducing stress and bringing a healthier mind-body balance into your life. Particularly if you have a lot of fear about childbirth and want a good bit of time to prepare emotionally for the experience, or if you are experiencing a challenging pregnancy, perhaps one that is complicated by a health condition, either yours or your baby's, or if you and your partner have had a difficult or even traumatic previous birth experience, you may truly benefit from beginning a mindfulness practice early in pregnancy, possibly in conjunction with other therapies.

If we think of mindfulness meditation as something we do to cultivate a healthy mind-body balance, then wherever you are in your pregnancy is a good time to begin a mindfulness practice. Like today. Like right now.

WHEN TO PRACTICE

After a period of experimentation, many people find that early morning is an optimal time to practice. The mind is alert, the body is usually at ease, and the busyness of the day is still ahead. Some people set their alarm to wake up a bit earlier to make time for practice. Of course this may mean going to bed earlier, which can entail some reevaluation of how you are spending your evenings. This in itself can be quite helpful at this transitional time, when your priorities are definitely changing. Pregnancy affords us an opportunity to reconsider and reevaluate what is really most important in our lives now.

It's not necessary, and it may not be realistic, for you and your partner to always practice together. Each of us needs to take responsibility for finding our own time for meditation. However, meditating together can be wonderfully nourishing, and you and your partner may often be able to find times for practicing together, perhaps on weekends. It is quite wonderful that each of you has a support system right in your home, and when motivation to practice may be flagging for one of you, it can be a real blessing to have encouragement from the other.

Personally, I find that practicing in the morning sets a certain tone for the day. For me there is something special about practicing in the early morning hours when the house is quiet and everything outside is still. Maybe it takes me back to all those early morning hours I spent with laboring women, but to close my eyes when it's still dark outside and then open them thirty or so minutes later to find a sky turning pale blue as the sun begins to rise reminds me of the wonder that there is a fresh new day ahead and curious about how it will unfold. Tapping into feelings of gratitude for just being alive, I set my intention to live this day being as fully present as I can be.

WHERE TO PRACTICE

It can be helpful to choose a particular place in your home for your regular practice. Most of us don't have the luxury of being able to set aside a whole room to practice in, but dedicating a place somewhere in your home says something to you, and perhaps to each other, about the commitment you are making to practice. It says that meditation, which is about finding your home within, is important enough that you are going to dedicate space to it where you live, at least for the next nine weeks.

Choose a place that's warm and comfortable, ideally a place where you can close a door or at least where you will not be disturbed. This is where you'll put your meditation cushion (if you are going to use one), or a chair that you find comfortable, your yoga mat, and any pillows or blankets for your comfort when you lie down. If you will be using the audio guided meditations, put whatever technology you will need in your practice space as well. When you are ready to practice, turn off your cell phone, and take the house phone out of the room if you can.

HOW LONG TO PRACTICE

The week-by-week guide on the next several pages is based on the commitment to practice thirty minutes a day, six days a week, just as the expectant couples do with the audio meditations in the MBCP course. This is optimal, but of course life being what it is, things may come up that make it difficult or even impossible to practice on a particular day. Do your best with the formal practice, for there is simply no substitute for what you can learn from it. And of course if you want to practice *more* than thirty minutes a day, don't hesitate!

Also remember that any moment in your life is a moment when you can be awake and fully present. Even one breath taken mindfully can shift a mood, an interaction, or even the flow of a whole day. Informal practice, which in the MBCP course starts explicitly in the second week and was the topic of Chapter 11, "Mindfulness in Everyday Life," is exceedingly important, especially once your baby is born. As Jon Kabat-Zinn puts it, "The real practice is your life."

Each of the formal practices you have read about has its gifts and its challenges, and each is important. Though initially you may find that you don't like a particular practice, stick with it. Liking or not liking is really not the point—there are bound to be moments of not liking during childbirth and parenting too. Those of us who teach mindfulness in this way often tell participants, "You don't have to like it, you just have to do it." That is certainly true about childbirth! Staying with a practice that is challenging rather than skipping it or letting it go after one or two tries can offer some of the greatest gifts of all, especially since one of our intentions here is to increase our capacity to be with the challenging and the difficult.

One practice is not better than another, and each is another resource for you to draw on. For example, you may find you prefer yoga to the Body Scan; however, there may be situations, such as being confined to bed, when yoga practice is just not an option. Then you'll have another practice to pull from your inner toolbox. When the nine weeks have passed, you will have learned many practices and be able to choose wisely which practice, or combination of practices, can serve you best at any particular time.

TAKING TIME TO NURTURE YOURSELF

The pregnant body often asks, if not demands, that you slow down. Remember, it is not in any way selfish for you to take time to learn the inner skills needed for becoming more balanced and centered, less stressed, and more in tune with Horticultural Time. Ultimately, as we saw during the Loving-kindness meditation, you may come to deeply realize that you are practicing not only for yourself, but for the benefit of your baby, your partner, everyone in your life and beyond.

AN OUTLINE OF THE MBCP PROGRAM

WEEK 1

Formal Practice

This week, begin the Awareness of Breathing meditation described in Chapter 4, "The Breath: A Friend for Life," for five to fifteen minutes every day. The audio guided meditation, if you are using it, has practices of varying lengths. Remember, *any* amount of time you devote to practice can bring benefit.

Informal Practice

Begin the Being with Baby practice, also described in Chapter 4. Continue this informal mindfulness practice from now until your baby is born. If your partner is also learning mindfulness practice, he or she can do this practice with you for several minutes at least once a day, perhaps when you are in bed at night, or first thing in the morning. The practice can be done whether your baby is moving or not.

If you didn't practice the Raisin Meditation when you read Chapter 3, "The World in a Raisin," please do so this week, both parts one and two.

Reread Chapter 2, "Inner Preparation for Childbirth and Beyond," for a review of the eight foundational attitudes of mind you will be cultivating in the weeks to come. You might consider posting a list of these qualities somewhere in your home—on your refrigerator or a kitchen bulletin board—as a reminder of your commitment to being more present and aware in your life.

WEEK 2

Formal Practice

For your formal practice this week, you are invited to practice the Body Scan for thirty minutes every day for the next six days. Please reread Chapter 5, "Practicing Embodiment: The Body Scan," for specific instructions and answers to questions that might come up as you practice.

Informal Practice

For your informal practice this week, please eat one meal mindfully, just as you ate the raisin—really seeing, smelling, and tasting your food, moment by moment, bite by bite. Include reflections on interconnectedness in your eating meditation. Bring awareness to the food choices you make throughout the week, perhaps asking yourself periodically, "Have I taken in all the vitamins and nutrients that my baby and I need today?"

- Continue the Awareness of Breathing sitting practice for five to fifteen minutes every day.
- Continue the Being with Baby practice throughout your day whenever you feel the baby moving.

WEEK 3

Formal Practice

Practice the Body Scan again six days this week.

Informal Practice

For your informal practice, reread Chapter 11, "Mindfulness in Everyday Life." Choose one or more of the activities listed there, such as brushing your teeth, taking a shower, shaving, washing the dishes, cooking, or driving, and commit to practicing this activity mindfully every day.

- Continue the Awareness of Breathing sitting meditation for five to fifteen minutes every day.
- Continue the Being with Baby practice.

PLEASANT EVENTS CALENDAR

This week, set your intention to become aware of one pleasant calm-and-connecting event in your life per day *as it is happening,* noticing how your body feels and what thoughts and emotions are present in those moments. To aid you in this practice, you can fill out one entry per day using the Pleasant Events Calendar found in Appendix C. At the end of the week, read the calendar and ask yourself: Am I more aware of pleasant events in my life as they are happening? Where in my body do I experience pleasant sensations or emotions? Am I slowing down enough to fully take in moments of happiness, calm, and connection, moments of ease and peace? Am I appreciating the beauty of my surroundings (especially in the natural world) each day? Am I appreciating the wonder of my body and its capacity to grow another human being within it?

Reread Chapter 6, "The Dynamic Duo: Pain and Fear." This will remind you of the mind-body connection during childbirth and why you have made the commitment to learn mindfulness practice as a way to prepare for childbirth and parenting.

WEEK 4

Formal Practice

Alternate the yoga sequence found in Chapter 8, "The Yoga of Childbirth." with the Body Scan, practicing one on the first day and the other on the next, for six days this week. During yoga practice, see if you can just be with whatever sensations are present, even if they are unpleasant or challenging. You can also practice breathing into the sensations and softening into the pose, going deeper as you breathe out. Each time the mind wanders during your yoga practice, bring awareness back to the sensations in the body or the breath. Remember to use your breath as an anchor to the present moment *between the poses,* just as you will in the moments between the contraction-expansions during labor. It can be helpful to reread Chapter 8 on practicing yoga mindfully.

Continue your Awareness of Breathing sitting practice for five to fifteen minutes each day. Begin with focusing on the breath, then expand awareness to the sensations in your body and your body as a whole, as described in Chapter 9, "Deepening and Expanding Your Practice."

Alternatively or additionally, experiment with the Three-Minute Breathing Space described in Chapter 4 at least two times during your day. Though we call it the Three-Minute Breathing Space, this practice can be done for a much shorter time. Even thirty seconds of this practice interspersed throughout your day, especially if it is a stressful one, can make a big difference.

Formal Pain Practice

Reread Chapter 7, "Mindfulness Practices for Being with Pain." Practice the mindful pain practices sequence from that chapter, optimally with your partner or a support person, at least one time this week. (You will add the touch practices with your partner and sounding next week.)

Informal Mindfulness Practice

During this week, begin to bring awareness directly to your stress reactions—the times of the contractions of life. Can you be with your experience in the present moment, even if it is painful, observing the arising and eventual passing, without trying to change it in any way? Can you begin to be with resistance, the not-liking, or the judging mind, if it is there? Explore feelings of blocking, numbing, shutting off, or wanting to get away from what is happening in the present moment.

Informal Pain Practice

Bring attention to any physical discomforts you may experience during the day, such as back pain, sciatica, shortness of breath, or heartburn. See if you can just be with whatever sensations are present, even if they are unpleasant or challenging, just as you have been learning to do in the Body Scan, yoga practice, and formal pain practices. Observe what the mind is saying, especially any story you are constructing about yourself, as you experience unpleasant physical sensations.

- Continue the Being with Baby practice.
- Continue to cultivate mindfulness in your activities of daily life.

UNPLEASANT EVENTS CALENDAR

Just as you did with the Pleasant Events Calendar last week, set your intention *to become aware of one unpleasant, stressful, or contracting event in your life per day as it is happening*. To aid you in this practice of bringing awareness to the more challenging moments of your day, use the Unpleasant Events Calendar found in Appendix C, entering one event per day. See if you can be aware of how an event you perceive as unpleasant or stressful triggers a contraction in the body, a negative or unpleasant emotion such as fear or anger, a narrowing of attention or contraction of the mind, and the replaying or rehashing of negative thoughts.

During these unpleasant moments of stress or contraction, can you cradle the whole of whatever pain you are experiencing—your thoughts, your emotions, and sensations in your body—in mindful awareness? Can you use your breath as an anchor to the present moment, riding the waves of all the components of an unpleasant experience? In these moments can you ask yourself, "Who or what is contracting?" We are learning to hold the contractions of life in the same way as we are learning to hold the contractions of labor—in mindful awareness.

WEEK 5

Formal Practice

Continue to alternate between the yoga sequence and the Body Scan for six days this week. If you are attending a prenatal yoga class, use it as another opportunity to practice mindful awareness. If you are doing any other form of physical activity, such as walking or swimming, see if you can do that mindfully too, bringing full awareness to the breath and the physical sensations arising and passing as you move.

If you have been sitting for less than fifteen minutes, lengthen your Awareness of Breathing practice to fifteen minutes this week. Begin by focusing on the breath, gradually expanding awareness to sensations in the body, to the body as a whole (as in the Body Scan), and then to sounds as they arise and pass, as described in Chapter 9.

Formal Pain Practice

Choose any of the pain practices you have found helpful so far, or ones you would like to experiment with from Chapter 7, "Mindfulness Practices for Being with Pain," and practice them for at least thirty minutes one time this week, adding the touch practices with your partner and sounding. Be sure to take turns during the pain practice so that each of you has the opportunity to learn these important life skills.

Informal Practice

Bring awareness to moments of reactivity in your daily life, and explore options for responding with greater mindfulness and creativity in the present moment. Practice opening up space for the mindful pause, the moment of responding rather than reacting. Use the breath to slow things down.

- Continue the Being with Baby practice.
- Continue to cultivate mindfulness in your activities of daily life. Add mindful pooping practice, as described in Chapter 7, to your informal daily mindfulness practice.
- Continue to bring the Three-Minute Breathing Space into your daily life— once an hour, three times a day, whenever you can remember to do it.
- Continue to use your mindfulness practice when physical discomforts arise in everyday life.

WEEK 6

Formal Practice

This week alternate between thirty minutes of Sitting Meditation, as described in Chapter 9, and either the Body Scan or yoga practice. In Sitting Meditation, add awareness of thoughts and emotions as objects of awareness, eventually shifting into the practice of Choiceless Awareness. Letting go of all objects of attention (the breath, body sensations, the body as a whole, sounds, thoughts, and emotions), just sit in open awareness, paying attention to whatever is predominant in your experience at any given moment. If at any time you get lost or confused during Choiceless Awareness, just return to the basic Awareness of Breathing meditation.

Formal Pain Practice

You are ready to move into the more advanced pain practice described in Chapter 7. Do one formal pain practice session (or more) this week, with your partner or other support person. Using Awareness of Breathing, touch, sounding, movement, various positions—whatever you have found helpful in your pain practice so far—immerse first one hand and then eventually both hands into a bowl of ice water. Use your creativity to explore what might work best for you during moments of intense physical sensations. Use the breath as your anchor between the intense physical sensations. During your pain practice, ask yourself, "Is that which is observing the pain, in pain?" If not, then dwell where there is no pain as best you can.

Informal Practice

Continue to bring awareness to pleasant events and to the contractions of life, the stress reactions that may happen during the week, exploring options for responding with greater mindfulness and creativity in the present moment, as we have been learning to do. Bring awareness to any pattern of fearful or negative thoughts about the future. Is there a particular situation or context that triggers these thoughts or emotions? How do your thoughts contribute to stress? To fear? To anger? Can you stop long enough to find the breath and the mindful pause right in the midst of a storm of reactivity?

- Continue the Being with Baby practice.
- Continue to cultivate mindfulness in your activities of daily living, including mindful pooping.
- Continue to use the Three-Minute Breathing Space as a way to integrate formal and informal practice into moments of everyday life. It is particularly helpful to use the breathing-space practice when you become aware of going too fast or are experiencing an increased level of stress.
- Continue your informal pain practice, using times of physical discomfort as opportunities to practice your ever-growing mindfulness skill of being with what is.
- If you are not going to do a full day of practice as described on the next page, practice the inquiry on fear and happiness sometime this week.

Reread Chapter 16, "Causes and Conditions: Navigating What Is." Arrange for your hospital tour if you haven't yet taken one, and ask the questions that need to be asked when you are there. Begin interviewing doulas if you intend to hire one, and begin to mindfully communicate with those on your birth team how you are approaching your birth experience and what you think you may need from them. It could be helpful for those on your birth team to read Chapter 6, "The Dynamic Duo: Pain and Fear," and Chapter 16.

Begin to interview healthcare providers for your baby—a family physician, a pediatrician, a family or pediatric nurse practitioner. Essential is finding a healthcare provider who inspires trust and sees you as a partner in the decision-making process about your baby's health.

Read one book on the drugs, medications, procedures, and technology that are commonly used in a hospital setting during childbirth if you haven't already done so. (See Appendix B for recommended books and resources.) Read mindfully, noticing any thoughts or emotions that arise as you read the information. Ask yourself, "Is there anything more I need to find out about in relation to the who, what, where, and how surrounding my birthing experience?"

BETWEEN WEEK 6 AND WEEK 7: A DAY OF MINDFULNESS PRACTICE

On the Saturday or Sunday between Week 6 and Week 7, the MBCP expectant parents come together for a day of silent meditation practice as described in Chapter 12, "A Day of Mindfulness Practice." Ideally you and your partner (and other couples if you are practicing with them) would also choose to deepen your practice by giving yourselves the gift of a day or at least a morning (through lunch) of silent meditation when you seamlessly practice all the formal meditations you have learned so far. After all, paying attention to your moment-to-moment experience as it unfolds is what you will be doing for an unknown number of hours when you are in labor, so practicing for an extended period of time is excellent preparation for childbirth.

If you do decide to have a silent morning or full day of practice, reread Chapter 12 and learn the formal Walking Meditation as described in Chapter 10, "When You're Walking, Just Walk. . . . " Practice it at least once before your weekend day of silence. You can also practice the Speaking and Listening Inquiry on fear and happiness during this day of silent practice.

There are many ways to organize a day of silence, but here is an example of a schedule that is similar to the all-day session in the MBCP course that might work well for you. Of course, feel free to modify it, including the starting and ending times. Decide beforehand how you want to do this. Either prepare lunch ahead of time, or have the ingredients ready for mindful meal preparation, and turn off all electrical devices that have an on-off switch (cell phones and so forth).

9:00–9:05 A.M. Share with each other how you are feeling about spending a day (or morning) in silence together. What are your intentions for the day?

9:05–9:30 A.M. Sitting Meditation

9:30 A.M. Yoga practice

10:00 A.M. Body Scan

10:30 A.M. Walking Meditation, indoors or out

11:00 A.M. Sitting Meditation

11:30 A.M. Yoga or Walking Meditation

12:00 P.M.–1:15 P.M. Mindful lunch

    If possible, eat outdoors. Notice the trees, the sky; feel the sun or breeze on your skin.

1:15 P.M.–2:00 P.M. Rest. Take a nap, or continue with Walking or Sitting Meditation.

    If you want only a half day of practice, this would be an ideal time to end. If you want a full day of practice, you could continue as follows:

2:00 P.M. Walking Meditation

2:30 P.M. Speaking and Listening Inquiry on fear and happiness

    This practice is outlined in Chapter 6, "The Dynamic Duo," Part 2.

3:30 P.M. Walking Meditation

3:50 P.M. Sharing

4:00 P.M. Closing

Whenever you decide to end your practice for the day, take time to share your experiences with each other, perhaps focusing on one or more of the following questions—the same questions the expectant parents in the MBCP course share: What touched you? What was challenging for you? What, if anything, was inspiring? What was the highlight of the day? What new insight did you gain (if any)? Perhaps read a poem or something one of you has written to end this time of formal practice.

WEEK 7

Formal Practice

This week alternate between your thirty-minute Sitting Meditation—especially Choiceless Awareness—and either the Body Scan or yoga practice. Experiment with Choiceless Awareness, letting go of all objects of attention (the breath, body sensations, the body as a whole, sounds, thoughts, and emotions). Just sit in open awareness, paying attention to whatever is predominant in your experience at any given moment. If at any time during Choiceless Awareness you get lost or confused, just return to the basic Awareness of Breathing meditation.

    Although this is the assignment for this week, it may be that after all these weeks of practice you are beginning to make the practice your own, crafting your meditation time according to what fits for you and your mind-body on any particular day. For example, you may find yourself combining practices, such as practicing ten minutes of yoga followed by twenty minutes of sitting practice to make up your thirty minutes of formal practice on a particular day, while on another day you may find you really need the enlivening energy of thirty minutes of yoga practice or the grounding, stability, and peace that can be found in thirty minutes of formal sitting practice. Please do what works for you, but do keep your commitment to the thirty minutes a day of formal practice.

In addition, this week please reread Chapter 14, "It's All About Kindness," and begin to incorporate Loving-kindness meditation into your formal practice. You might want to begin and/or end each of your meditation sessions with a few minutes of Loving-kindness practice, sending good wishes to your baby, yourself, and those near and dear to you. You could end there, or continue widening the circle of Loving-kindness to include all children, all parents, and all beings who have ever been babies and children—which, as we know, is all of us. Or you could choose to practice Loving-kindness for a full thirty minutes as your formal practice for the day. Like giving birth, there is no one right way—and you are finding yours.

➤ MINDFUL SPEAKING AND LISTENING INQUIRY ➤

Using the Speaking and Listening Inquiry form that you learned in relation to fear and happiness, practice the Speaking and Listening Inquiry on Families of Origin at least once this week; you will find it at the end of Chapter 13, "Befriending: Mindfulness in Relationship."

Informal Practice

- Continue the Being with Baby practice, perhaps adding phrases of Loving-kindness during those moments when you bring your attention to the movements of your baby.
- Continue to bring awareness to the routine activities of daily living in preparation for continued practice after the baby is born.
- Continue to use the Three-Minute Breathing Space in daily life, particularly when you are feeling stressed.
- Continue informal pain practice, using times of physical discomfort as an opportunity to prepare for your birth experience.

Reread Chapter 17, "Your Baby, Your Mindfulness Teacher." Bring awareness to how you are thinking about the early weeks after giving birth. Are you wisely creating a way for your newly birthed family to be cared for during the postpartum period?

Begin to read a book or educate yourself about breastfeeding. (See Appendix B for suggested resources.)

WEEK 8

Formal Practice

If you have been using the audio guided meditations for your formal practice, experiment with not using them at all this week. Choose whatever formal practice you feel is appropriate for you, and practice for thirty minutes, six days this week. In addition to your formal practice, consider sending the phrases of well-wishing and friendliness in Loving-kindness practice to yourself, especially when you are caught in a painful mind state or negative emotion. This is a healthy habit of mind to cultivate before your baby is born, bringing with her or him all the joys and challenges of caring for a newborn.

Informal Practice

Bring awareness to what you are taking into your body through your senses—eating, reading, watching TV, searching the Internet, listening to the radio. How much time are you spending looking at your cell phone, texting, or posting to Facebook? How might this relate to stress? How might this relate to your capacity to be present in the home you and your partner are creating for yourselves and your baby? What might it be like for you and your partner to make a commitment to a "no technology day" once a week?

- Continue to bring awareness to the routine activities of daily living in preparation for continued practice after this formal structured learning time is over—and for the time after your baby is born.
- Continue the Being with Baby practice, adding phrases of Loving-kindness practice during the moments when you bring your attention to the movements of your baby during your day.
- Continue to practice the Three-Minute Breathing Space and perhaps Loving-kindness practice throughout your day.
- Continue informal pain practice, using times of physical discomfort as an opportunity for preparing for your birth experience.
- If you or you and your partner feel the need for more formal pain practice, by all means, just do it!

Reread Chapter 18, "Breastfeeding: A Dance of Connection." If you have not yet acquired and begun reading a book on breastfeeding as suggested last week, do so this week. Consider going to a La Leche League meeting or a breastfeeding support group while you are still pregnant. Locate a lactation consultant in your community. Have her number on hand before you give birth, in case you need her assistance once your baby is born.

WEEK 9

Formal Practice

Now that you have completed the nine-week course, the challenge is to continue your daily practice in the days and weeks before giving birth, during labor and delivery, in the days, weeks, months, and years of parenting—and indeed for all the moments of the rest of your life. This week, do whatever practice or practices you have found most beneficial, making the practices your own. Reflect on how you and your partner might support each other in continuing your regular formal meditation practice.

Reread Chapter 19, "Endings and Beginnings: A Last Class." Do the same meditative reflection the expectant parents in the MBCP course do when they drop a stone into the well. Take turns sharing with your partner whatever comes up for you.

Formal Pain Practice

Continue to do some formal pain practice until you give birth. Notice resistance or the tendency to avoid this practice; if that's present for you, notice it and do some pain practice anyway. I suspect you'll be glad you did.

Informal Practice

Continue to cultivate mindfulness in all the moments of your daily life, bringing awareness to your routine activities (don't forget mindful pooping!). This is excellent preparation for all the routine activities that await you after your baby is born—nursing, diaper changing, dressing and undressing your baby—which are not routine activities at all! They're you and your baby's life!

- Continue the Being with Baby practice, adding phrases of Loving-kindness as you care to.
- Continue to practice the Three-Minute Breathing Space and Loving-kindness practice as you care to throughout your day.

Reread anything in this book you found helpful or useful.

Explore the recommended books and websites in Appendix B. Highly recommended is *Everyday Blessings: The Inner Work of Mindful Parenting* by Myla and Jon Kabat-Zinn.

Investigate meditation communities in your area.

We can never be born enough. We are human beings; for whom
birth is a supremely welcome mystery, the mystery of growing:
which happens only and whenever we are faithful to ourselves.

e. e. cummings

Epilogue

IT'S 6:30 A.M. and the early morning fog outside the window seems to add to the hush of the house. Ry, my two-year-old grandson, and I are contentedly sitting on the floor putting the last pieces of a farm animal puzzle into place. Everyone else—my son Ted, my daughter-in-law Naomi, and Ry's older brother, Niko—is still asleep. I'm happy that Ry and I can share this special time together and that Ted and Naomi can sleep in this morning; they certainly need the extra rest. Ry is in a bright, cheerful mood. As he puts the last puzzle piece into place, the one that completes the head of a cow, he throws his arms into the air and with complete satisfaction announces, "Done! I did it!"

"Hooray!" I respond. "Yes, you did it!"

"I'm hungry," Ry suddenly declares.

"Do you want some breakfast?" I ask.

"Yes," he says as he toddles over to his high chair and climbs into it. After a brief conversation to sort out which cold cereal he wants—this morning it's a combination of Cheerios and granola—he settles happily into the task of feeding himself. Within minutes he says, "Grandma, I want some orange juice."

Under ordinary circumstances this would be a simple enough request, but not today. You see, yesterday Ry had diarrhea, enough so that by bedtime he had developed a painful diaper rash. Since he was obviously not sick, the family consensus had it that the most likely cause was the large amount of fruit he had enjoyed throughout the day. We had decided that today would be a "no fresh fruits or vegetables" day. (Milk was definitely off the list as well.) So the dilemma of the present moment is this: How does Grandma Nancy respond to the request for orange juice?

I take a breath and say, "Ry, remember how much you pooped yesterday? And how much your bum hurt? Well, we don't want you to get a sore bum again today, so you can't have any orange juice. I can give you some water. . . ."

As I say this I am perfectly aware that, first of all, water is a pretty lame substitute for fresh orange juice and, second, that my rationale for denying Ry orange juice—the connection between orange juice and pooping and his sore bum yesterday—makes absolutely no sense whatsoever to his two-year-old mind. As any neuroscientist worth their salt would tell you, his prefrontal cortex just isn't myelinated enough yet to sort through what I'm talking about. All Ry knows is that he is thirsty, that he desires to rid himself of this uncomfortable body sensation called thirst with a desired pleasant experience (delicious orange juice), and that I, his trusted grandmother and the potential instrument for fulfilling his desire, am not cooperating.

Ry immediately begins to cry.

"I want orange juice!" he wails loudly.

A totally human reaction on his part, I think to myself. Desire arising, desire thwarted, sadness arising.

And then comes the cry, "I want my mommy." How intelligent my grandson is! Desire thwarted by Grandma, he tries another option for fulfilling his desire—his mother, who he expects, based on his past experience, will not only comfort him in his sadness but might actually give him some orange juice!

I become aware of a growing tension in my belly and a tightness in my chest in response to his cries. I know that one solution to the situation would be to just give him the orange juice. That would stop his crying for sure, and, like Ry, I too would be able to get rid of a very uncomfortable feeling in my body. But I'm supposed to be the adult here, and my job is to hold the larger picture of his health and wellbeing despite the agitation, discomfort, and unhappiness I too am feeling.

I bring my attention to my breath as I watch my mind race. Oh, no, I think to myself, I don't want him to go running into Ted and Naomi's room and wake them up. I want them to be able to sleep! And I don't want to prove myself a failure as a grandmother who can't handle this situation! The cries are getting louder as the thought arises again: Well, maybe just a little orange juice won't hurt.

"I want my mommy!" The wail continues. And I take a breath.

"How about some water with a splash of orange juice in it?" I offer, pleased to have come up with what, at least in my opinion, is a nice middle-way solution. I pour half a cup of water into his plastic cup and splash a teeny tiny bit of orange juice into it, just enough to barely turn it a light orange color.

"Noooo," he wails. "I don't want water with orange juice! I want orange juice!"

The tears, which are surprisingly voluminous, flow freely down his cheeks. Passionately attached to what he wants, he is totally and completely awash in suffering. My heart goes out to him. The tension, mostly in my belly, is stronger now. I am really having a contraction, he really can't have orange juice, and I really don't want Ted and Naomi to wake up!

I pull up a chair close to his and sit down beside him. Looking gently and directly into his tearful eyes, I begin to speak. I have no idea what I am going to say, but words come tumbling out.

"Ry, I'm so sorry that I can't give you some orange juice and that it is making you so sad. It is making me sad too. What is happening right now is that you are stuck in desire, grasping and clinging to your wanting the pleasant experience of orange juice." I can't believe I am sitting here about to explain mindfulness to a two-year-old, but that's what is happening. I don't know what else to do.

"I feel exactly like you do sometimes, when I really, really want something and I can't have it. But then I use my mindfulness practice to let go of my wanting and my attachment. But you see," I continue, "you are only two years old, and your brain's capacity to let go is not so well developed yet. I wish I could tell you to just pay attention to your breath and be with your sadness and know that eventually it will pass, but that wouldn't do any good right now. You are really thirsty, and just desperate to quench your thirst. A solution to your thirst is right here in this cup—water with a splash of orange juice in it (I point toward the cup), but you can't see that. You are so attached to the orange juice–only solution that you can't let go. Your mind, your attachment to what you want and can't have in this very moment, is making you suffer." He continues to cry, but he is watching me intently. He is definitely listening.

"It's just like the story of the monkey and the banana." I'm definitely on a roll here, I think to myself. I wonder where we're going to end up.

"Do you know the story of the monkey and the banana? The hunters want to catch a monkey, so they put a banana inside a coconut and tie the coconut to a tree. The coconut has a hole in it just big enough for the monkey to put his hand inside and take it out again, except when he is grasping the banana. Then his hand is too big to get out through the hole. If the monkey wants to get away, all he has to do is let go of the banana and run. But the monkey is just too attached to the banana to let it go. And so he is caught. Totally stuck. Just like you are right now. I see how much you want the orange juice and how much you are suffering, and I'm so sorry."

With that statement I gently pick him up from his high chair. No more cereal will be eaten until this emotional storm has passed. I carry him over to the couch, where, to my great good fortune, his blankie is waiting. Ry simultaneously reaches for his blankie and puts his thumb into his mouth. Mercifully, the cries subside and the tension in my belly lessens. I hold him on my lap, and we quietly sit together. I feel his warm body relax into mine. I breathe in the sweet smell of his hair, which I shampooed the night before. A feeling I can only call love pours through my body. When I observe the feeling more closely, it seems to emanate from somewhere deep in my chest. Around my heart.

"Would you like me to read you a story?" I inquire, reaching for the copy of *Hand, Hand, Fingers, Thumb* that's lying on the couch. He nods, and I begin reading.

Hand, hand, fingers, thumb,
One thumb, one thumb drumming on a drum. . . .

After a complete rendition of *Hand, Hand, Fingers, Thumb*, Ry states once again, "I'm hungry."

"Would you like to go back and eat your cereal?" I ask.

"Yes," he replies.

"Okay," I say.

"And I want some water with a splash of orange juice in it," he adds.

"Okay. I'm happy to get you some," I say in quiet amazement.

Amazing, utterly and completely amazing, I think to myself. He did it. He let it go. It was hard work, but he got there. In this moment, he is free. And, thankfully, so am I.

Mindfulness-Based
Childbirth and Parenting (MBCP)
and Integrative Medicine
A Little More Background

IT'S SPRING 2006, and I'm sitting at a big round dining table, the kind you find in Chinese restaurants where whole families gather to enjoy a meal together. It's lunchtime at the Crowne Plaza Hotel in Worcester, Massachusetts, the site for the Fourth Annual Scientific Conference of the Center for Mindfulness at the University of Massachusetts Medical Center. The conference is titled "Investigating and Integrating Mindfulness in Medicine, Health Care, and Society." A woman with a lovely smile and short gray hair like my own sits down at the table next to me.

Within minutes we find ourselves animatedly chatting about children (she has four and so do I) and grandchildren (she has six and I have two), and soon we are doubled over in gales of laughter, sharing the pitfalls and joys of parenting grown children who have children of their own. "This parenting business is never over, no matter how old they get," she says, laughing as she shakes her head. "Or no matter how old *we* get!" I reply.

At the end of our meal, as we get ready to go to the main hall for the keynote address (I will soon discover that she is the one *giving* the address), she says, "So tell me, what do you do?"

"I teach a course called Mindfulness-Based Childbirth and Parenting, a childbirth preparation course for expectant parents. It's an adaptation of the traditional MBSR course," I reply simply.

"Oh, we might be interested in something like that. Why don't you get in touch with me when you get back home?" And with that, she hands me a business card that says, "Susan Folkman, PhD, Director, Osher Center for Integrative Medicine, UC San Francisco Medical Center."

And so began a new and quite remarkable phase in the unfolding journey of MBCP. By the time I got in touch with Susan a week or so later, I had learned that she was one of the academic world's leading theoreticians and researchers on stress and coping. She connected me with Dr. Kevin Barrows, a gifted family practice physician and integrative medicine specialist who had started the MBSR program in the founding years of the Osher Center. Now clinical director and head of group programs at the Osher Center, Dr. Barrows proved to be the perfect midwife for bringing the MBCP program out of my living room and into a setting where it could expand beyond the classroom and into professional training and research.

Within a year I had joined the Osher Center's teaching staff and was teaching the MBCP course there, making it the first integrative medicine center in the country to address the health and wellbeing of expectant families. A few months later my colleague and friend Larissa Duncan, PhD, a brilliant developmental psychologist with a deeply caring heart and extraordinarily well trained mind, joined me at the Osher Center. Larissa's task was to build a research program dedicated to investigating the impact of mindfulness practice on the health and wellbeing of families in this transformative period in their lives. A year and a half later, in 2009, I was able to begin a Mindfulness-Based Childbirth and Parenting Professional Development and Teacher Training Program (PDTT) for those in the field of perinatal medicine who want to become MBCP instructors or in some way bring mindfulness skills into their own lives and the lives of the couples and families they serve.

For me, teaching at the Osher Center was a kind of homecoming. Located in a building right across the street from the hospital where I first assisted laboring women and their families in the Alternative Birth Center more than three decades ago, I had come full circle. Remarkable changes have taken place in medicine since I was in clinical practice there, changes reflected in the environment itself. The barren concrete courtyard where I used to send birthing women in early labor to walk with their partners has been transformed into a peaceful garden, where a gravel path meanders among pink roses, lush ferns, and arching trees as benches invite the visitor to sit in the warm sun or eat a quiet lunch in the shade. The space has become a place where patients challenged with illness can stroll, sit, reflect, and encourage the body's natural healing—and where hospital staff can find some moments of calm in a hectic workday. The existence of the garden itself gives me hope that perhaps we are slowly coming to recognize that medical care can (and indeed must) include caring for and supporting the whole person, drawing on the natural, inherent wisdom of the mind, body, and heart.

INTEGRATIVE MEDICINE

Known by various names over the years—mind-body medicine, complementary and alternative medicine (CAM), behavioral medicine, and holistic medicine—integrative medicine is a relatively new branch of medicine based on research showing that how we think, feel, and behave significantly affects both our physical and mental health and wellbeing. Over the past two decades the field has grown exponentially, and there is now an Academic Consortium on Integrative Medicine with representatives from more than forty medical schools at major universities across the United States and Canada. Many of these institutions have integrative medicine centers that offer patients a wide variety of healing modalities from acupuncture, massage, and Ayurvedic medicine to classes in yoga, tai chi, and qigong—healing modalities that would have been unthinkable within major academic medical centers only a few decades ago. Given the well-documented benefits of mindfulness meditation, particularly the Mindfulness-Based Stress Reduction program, MBSR classes are now a core offering in any integrative medicine program.

The very existence of the field of integrative medicine is evidence of a radical shift taking place in mainstream medicine today. Conventional Western medicine is based for the most part on a several-hundred-year-old paradigm in which the body and mind are seen as separate. Approaching the body as an entity that needs to be fixed or as a body with a disease that needs to be conquered or killed, this conventional view relies on a complex array of drugs, procedures, machines, and surgery to make people well.

This fix-it approach can seem dazzling, even miraculous to any of us who have been its beneficiaries—whether it's the replacement of a body part or a drug that stopped an infection or helped bring the mind back into balance. It can seem particularly miraculous in perinatal medicine for those who have been the lucky recipients of fertility treatments, who have been able to deliver a healthy baby despite a preexisting health challenge such as severe diabetes, who have had a cesarean birth for a baby that was too big to be born vaginally, who have had a postpartum hemorrhage stopped with drugs or surgery or both, or whose child is happy and healthy despite being born well before their due date. There is no question that many people, including many women and babies, who would not be here a mere fifty years ago are alive today because of the fix-it paradigm.

However, it is also coming to be recognized that this fix-it paradigm has definite limitations. There are entire realms of health and wellness where this conventional Western paradigm does not serve, particularly when so many of the ills we suffer from today can be traced to the simple lifestyle choices we make with regard to diet, exercise, and the way we manage or, more accurately, don't manage stress. Nor does it serve us when a healthy woman is pregnant with a seemingly healthy baby.

The field of integrative medicine offers a different and complementary paradigm to the fix-it one, a paradigm that *sees the patient as a whole being, a person who has tremendous inner resources for their own health and wellbeing and who, in a partnership of mutual trust and respect with their healthcare provider, can and needs to be a full participant in their health care.* This approach provides a much-needed balance to the conventional medical paradigm, one that all too often leaves patients no better or sometimes worse off than when they initially sought care. Implicit in an integrative medical approach is prevention and health promotion across the full span of life.

INTEGRATIVE MEDICINE, PREGNANCY, CHILDBIRTH, AND THE TRANSITION TO PARENTING

The field of integrative medicine provides a perfect home for the Mindfulness-Based Childbirth and Parenting program. Given that pregnancy is fundamentally a normal, healthy condition of the female body, and since mindfulness training promotes skills that are invaluable to our health and wellbeing across the life cycle, it makes perfect sense to use an integrative approach for families living through this normal healthy life transition. As colleagues in Britain wrote in a study for their National Health Service: "Giving every child the best start in life is crucial to reducing health inequalities across the life course. The foundations for virtually every aspect of human development—physical, intellectual and emotional—are laid in early childhood. What happens during these early years *(starting in the womb)* [italics mine] has lifelong effects on many aspects of health and wellbeing—from obesity, heart disease and mental health, to educational achievement and economic status."[1]

Having a place where mindfulness skills can be learned in this formative stage of family life, skills that can enhance the health and wellbeing of parents and their unborn baby, is certainly a bright spot in a domain of health care that is sorely in need of rebalancing. As we learned in Chapter 16, despite all the money we spend on maternal and child health, the data show that as a society we are not doing so well at all. Using the tremendous rise in cesarean births as an example, we have to ask whether we are making a process that is usually very simple for the majority of mothers and babies into something terribly complex for all. Reproducing and birthing our own species *is* relatively simple—that is, when all is well, which it usually is—and an integrative medicine approach can help optimize this healthy state.

Mindfulness in this context helps support and strengthen our body and mind's innate inner resources, developing lifetime awareness skills that will help us all make the best lifestyle choices we can regarding the food we eat, the exercise we get, the need to reduce stress and live as best we can in a healthy mind-body balance—all of which will affect our baby and the kind of environment we create for our child or children to grow in.

Yet with its inherent unknowns, pregnancy and childbirth can at times become terribly complicated and scary. In the process of reproducing and giving birth to our young, we are dealing with a paradox: we are working with nature—and unfortunately nature, viewed through the lens of our oh-so-human desires, is not always perfect. It is at those times that we most definitely need our mindfulness practice *and* the finely honed skills of those who practice obstetrics in the fix-it paradigm. The situation calls not for either/or but for both—and the wisdom to know which and when each approach is applicable and appropriate.

The seeds for integrating these two paradigms in the field of perinatal medicine, which covers the period of time surrounding pregnancy, childbirth, and early parenting, have actually been in existence for a long time. Within the conventional medical system, many midwives, nurses, and a myriad of other health professionals—from doulas to lactation consultants, childbirth educators, and infant massage instructors, to name just a few—*already are* integrative medicine practitioners. For them, given that they already see the people they serve as physical, psychological, social, and spiritual beings living within their family and community context, an integrative medicine approach during the perinatal period is a no-brainer. These professionals are joined by a growing number of physicians who are bringing complementary modalities into their practices, healers who already specialize in one or more complementary modalities, and psychologists and other mental health professionals who are coming to understand the profound benefits of mindfulness practice for the mental and physical health and wellbeing of their clients.

In many countries of the world that are doing much better than the United States in the domain of maternal-child health, it is midwives and nurses who predominantly care for the normal, healthy pregnant woman, her newborn, and her family during the perinatal period. Training many more of these midwife and nurse providers to care for the healthy pregnant woman, baby, and family while working in collaboration with their obstetrician specialist colleagues is a positive development in many places in the United States.[2] Of course ensuring that training in mindfulness skills is an essential element in *any* training program for healthcare providers—nurses, midwives, or physicians—for managing their own stress will enhance the health and wellbeing not only of families but of society as a whole.[3]

A RESEARCH PROGRAM

One of the greatest delights in bringing the Mindfulness-Based Childbirth and Parenting program to the Osher Center has been the opportunity to systematically investigate whether what I was observing in the classroom over the years would be borne out in studies of expectant parents who learn mindfulness skills in this transformative period of their lives. A true kindred spirit, Larissa Duncan, PhD, had taught and researched the impact of mindfulness skills in a program for teens and their parents in Pennsylvania.[4] In that work Larissa repeatedly heard the parents express regret at not having learned these skills earlier and had missed out on being present during the first decade or more of their children's lives. Given Larissa's own mindfulness practice and her passion for decreasing suffering in families, she knew she had to look further upstream. Teaching mindfulness skills to parents before their babies were born was as far upstream as she could get, so when a door opened for us to work together at the Osher Center, she bravely stepped through it.

Our first pilot study, published in 2010 and described briefly in Chapter 6, brought promising results. Work is currently under way to look at the effectiveness of mindfulness training in relation to the perception of pain during childbirth, using the same exercises that are described in Chapter 7, "Mindfulness Practices for Being with Pain." We are also conducting an observational study to explore the effects of MBCP on children born to parents who have chosen to take the MBCP program as their way to prepare for childbirth. This study will help us begin to understand the impact of mindfulness skills on such things as children's emotional regulation, the adjustment of mothers and partners to parenting, and the changes in their relationship to each other in this early time of family making.

Another bright spot in our MBCP research program is our Centering-Pregnancy with Mindfulness Skills study. In a collaborative project with the Centering Healthcare Institute (CHI), we are weaving mindfulness skills from the MBCP program into the ten prenatal sessions that run throughout pregnancy in the Centering Pregnancy model of care. In this way some of the most vulnerable and highly stressed among us—low-income pregnant women and their families—are able to bring the benefits of mindfulness practice into their lives.[5]

Yet another collaborative effort is our work with colleagues at the Oxford Mindfulness Center (OMC) at Oxford University. Under the amazing leadership of Professor Mark Williams, who leads the OMC, a project has begun to offer MBCP to expectant families in the United Kingdom. This project will focus on both training British midwives to be able to offer the MBCP program to the pregnant women and partners they care for as well as studying the benefits of MBCP for parents at risk for depression and anxiety. The remarkable Maret Dymond, PhD, is leading these efforts.[6]

It will take time, patience, and the work of many before the growing body of research reaches a tipping point where we can say with certainty that mindfulness practice during pregnancy does indeed contribute to healthier pregnancies, more positive childbirth experiences, healthier couple relationships, more attuned parenting, and by extension, happier, healthier, and calmer babies, children, and families. However, I strongly suspect that someday we may be able to say such words with demonstrable confidence.

For now, what seems to be true is that leading a less stressful, calmer, and happier life during pregnancy is beneficial for our own mental and physical health and wellbeing and for the mental and physical health and wellbeing of our babies. Mindfulness practice, and the inner skills we cultivate through it, offers great potential to grow and nurture ourselves as we grow and nurture the next generation.

Resources

THE BOOKS and websites listed below are intended to provide you with a few trusted sources for additional information about pregnancy, childbirth, and early parenting. Though there are many excellent resources beyond those listed here, in the interest of decreasing stress and information overload and allowing time for mindfulness practice, I suggest you use these when seeking information; they may be all you need. Remember, looking toward a balance between information from the outside and your own inner wisdom cultivated through mindfulness practice can be a helpful direction. Keep it simple, or as simple as you can.

BOOKS

Pregnancy and Childbirth

Boston Women's Health Book Collective. *Our Bodies, Ourselves: Pregnancy and Birth*. New York: Touchstone, 2008.

Dick-Read, Grantly. *Childbirth Without Fear: The Principles and Practice of Natural Childbirth*, London: Pinter & Martin, Ltd., 2004.

Gaskin, Ina May. *Ina May's Guide to Childbirth*. New York: Bantam Books, 2003.

Klaus, Marshall H., John H. Kennell, and Phyllis H. Klaus. *The Doula Book: How a Trained Labor Companion Can Help You Have a Shorter, Easier, and Healthier Birth*. USA: Perseus Publishing, 2012.

Lothian, Judith, and Charlotte DeVries. *The Official Lamaze Guide: Giving Birth with Confidence*. New York: Meadowbrook Press, 2010.

Simkin, Penny. *The Birth Partner: A Complete Guide to Childbirth for Dads, Doulas, and All Other Labor Companions*. Massachusetts: Harvard Common Press, 2008.

Breastfeeding

Gaskin, Ina May. *Ina May's Guide to Breastfeeding*. New York: Bantam Books, 2009.

Huggins, Kathleen. *The Nursing Mother's Companion*. Massachusetts: Harvard Common Press, 2010.

La Leche League International. *The Womanly Art of Breastfeeding*. New York: Ballantine Books, 2010.

Mohrbacher and Kendall-Tackett. *Breastfeeding Made Simple: Seven Natural Laws for Nursing Mothers*. Oakland: New Harbinger Publications, 2010.

Sears, William, and Martha Sears. *The Breastfeeding Book: Everything You Need to Know About Nursing Your Child from Birth Through Weaning*. New York: Little, Brown and Company, 2000.

Parenting

Kabat-Zinn, Myla, and Jon Kabat-Zinn. *Everyday Blessings: The Inner Work of Mindful Parenting*. New York: Hyperion, 1997.

Klaus, Marshall, and Phyllis Klaus. *Your Amazing Newborn*. Massachusetts: Perseus Books, 1998.

Martin, William. *The Parent's Tao Te Ching: Ancient Advice for Modern Parents*. New York: Marlowe and Co, 1999.

McClure, Vimala. *Infant Massage: A Handbook for Loving Parents*. New York: Bantam Books, 2000.

Nugent, Kevin. *Your Baby Is Speaking to You: A Visual Guide to the Amazing Behaviors of Your Newborn and Growing Baby*. New York: Houghton Mifflin Harcourt, 2011.

Sears, William, and Martha Sears. *The Baby Book: Everything You Need to Know About Your Baby—From Birth to Age Two*. New York: Little, Brown and Company, 2003.

Siegel, Daniel J., and Tina Payne Bryson. *The Whole-Brain Child: 12 Revolutionary Strategies to Nurture Your Child's Developing Mind, Survive Everyday Parenting Struggles, and Help Your Family Thrive*. New York: Delacorte Press, 2011.

Small, Meredith F. *Our Babies, Ourselves: How Biology and Culture Shape the Way We Parent*. New York: Anchor Books, 1998.

Other Books of Interest

Block, Jennifer. *Pushed: The Painful Truth About Childbirth and Modern Maternity Care.* Boston: Da Capo Press, 2007.

Hrdy, Sarah Blaffer. *Mothers and Others: The Evolutionary Origins of Mutual Understanding.* Massachusetts: Belknap Press, 2011.

Paul, Annie Murphy. *Origins: How the Nine Months Before Birth Shape the Rest of Our Lives.* New York: Free Press, 2010.

Pollan, Michael. *Food Rules: An Eater's Manual.* New York: Penguin Books, 2009.

Uvnäs Moberg, Kerstin. *The Oxytocin Factor: Tapping the Hormone of Calm, Love, and Healing.* Boston: Da Capo Press, 2003.

Walser, Robyn, and Darrah Westrup. *The Mindful Couple: How Acceptance and Mindfulness Can Lead You to the Love You Want.* Oakland: New Harbinger, 2009.

PREGNANCY, CHILDBIRTH, AND PARENTING: ONLINE RESOURCES

The official website for the Mindfulness-Based Childbirth and Parenting program and the book *Mindful Birthing: Training the Mind, Body, and Heart for Childbirth and Beyond:* www.mindfulbirthing.org

Here you can find:

- The audio guided meditations used in the MBCP course
- Locations of MBCP courses
- Information about the MBCP Teacher Training Program
- 🔖 A link to the Mindfulness for Pregnancy App

American College of Nurse-Midwives (ACNM): www.mymidwife.org
- For information about pregnancy, childbirth, postpartum, breastfeeding, and general women's health to help you make informed and educated decisions during pregnancy and beyond.

Centering Healthcare Institute: www.centeringhealthcare.org
- For information about this pioneering group care model promoting the overall health of mothers, babies, and families across the life cycle.

Childbirth Connection: www.childbirthconnection.org
- An excellent resource for evidence-based information about maternity care practices in the United States and resources about pregnancy, childbirth and the postpartum period.

Greater Good Science Center: http://greatergood.berkeley.edu/
- The Greater Good Science Center (GGSC) studies the psychology, sociology, and neuroscience of wellbeing, teaching skills that foster a thriving, resilient, and compassionate society.
- For the GGSC's parenting program created by Christine Carter, PhD, go to the "Raising Happiness" page.

Infant Massage DVD BabyBabyOhBaby: www.babybabyohbaby.com
- Video instructions for infant massage.

Metta Programs: http://www.metta.org/
- For information about teaching Loving-kindness practice to children, go to the "Loving-kindness Practice with Children" page.

Postpartum Support International: www.postpartum.net
- For information, direct support, and help finding professional care for mental health during pregnancy and the postpartum period.

Secrets of Baby Behavior: www.secretsofbabybehavior.com
- Evidence-based information sponsored by the UC Davis Human Lactation Center. Covering such topics as infant crying, infant sleep, normal infant growth and development, and breastfeeding.

MINDFULNESS MEDITATION: SUGGESTED READING

There are many outstanding meditation teachers, and a wealth of new books about mindfulness and meditation are being published all the time. The selection below is only a small representation; it is intended as a starting point for a lifelong journey of exploration. It is worth mentioning that Jon Kabat-Zinn's book *Mindfulness for Beginners* has an extensive list of suggested readings. There are also many audio programs and resources on the Internet to help you begin and maintain a meditation practice.

Brach, Tara. *Radical Acceptance: Embracing Your Life with the Heart of a Buddha*. New York: Bantam Books, 2003.

Chödrön, Pema. *Comfortable with Uncertainty: 108 Teachings on Cultivating Fearlessness and Compassion*. Boston: Shambhala, 2003.

Goldstein, Joseph, and Jack Kornfield. *Seeking the Heart of Wisdom: The Path of Insight Meditation*. Boston: Shambhala, 1997.

Gunaratana, Bhante. *Mindfulness in Plain English*. Massachusetts: Wisdom Publications, 2002.

Hanh, Thich Nhat. *Peace Is Every Step: The Path of Mindfulness in Everyday Life*. New York: Bantam Books, 1991.

Hanh, Thich Nhat. *The Miracle of Mindfulness: An Introduction to the Practice of Meditation*. Boston: Beacon Press, 1976.

Kabat-Zinn, Jon. *Mindfulness for Beginners: Reclaiming the Present Moment—and Your Life*. Sounds True, Inc. Boulder, CO, 2012.

Kabat-Zinn, Jon. *Wherever You Go There You Are: Mindfulness Meditation in Everyday Life*. New York: Hyperion, 1994.

Kornfield, Jack. *A Lamp in the Darkness: Illuminating the Path Through Difficult Times*. Sounds True, Inc. Boulder, CO 2011.

Salzberg, Sharon. *Lovingkindness: The Revolutionary Art of Happiness*. Boston: Shambhala, 1995.

Salzberg, Sharon. *Real Happiness: The Power of Meditation*. New York: Workman Publishing, 2011.

Stahl, Bob, and Elisha Goldstein. *A Mindfulness-Based Stress Reduction Workbook*. Oakland: New Harbinger, 2010.

Suzuki, Shunryu. *Zen Mind, Beginner's Mind*. Boston: Shambhala, 1973.

Williams, Mark, and Danny Penman. *Mindfulness: An Eight-Week Plan for Finding Peace in a Frantic World*. New York: Rodale, 2011.

MINDFULNESS MEDITATION: ONLINE RESOURCES

Center for Mindfulness in Medicine, Health Care, and Society: www.umassmed.edu/cfm
- To learn more about Mindfulness-Based Stress Reduction (MBSR) or to find a MBSR course.

Mindfulness-Based Cognitive Therapy for Prevention of Depression Relapse (MBCT): www.mbct.com
- To learn more about the theory and effectiveness of this program or to find a MBCT course.

Oxford Mindfulness Centre: http://oxfordmindfulness.org/
- For information about MBCP courses and other mindfulness programs in the United Kingdom.

Association for Mindfulness in Education: www.mindfuleducation.org
- An association of organizations and individuals working to bring mindfulness training into K–12 education.

Inquiring Mind: http://www.inquiringmind.com
- A helpful guide for finding a retreat center, meditation classes, or a local meditation group.

Mindfulness Research Monthly (MRM): http://www.mindfulexperience.org
- A monthly online newsletter of current mindfulness research.

Pleasant and Unpleasant Events Calendars

	What was the experience?	How did your body feel during this experience?	What thoughts or images accompanied this experience?	What moods, feelings, and emotions accompanied this experience?	What thoughts are in your mind as you record this?
Example	I felt the baby moving just under my ribs.	There was stretching and pressure.	I thought, "Hello, baby. How are you doing in there?" I imagined the baby not having a lot of room to move.	I was pretty happy to feel the baby. I felt I wasn't alone. I felt amazed that I'm pregnant.	Excitement about meeting this little person and becoming a mother—and a little scared about it too.
Monday					
Tuesday					

Wednesday				
Thursday				
Friday				
Saturday				
Sunday				

UNPLEASANT EVENTS	What was the experience?	How did your body feel during this experience?	What thoughts or images accompanied this experience?	What moods, feelings, and emotions accompanied this experience?	What thoughts are in your mind as you record this?
Example	I felt the baby moving just under my ribs.	Sharp pain, discomfort, like my rib was getting bruised. It made me tense up.	I wondered what the baby was doing in there and was it a foot or an elbow that I felt.	I'm tired of being pregnant; I want this to be over. I felt worried about how the baby is going to get out!	I feel guilty that I was so crabby this afternoon, and I'm still nervous about labor and becoming a mom!
Monday					
Tuesday					

Wednesday				
Thursday				
Friday				
Saturday				
Sunday				

APPENDIX D

Mindfulness Practices

Notes

INTRODUCTION

1. Jon Kabat-Zinn, *Coming to Our Senses* (New York: Hyperion, 2005), 108.

CHAPTER 1: EVERYTHING'S CHANGING!

1. Used with permission from Mark Williams and Danny Penman, *Mindfulness: An Eight-Week Plan for Finding Peace in a Frantic World* (New York: Rodale, 2011), 6. For primary references, see 253–55.

CHAPTER 2: INNER PREPARATION FOR CHILDBIRTH AND BEYOND

1. I first heard about Horticultural Time from Professor Mark Williams, director of the Oxford Mindfulness Centre. Professor Williams acknowledges Sister Rosemary of the Convent of the Incarnation, Oxford, England, as the source of the concept.

CHAPTER 4: THE BREATH

1. Sharon Begley, *Train Your Mind, Change Your Brain: How a New Science Reveals Our Extraordinary Potential to Transform Ourselves* (New York: Ballantine Books, 2007).

2. The Three-Minute Breathing Space was originally developed by Zindel V. Segal, J. Mark G. Williams, and John D. Teasdale in their program *Mindfulness-Based Cognitive Therapy for Depression: A New Approach to Preventing Relapse* (New York; Guilford Press, 2002). It can also be found in J. Mark G. Williams, John D. Teasdale, Zindel V. Segal, and Jon Kabat-Zinn, *The Mindful Way Through Depression: Freeing Yourself from Chronic Unhappiness* (New York: Guilford Press, 2007). This particular adaptation is from Mark Williams and Danny Penman, *Mindfulness: An Eight-Week Plan for Finding Peace in a Frantic World* (New York: Rodale, 2011).

CHAPTER 5: PRACTICING EMBODIMENT

1. Kathryn Lee, "Sleep in Late Pregnancy Predicts Length of Labor and Type of Delivery," *American Journal of Obstetrics and Gynecology* 191, no. 6 (December 2004): 2041–46.

CHAPTER 6: THE DYNAMIC DUO

1. Kerstin Uvnäs Moberg, *The Oxytocin Factor: Tapping the Hormone of Calm, Love, and Healing* (New York: De Capo Press, 2003.) This groundbreaking book is important for understanding the underlying physiological mechanisms of our nervous system that support vibrant health and wellbeing. The description of the calm-and-connection system is drawn in part from Dr. Moberg's book, and I owe her a debt of gratitude for having written it. It is this mind-body calm-and-connection system that we cultivate and strengthen in our mindfulness practice.

2. Oxytocin is only one factor that initiates childbirth, which is a reason why an induction of labor using only Pitocin, the synthetic form of oxytocin, doesn't always work as quickly as one might wish and why additional drugs are sometimes used before an induction. For more information about the benefits and risks of induction, see the website of the American College of Nurse-Midwives, http://www.midwife.org.

3. Larissa Duncan and Nancy Bardacke, "Mindfulness-Based Childbirth and Parenting Education: Promoting Family Mindfulness During the Perinatal Period," *Journal of Child and Family Studies* 19 (2010): 190–202.

4. Rick Hanson, *The Buddha's Brain: The Practical Neuroscience of Happiness, Love, and Wisdom* (Oakland: New Harbinger Publications, 2009), 68.

5. Attempting to put something as complex as the interaction of our brain, body, and mindfulness into one illustration for you, the reader, was a complex undertaking; the degree to which I have provided a useful heuristic at this point in time will be determined by future research.

6. I originally learned this elegant Speaking and Listening Inquiry form from Saki Santorelli, EdD.

CHAPTER 7: MINDFULNESS PRACTICES FOR BEING WITH PAIN

1. Though childbirth educators have for decades used various ways of inducing discomfort as part of childbirth education (in my day partners would pinch the pregnant woman's Achilles tendon), I first observed and experienced the use of ice for inducing discomfort in two wonderful Birthing from Within workshops led by midwife Pam England. A bow of appreciation for that teaching and for her continuing innovative work.

2. This is not true if you have back labor. With back labor, the back of your baby's head rather than your baby's face presses against your sacrum. Because of this, a woman with back labor will continue to feel sensations in her back (though usually of less intensity) in the otherwise calm and peaceful time between contraction-expansions. Back labor occurs in about 10 percent of childbirths.

3. Sharon Salzberg, *Real Happiness: The Power of Meditation* (New York: Workman Publishing, 2011), 63.

4. A great deal more could be written about the positive physical and emotional healing aspects of touch, including infant massage. See Appendix B for resources.

CHAPTER 10: WHEN YOU'RE WALKING, JUST WALK;
WHEN YOU'RE BIRTHING, JUST BIRTH

1. This Walking Meditation is adapted with permission from J. Mark G. Williams, John D. Teasdale, Zindel V. Segal, and Jon Kabat-Zinn, *The Mindful Way Through Depression: Freeing Yourself from Chronic Unhappiness* (New York: Guilford Press, 2007), 91–93.

CHAPTER 11: MINDFULNESS IN EVERYDAY LIFE

1. Michael Pollan, *Food Rules: An Eater's Manual* (New York: Penguin Books, 2009).

CHAPTER 12: A DAY OF MINDFULNESS PRACTICE

1. Pema Chödrön, *The Places That Scare You: A Guide to Fearlessness in Difficult Times* (Boston: Shambhala, 2001), 36.

CHAPTER 13: BEFRIENDING

1. Albert Einstein, from a 1950 letter, quoted in Walter Sullivan, "The Einstein Papers: A Man of Many Parts," *New York Times,* March 29, 1972, 22M.

2. Myla and Jon Kabat-Zinn, *Everyday Blessings: The Inner Work of Mindful Parenting* (New York: Hyperion, 1997), 28.

3. D. W. Winnicott, MD, was a renowned British pediatrician and psychoanalyst who developed the concept of the "good enough mother." This concept was taken a step further by the American child psychologist Bruno Bettelheim in his book *A Good Enough Parent* (New York: Knopf, 1987). The concept acknowledges that real-life everyday parenting is both complex and challenging and that no one can ever be a "perfect parent."

CHAPTER 14: IT'S ALL ABOUT KINDNESS

1. Myla and Jon Kabat-Zinn, *Everyday Blessings: The Inner Work of Mindful Parenting* (New York: Hyperion, 1997), 160–61.

CHAPTER 16: CAUSES AND CONDITIONS

1. The statistics in the above paragraph are summarized in the presentation *Evidence-Based Practice: Pearls of Midwifery: A Presentation by the American College of Nurse-Midwives* from the American College of Nurse-Midwives (2010), http://www.midwife.org/pearlsfor women. See this presentation for primary resources.

2. M. Z. Oestergaard et al., on behalf of the United Nations Inter-agency Group for Child Mortality Estimation and the Child Health Epidemiology Reference Group, "Neonatal Mortality Levels for 193 Countries in 2009 with Trends since 1990: A Systematic Analysis of Progress, Projections, and Priorities," *PLoS Medicine* 8, no. 8 (August 2011), http://www. plosmedicine.org/article/info%3Adoi%2F10.1371%2Fjournal.pmed.1001080.

3. For more information about the history and culture of childbirth in the United States, see Jennifer Block, *Pushed: The Painful Truth about Childbirth and Modern Maternity Care* (New York: Da Capo Press, 2007).

4. Evidence-based practice (EBP) is an approach in medicine that began about 1992. It is based on the understanding that patient care "involves complex and conscientious decision-making which is based not only on the available evidence but also on patient characteristics, situations, and preferences. It recognizes that care is individualized and ever changing and involves uncertainties and probabilities." http://en.wikipedia.org/wiki/ Evidence-based_practice

An excellent online resource for evidence-based recommendations relating to childbirth is Childbirth Connection, especially the page "Understanding and Navigating the Maternity Care System" at http://www.childbirthconnection.org.

5. BRANN is adapted from Mary Nolan, "Childbirth Education: Politics, Equality and Relevance," in *Essential Midwifery Practice: Intrapartum Care,* edited by Denis Walsh and Soo Downe (Oxford: Blackwell, 2010), 31–44.

6. Statistics on midwife-assisted births come from Joyce A. Martin et al., "Births: Final Data for 2009," *National Vital Statistics Reports* 60, no. 1 (November 3, 2011); American College of Nurse-Midwives, Core Data Survey, 2010, http://www.midwife.org/Essential-Facts-about-Midwives. CNMs, CMs, and other midwives also attend deliveries at home and in freestanding birth centers. Less than 1 percent of the 4.2 million annual births in the United States take place at home or in birth centers, though this appears to be changing in some areas of the country.

7. The quality of available data regarding the safety of home birth remains a subject of some controversy. The official opinion of the Committee on Obstetric Practice of the American College of Obstetrics and Gynecology is that hospitals and birth centers are the safest places to give birth, but "[the committee] respects the right of women to make a medically informed decision." See ACOG Committee on Obstetric Practice, "Opinion No. 476: Planned Home Birth," *Obstetrics and Gynecology* 117, suppl. 2, pt. 1 (February 2011):425–28; erratum in *Obstetrics and Gynecology* 117, suppl. 5 (May 2011): 1232.

A recent hopeful development is the consensus statement of the 2011 Home Birth Consensus Summit, which provides a platform for improving home birth services as well as the entire maternity care system in the United States. For more information regarding this important gathering, go to http://www.homebirthsummit.org/summit-outcomes.html.

8. A doula is usually not needed if you are planning to give birth at home. If you are planning to birth in a birthing center, discuss the need for a doula with your healthcare provider.

9. For more information about doulas, see Marshall H. Klaus, John H. Kennell, and Phyllis H. Klaus, *The Doula Book: How a Trained Labor Companion Can Help You Have a Shorter, Easier, and Healthier Birth* (New York: Perseus Publishing, 2012). Also visit the website of DONA International, http://www.dona.org.

10. "Given that available data do not show a clear benefit for the use of EFM over intermittent auscultation, either option is acceptable in a patient without complications"; see "Intrapartum Fetal Heart Rate Monitoring," *ACOG Practice Bulletin*, no. 106 (July 2009): 5. Also see American College of Nurse-Midwives, "Intermittent Auscultation for Intrapartum Fetal Heart Rate Surveillance," *Journal of Midwifery and Women's Health* 55, no. 4 (July–August 2010): 397–403.

11. O. Andersson, L. Hellström-Westas, D. Andersson, and M. Domellöf, "Effect of Delayed Versus Early Umbilical Cord Clamping on Neonatal Outcomes and Iron Status at 4 Months: A Randomised Controlled Trial," *British Medical Journal* 343 (November 15, 2011), http://www.bmj.com/content/343/bmj.d7157.

12. J. Mercer et al., "Evidence-Based Practices for the Fetal to Newborn Transition," *Journal of Midwifery and Women's Health* 52 (2007): 262–72; S. Velaphi and D. Vidyasagar, "The Pros and Cons of Suctioning at the Perineum (Intrapartum) and Post-Delivery with and without Meconium," *Seminars in Fetal & Neonatal Medicine* 13 (2008): 375–82.

13. For the full World Health Organization/UNICEF Baby-Friendly Hospital Initiative, a program that outlines evidence-based best practices for newborns and is endorsed by the American Academy of Pediatrics (AAP), see "The Baby-Friendly Hospital Initiative" page of the UNICEF Home website, http://www.unicef.org/programme/breastfeeding/baby.htm. Also see the AAP policy statement: "Avoid procedures that may interfere with breastfeeding or that may traumatize the infant, including unnecessary, excessive, and overvigorous suctioning of the oral cavity, esophagus, and airways to avoid oropharyngeal mucosal injury

that may lead to aversive feeding behavior"; see "Breastfeeding and the Use of Human Milk," *Pediatrics* 115, no. 2 (February 2005): 496–506, http://aappolicy.aappublications.org/cgi/content/full/pediatrics;115/2/496.

CHAPTER 17: YOUR BABY, YOUR MINDFULNESS TEACHER

1. Kevin Nugent, *Your Baby Is Speaking to You* (New York: Houghton Mifflin Harcourt, 2011), xv.

2. Marshall Klaus and Phyllis Klaus, *Your Amazing Newborn* (New York: Perseus Books, 1998).

3. For postpartum depression in new fathers, see the website PostpartumMen, http://www.postpartummen.com.

4. Zindel V. Segal, J. Mark G. Williams, and John D. Teasdale, *Mindfulness-Based Cognitive Therapy for Depression: A New Approach to Preventing Relapse* (New York: Guilford Press, 2002). On the effectiveness of the MBCT course in prevention and treatment of depression, see W. Kuyken et al., "Mindfulness-Based Cognitive Therapy to Prevent Relapse in Recurrent Depression," *Journal of Consulting and Clinical Psychology* 76 (2008): 966–78, and Z. Segal et al., "Antidepressant Monotherapy Versus Sequential Pharmacotherapy and Mindfulness-Based Cognitive Therapy, or Placebo, for Relapse Prophylaxis in Recurrent Depression," *Archives of General Psychiatry* 67 (2010): 1256–64.

5. For more information about the MBCT program adapted into a prevention program for women at risk for postpartum depression, contact Sona Dimidjian, PhD, sona.dimidjian@colorado.edu, or Sherryl Goodman, PhD, psysg@emory.edu.

CHAPTER 18: BREASTFEEDING

1. To view the full American Academy of Pediatricians report "Breastfeeding and the Use of Human Milk," *Pediatrics* 129, no. 3 (March 2012): e827–e841, go to http://pediatrics.aappublications.org/content/early/2012/02/22/peds.2011-3552.full.pdf+html.

2. For more information about Biological Nurturing, go to the Biological Nurturing website, http://www.biologicalnurturing.com.

3. Suzanne Colson, "Bringing Nature to the Fore," *The Practicing Midwife* 8, no. 11 (December 2005): 14–19.

CHAPTER 20: LIFE AFTER BIRTH

1. Myla and Jon Kabat-Zinn, *Everyday Blessings: The Inner Work of Mindful Parenting* (New York: Hyperion, 1997), 13.

APPENDIX A : MINDFULNESS-BASED CHILDBIRTH AND PARENTING (MBCP) AND INTEGRATIVE MEDICINE

1. Michael Marmot and the UCL Institute for Health Equity, *Fair Society, Healthy Lives: Strategic Review of Health Inequalities in England Post 2010* (London: Marmot Review, 2010), 23, http://www.ucl.ac.uk/marmotreview.

2. As the specialties of obstetrics and gynecology have become more complex, some physicians are coming to see that collaboration with their nurse-midwife and midwife colleagues is not only desirable but necessary to ensure the highest quality of care needed for the normal healthy pregnant woman, her baby, and family. Such collaboration ensures that a pregnant woman, her baby, and family will first be cared for by the midwife, who is expert

in the normal pregnancy and childbirth and often knowledgeable in a wide range of complementary modalities to support the normal process. In a collaborative relationship, the expertise of the obstetrical specialists, the highly trained and much-needed experts in the fix-it paradigm, is called upon when necessary and appropriate. See Margaret Hutchison et al., "Great Minds Don't Think Alike: Collaborative Maternity Care at San Francisco General Hospital," *Obstetrics and Gynecology* 188, suppl. 3 (September 2011): 678–682.

3. Michael S. Krasner, Ronald M. Epstein, Howard Beckman et al., "Association of an Educational Program in Mindful Communication with Burnout, Empathy, and Attitudes Among Primary Care Physicians," *Journal of the American Medical Association* 302, no. 12 (2009): 284–93.

4. For more information about the Strengthening Families Program, see L. G. Duncan, J. D. Coatsworth, and M. T. Greenberg, "A Model of Mindful Parenting: Implications for Parent-Child Relationships and Prevention Research," *Clinical Child and Family Psychology Review* 12 (2009): 255–70.

5. The ultimate goal of Centering Healthcare is a fundamental redesign of our health delivery system, a redesign that would make healthcare more educational, economical, health promoting, and compassionate—a true healthcare delivery system rather than a disease-care system. Learning through connection with others and honoring the inner wisdom of those seeking care, this model fosters responsibility for one's optimal health and wellbeing in partnership with healthcare providers. http://www.centeringhealthcare.org.

6. For further information, contact Maret Dymond, PhD, lead clinical psychologist in Mindfulness-Based Childbirth and Parenting at the Oxford Mindfulness Centre, University of Oxford, UK: maret.dymond@psych.ox.ac.uk.

Credits

Index

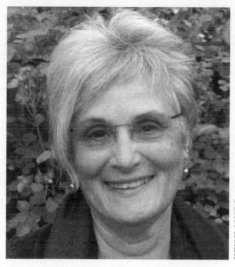

Nancy Bardacke, RN, CNM, MA

Nancy Bardacke, midwife, mindfulness teacher, and founding director of the Mindfulness-Based Childbirth and Parenting (MBCP) program, has been assisting birthing families since 1971. In her many years working as a midwife, Nancy has attended births in homes, birth centers, and hospitals. A longtime meditation practitioner, she began her professional training in Mindfulness-Based Stress Reduction (MBSR) with Jon Kabat-Zinn, PhD, in 1994. After teaching MBSR for a number of years, Nancy began adapting it to the needs of pregnant women and their partners, creating the MBCP program. Since 1998 the MBCP program has served more than a thousand expectant parents. In addition to leading the MBCP program at the Osher Center for Integrative Medicine at the University of California, San Francisco, Medical Center, Nancy offers mindfulness workshops for expectant parents and healthcare providers, as well as trainings for MBCP instructors in the United States and abroad.

www.mindfulbirthing.org

Scan this code with your smartphone to be linked to bonus materials for *Mindful Birthing* and other healthy living books and information.

You can also text MINDBODYBIRTH to READIT (732348) to be sent a link to the mobile website.